Evoked Potentials in Psychology, Sensory Physiology and Clinical Medicine

Evoked Potentials in Psychology, Sensory Physiology and Clinical Medicine

D. REGAN

LONDON
CHAPMAN AND HALL LTD.

First published 1972
by Chapman and Hall Ltd
11 New Fetter Lane, London EC4P 4EE
Printed in Great Britain by
Richard Clay (The Chaucer Press), Ltd
Bungay, Suffolk

SBN 412 10920 4

TO MARIAN, DOUGLAS AND HOWARD

Contents

Preface

Only quite recently has it become technically possible to record, from electrodes attached to the scalp, the human brain's electrical responses to sensory stimulation.

The core of this book is a critical survey of endeavours to use these electrical responses (called evoked potentials) as tools in attempts to discover the ways in which the brain first processes incoming sensory information and then forms internal representations of features of the external world.

Buttressed by quantities of undeniably sloppy evoked potential research there are some who would dismiss out of hand the recording of evoked potentials as being comparable to 'holding an oscilloscope probe 6 feet in diameter up to a computer and pronouncing from the resultant waveform on the underlying structure and function'; many would contrast the scientific value of recording the activities of single nerve cells with microelectrodes. However, although it is certainly true that the brain may indeed function in a way which would not be susceptible to the approaches of the evoked potential researcher it might equally well resist the stratagems of the single-cell man. If, for example, the neural correlate of some sensation were the state of some large *population* of nerve cells, then the present-day researcher who records in great detail the activity of one single cell or of a very few cells would be faced with a major problem in trying to see the forest for the trees. At this time it is not possible to predict with any confidence whether single unit techniques will continue to flourish while evoked potential recording withers, or vice versa, or whether both types of study will continue to co-exist and provide complementary 'windows onto the brain'. There is some analogy here with a newspaper photograph which under high magnification seems to consist of a meaningless collection of dots. At the other extreme, when viewed from a large distance it looks like a greyish blob. Only when viewed from roughly norma viewing distance can the meaning be seen. Perhaps some progress may be made towards finding the 'correct reading distance' for the brain by some future amalgam of the microscopic single-nerve-cell approach and the large-scale approach of evoked potential recording.

Electrophysiological studies of those brain functions which are peculiar to man must necessarily involve human subjects. Furthermore, the reports and quantitative estimates of their sensations which can be provided by human subjects are more detailed, more certain and more easily obtained than corresponding behavioural data from animals. Human subjects, then, have overwhelming advantages in certain areas of brain research and the only practical means of access to the activities of nerve cells presently available in the intact (unexposed) human brain is evoked potential recording. 'But which nerve cells?' is still perhaps the most embarrassing question for the evoked potential researcher. The first and second chapters of this book discuss the efforts which have been made to identify neuroanatomical sites of evoked potential generators.

Quite apart from basic research into brain function, evoked potential techniques have promise as entirely noninjurious clinical procedures both for testing the sensory functions of infants and other noncooperative patients, and as a source of additional data on the sites of brain lesions in cases where conventional tests fail to provide clear diagnostic information.

Anyone who decides to use evoked potential recording in his research is hampered by the paucity of critical reviews of the field, and is faced with the prospect of working his way through a mass of often contradictory reports. One reason for writing this book was the hope that it might serve as an introductory guide both to research students entering the field, and to researchers working on other topics who need to assess whether evoked potential techniques might help them to solve their particular problem. Chapter 1 was written with research students in mind whose previous backgrounds were in the nonbiological sciences. Similarly, I hope that Chapter 5 may prove to be of some practical assistance to research workers whose previous training included little physics or engineering. Chapter 3 discusses the effects of psychological variables on evoked potentials from two viewpoints: in psychological research *per se*, and as complicating factors both in studies of sensory information processing and in studies of clinical problems. It is not too early to warn the reader that this area of research is notoriously confusing. Chapter 4, which is intended for the clinical research worker who wishes to assess whether evoked potential techniques are likely to be of value to him, consists of a review of clinical work to date and includes a number of cross-references both to fundamental research (Chapter 2) and to certain techniques (Chapter 5) whose clinical possibilities have not yet been exploited.

In the hope of achieving some balance in my treatment of controversial issues I sent preliminary drafts of individual Chapters to a number of research workers. I am grateful indeed for the time and effort which they devoted to patiently correcting many of my misconceptions and for many valuable suggestions. I thank most warmly Drs J. C. Armington, E. Callaway, F. W. Campbell, W. A. Cobb, O. D. Creutzfeldt, R. Elul, W. R. Goff, A. M. Halliday, M. R. Harter, J. R. Heron, D. A. Jeffreys, E. R. John, J. H. Kelsey, J. Kulikowski, D. M. MacKay, B. A. Milner, R. Näätänen, H. Oosting, L. A. Riggs, T. Shipley, A. D. Short, S. Sutton, W. R. Uttal, L. H. van der Tweel, H. G. Vaughan and M. Verzeano, and also those research students who gave a consumer's report, J. G. Axford, K. I. Beverley, P. G. H. Clarke and C. W. Tyler. I am especially indebted to Drs E. F. Evans and H. Spekreijse whose generosity and stamina extended to reading and criticising the entire manuscript. I owe many of the suggestions and comments incorporated in this book to discussions with Professor D. M. MacKay; a number of these are acknowledged, but in all probability many more are not. Errors and mis-statements which may still be found in the following pages are all my own work.

The list of references is no longer than is necessitated by the text. It is not meant to be exhaustive (but was certainly exhausting). Overwhelming fatigue set in before the planned glossary of terms was completed.

I thank the Medical Research Council for their support. The bibliographical service of the Brain Information Service, Los Angeles, was invaluable in the preparation of this book. The practical research work in which I have been involved owes much to the technical expertise of R. F. Cartwright.

This book could not have been written without the constant encouragement and practical assistance of my wife Marian, and her patient tolerance of the many irritations which, we found, accompany the writing of a book.

I am grateful for Dr B. A. Milner's assistance in correcting the proofs.

Finally, I must thank Julie Cave who cheerfully deciphered my handwritten manuscript, and often corrected the English in passing.

University of Keele
February 1971 D.R.

Author's Note

The numbers which occur in the text as superscripts refer to the General references listed on pages 259 to 304. However, superscript numbers prefixed by a capital S refer to the Supplementary footnotes added in proof and listed between pages 305 and 318.

1

The activities of single neurons and evoked potentials

1.1 General remarks: the neuron

This introduction is an outline account of the structure and functioning of a typical cortical neuron, and is intended for the reader with little or no background in biological science just as Chapter 5 is intended for the reader with little previous knowledge of physics or engineering. References [689, 702, 878, 86, 384, 442,] provide necessary background to this chapter. Readers who prefer to omit this introduction should start on page 12.

Brain tissue is composed of three constituents. These are glial cells, extracellular space and nerve cells (including fibres). Glial cells are electrically inexcitable and one function, suggested by their name (glue), might be to provide a mechanical frame for the brain although this is not certain and their role in brain activity is obscure. Extracellular space is not filled entirely by unstructured aqueous electrolyte, but on the contrary contains a substantial amount of organised macromolecular material.[753 p. 80]

A nerve cell (neuron) consists of a cell body (or soma) from which one or more of the following processes arise. A dendrite which may extend as far as 1 mm, transmits graded signals towards the cell body; the other type of process, an axon, normally transmits all-or-nothing signals (spikes)* away from the cell body. An axon may be enormously long in relation to its diameter, and in certain nerves may extend up to 1 m (Figs. 1.1 and 1.2).

In an electron micrograph the cell body of a neuron can be seen to be limited by a double membrane which encloses a number of distinguishable structures – a nucleus and nucleolus, mitochondria, lipochondria (Golgi substance), endoplasmic reticulum and ribosomes (Fig. 1.3). The double membrane which encloses the cell body also extends over the dendrites and axon. In addition to the double membrane the axon is enclosed, in a proportion of cases, by an insulating layer (myelin sheath) which is wrapped many times in a spiral fashion. The myelin sheath is a prominent feature of many axons; in the smaller fibres the sheath consists of one layer only and the

* The following terms are synonymous: spike, action potential spike, action potential, impulse, all-or-nothing signal and explosive electrochemical self-propagating impulse. 'Spike' is used throughout this chapter. To 'generate a spike' and to 'fire' are synonymous.

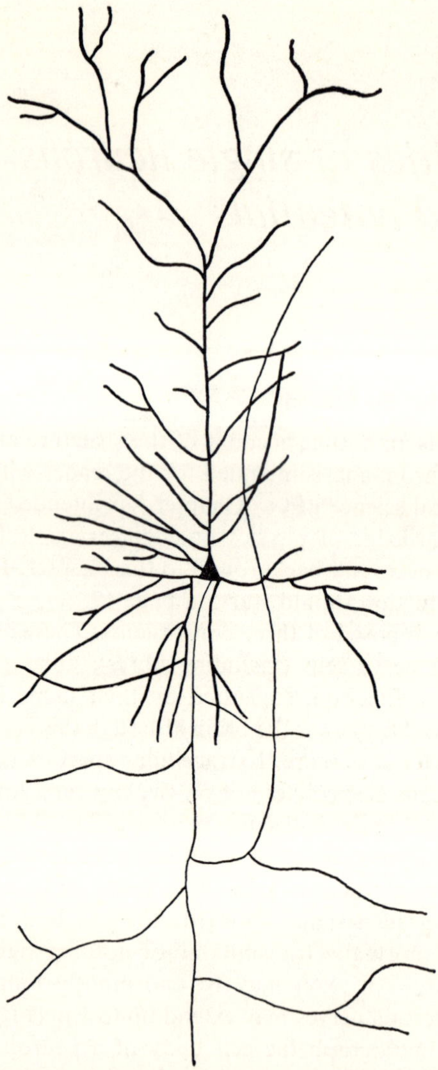

FIGURE 1.1 *Pyramidal cell from the third layer of the cortex. From G. von Bonin (1956).* Essay on the Cerebral Cortex. *Charles C. Thomas, Publisher, Springfield, Illinois.*

myelin is not evident under a light microscope. These two types of fibre are conventionally described as being myelinated and unmyelinated respectively.

Transmission between cells takes place at junctions called *synapses*. In most cases synaptic transmission seems to be chemically mediated. There may be a large number (thousands) of synapses on the body and dendrites of a single neuron. The activity of one type of synapse (excitatory) increases the probability that the cell will generate a spike, while the activity of a second type of synapse (inhibitory) decreases the probability of spike generation. Trans-

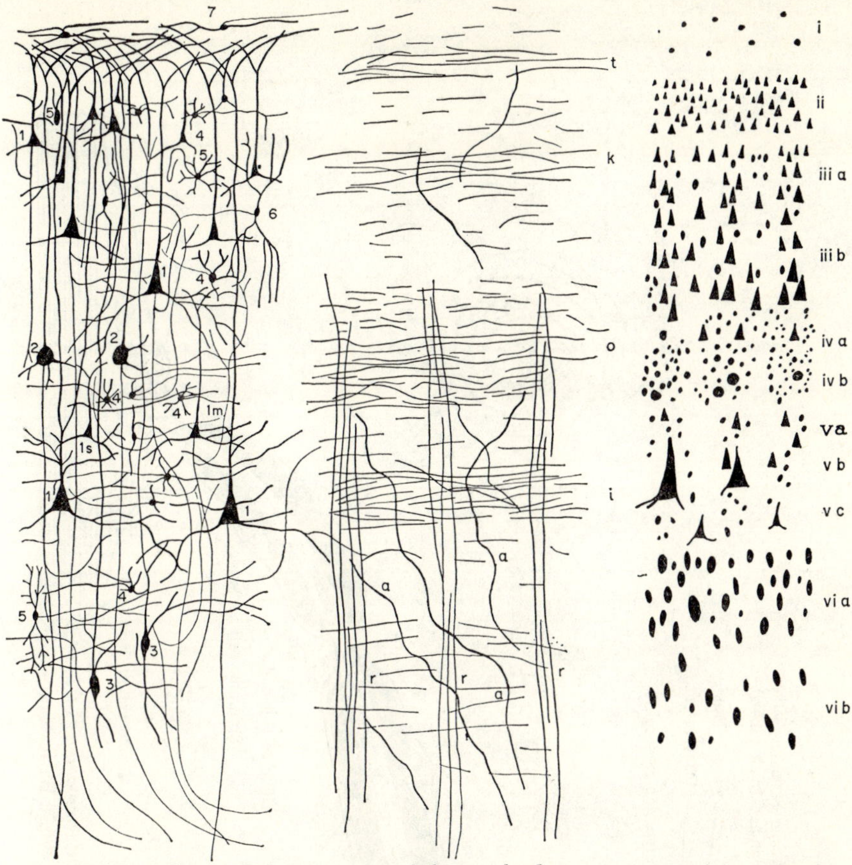

FIGURE 1.2 *Scheme of the structure of the cerebral cortex as seen in preparations after Golgi (outlines of neurons), Weigert (myelinated fibres) and Nissl (cell bodies).*

1 – pyramidal cell. 1m – 'medium pyramid'. 1s – 'short pyramid'. 2 – star pyramid. 3 – fusiform cell. 4 – star cell. 5 – spider cell. 6 – double bush cell. 7 – horizontal cell of Cajal.

a – oblique fibres. r – radii. t – tangential fibres. k – stripe of Kaes-Bechterew. o – outer. i – inner stripe of Baillarger.

The small roman numerals on the right margin indicate the different layers of the cortex. From G. von Bonin (1956). Essay on the Cerebral Cortex. *Charles C. Thomas, Publisher, Springfield, Illinois.*

mission across a synapse can occur in one direction only. As a consequence the neuron as a whole transmits signals in one direction only, that is, from dendrite to axon. [A spike initiated in an axon at a point some distance from the cell body will spread in both directions, so that one spike approaches the cell body from the 'wrong' direction (an antidromic spike). However, although the spike may invade the cell body and even the dendrites, it will not pass the synaptic junctions.]*

When a cell is sufficiently excited by incoming presynaptic spikes the

* An *orthodromic* spike approaches the cell body from the 'correct' direction.

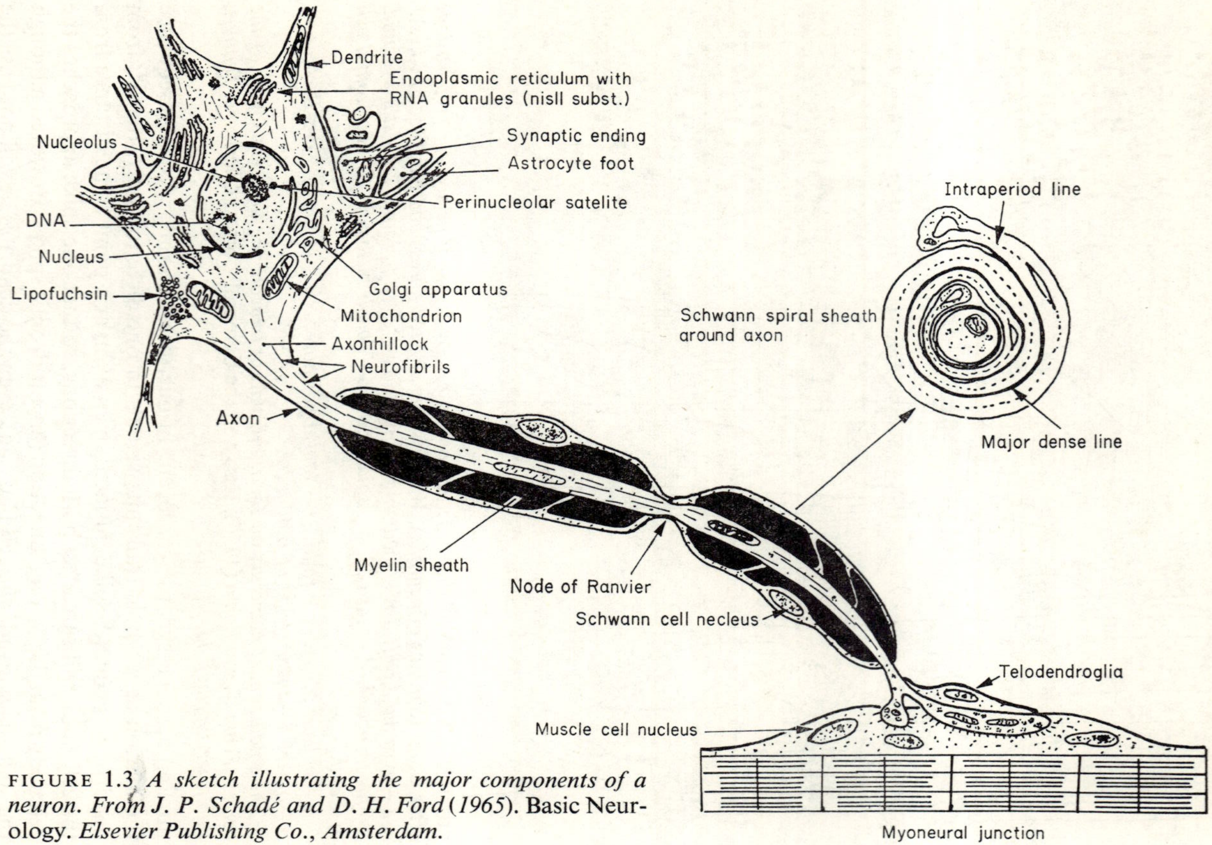

FIGURE 1.3 *A sketch illustrating the major components of a neuron. From J. P. Schadé and D. H. Ford (1965).* Basic Neurology. *Elsevier Publishing Co., Amsterdam.*

electrochemical change which spreads decementally along the dendrites and cell body initiates at some 'trigger' site an 'explosive' electrochemical self-propagating impulse (i.e. a second spike) which travels down the axon. This mode of nervous transmission by all-or-none spikes is well adapted for signalling over long distances since it can be rapid and the amplitudes of an individual spike do not attenuate (decrement) with distance travelled. The nature of synaptic transmission and spike initiation allows the cell body and dendrites to perform a function which has been described as 'weighing and integrating the incoming signals'.

Current notions of the way in which an all-or-nothing action potential arises and is propagated along an axon are as follows.

In the resting state there is a potential difference of roughly 70 mV across the membrane of a neuron, directed so that the interior of the axon is negative with respect to the fluid outside the membrane. This potential difference arises from the differences between the concentrations of ions in the aqueous solutions inside and outside the cell and is intimately related to properties of the cell membrane. The value of the resting potential difference appears to be controlled by potassium ions.[384 p. 41]

Sodium ions are roughly 12 times, and chloride ions roughly 30 times more concentrated in the fluid outside the cell than inside the cell. On the other hand potassium ions are roughly 40 times and organic anions roughly 20 times more concentrated inside the cell than in the fluid outside the cell. Fig. 1.4 illustrates the notion of how differences of ionic concentrations set up a standing potential difference across the cellular membrane. (This diagram should not be regarded as a realistic illustration of the detailed characteristics of a real membrane.)

At equilibrium the relationship between, on the one hand the external and internal concentrations of an ion, and on the other hand the potential difference across the cellular membrane can be deduced from the condition that the total potential energy difference per mole of the ion should be zero. The total potential energy per mole for any particular ion is the sum of the electrical and concentration energy differences across the membrane for that ion. This total potential energy difference per mole of ion is called the electrochemical potential difference. The Nernst equation expresses the condition that the electrochemical potential difference for any ion should be zero. For example the Nernst equation for potassium ions is:[384 p. 30]

$$V_k = \frac{RT}{F} \ln \frac{(\mathrm{K})_o}{(\mathrm{K})_i}$$

where V_k is the equilibrium concentration of the potassium ion defined in the sense 'internal potential minus external potential', R is the gas constant, T is the absolute temperature, F is the Faraday, and $(\mathrm{K})_o$ and $(\mathrm{K})_i$ are the potassium concentrations outside and inside the fibre.

The tendency for Cl^- ions to diffuse into the cell and K^+ ions to diffuse out of the cell along their concentration gradients is almost counterbalanced by the standing electrostatic field. Again, the tendency of organic anion (A^-) to diffuse out of the cell along the concentration gradient and along the electric field is opposed by the near-impermeability of the membrane to A^- ions. However, the effect of the standing electrostatic field is to destroy the Na^+ concentration gradient by accelerating diffusion through the membrane. An

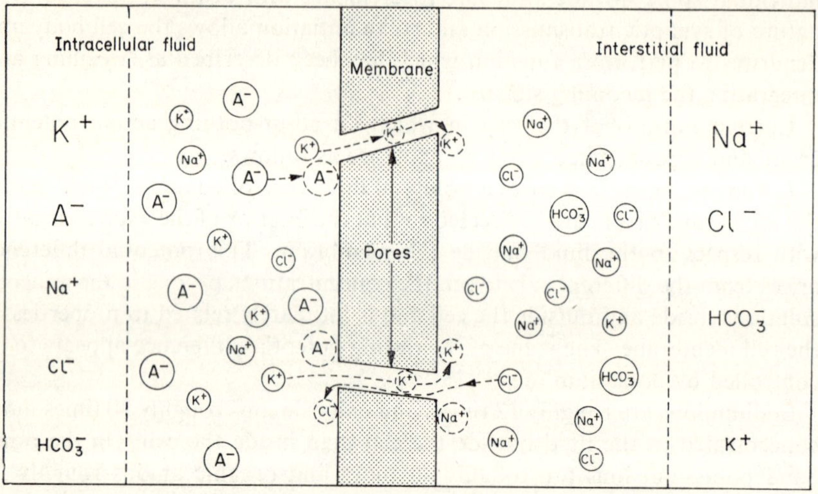

FIGURE 1.4 *Development of transmembrane voltage by an ion concentration gradient. Diagram of an intracellular fluid–membrane–interstitial fluid system. Membrane shown has some, but not all, properties of a real cell membrane. Hypothetical membrane is pierced by pores of such size that K^+ and Cl^- ions can move through them easily, Na^+ ions with difficulty, and A^- not at all. Sizes of symbols in left- and right-hand columns indicate relative concentrations of ions in fluids bathing the membrane. Dashed arrows and circles show paths taken by K^+, A^-, Na^+ and Cl^- ions as a K^+ or Cl^- travels through a pore. Penetration of the pore by a K^+ or Cl^- follows a collision between the K^+ or Cl^- and water molecules (not shown), giving the K^+ or Cl^- the necessary kinetic energy and proper direction. An A^- or Na^+ unable to cross the membrane is left behind when a K^+ or Cl^-, respectively, diffuses through a pore. Because K^+ is more concentrated on left than on right, more K^+ diffuses from left to right than from right to left, and conversely for Cl^-. Therefore, right-hand border of membrane becomes positively charged (K^+, Na^+) and left-hand negatively charged (Cl^-, A^-). Fluids away from the membrane are electrically neutral because of attraction between + and − charges. Charges separated by membrane stay near it because of their attraction. From T. C. Ruch, H. D. Patton, J. W. Woodbury and A. L. Towe (Eds.) (1961).* Neurophysiology. *W. B. Saunders Co., Publishers, Philadelphia.*

active sodium transport mechanism has been postulated to explain the maintainance of the Na^+ concentration difference in the face of Na^+ diffusion. Since energy is required to carry Na^+ from a region of lower to higher electrical potential, it follows that metabolic energy must be supplied to allow a net transport of Na^+ ions out of the cell. At the same time, metabolic energy must be supplied to produce a net transport of K^+ ions from the space outside the cell to the space inside the cell. The active mechanism responsible for this ionic transport is often referred to as the 'sodium-potassium pump'.

In the resting condition, then, the aqueous solution inside the cell is rich in potassium ions, the aqueous solution outside the cell is rich in sodium ions, and the interior of the cell is roughly 70 mV negative with respect to the fluid outside the cell. During an action potential the resting condition breaks down and is re-established within the span of a few milliseconds. The standing difference in sodium concentrations provides the e.m.f. which generates the action potential (i.e. the difference in sodium concentrations provides energy to the charges which cross the membrane during the action potential). The opposition of the Na^+ and K^+ concentration gradients allows the trans-membrane potential difference to reverse in sign during the action potential (and is the basis for inhibitory and excitatory postsynaptic potentials). A further result of the opposition of Na^+ and K^+ concentration gradients is to assist in speeding the return of the membrane to the resting state after the occurrence of an action potential.

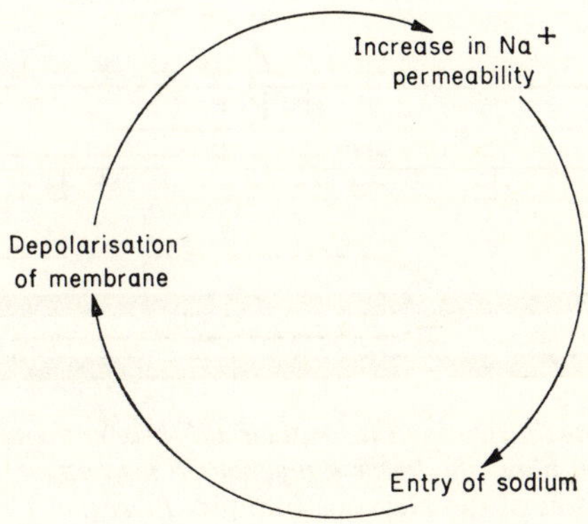

FIGURE 1.5

The resting conditions of the membrane break down when the potential difference across the membrane is reduced (*depolarisation*) to a certain critical value. This can be done either by spread from the cell body or dendrite of excitatory postsynaptic potentials, or (in laboratory conditions), by direct electrical stimulation of the axon. Once the potential difference across the membrane has been reduced to this rather sharply-defined critical value, an all-or-none impulse rapidly follows. 'Threshold' is the potential difference for which the inward Na^+ current just balances the outward K^+ current. Depolarisation beyond this point results in positive feedback: Na^+ ions enter at an accelerating rate and the transmembrane potential difference moves rapidly towards the equilibrium potential for Na^+ ions (Fig. 1.5). Since the concentration difference for K^+ ions is still maintained the interior of the cell is now positive with respect to the external fluid.

During the latter part of the action potential the permeability of the membrane to K^+ ions increases, so that after roughly 0·3 msec more K^+ ions leave the cell than Na^+ ions enter. At the same time the permeability of the membrane to Na^+ ions falls so that the potential difference across the membrane is rapidly restored to the resting condition. Before the cell is ready to sustain a further action potential there is an absolute refractory period. This is followed by a relative refractory period in which threshold is elevated and spikes, if generated, are abnormally small. The refractory period sets a limit to the firing frequency of an axon; in some nerves frequencies of 200 or even up to 1000 spikes per second have been recorded.

Although the difference of Na^+ concentration is the immediate source of energy during the action potential, only a very small change in Na^+ and K^+ concentration within the cell results from a single-action potential (e.g. for a 500 μm axon the internal concentration of K^+ is reduced by one-millionth part during a single action potential). The resting concentrations of Na^+ and K^+ are then restored by the action of the sodium-potassium pump which can therefore be regarded as the basic source of the energy of nervous conduction.

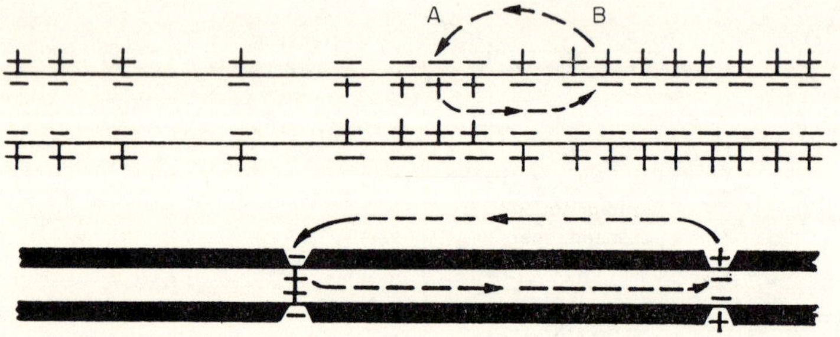

FIGURE 1.6 *Diagrams illustrating the local circuit theory; the upper sketch represents an unmyelinated nerve fibre, the lower a myelinated nerve fibre. From A. L. Hodgkin (1964).* The Conduction of the Nervous Impulse. *Liverpool University Press.*

The local flow of current due to the rapid changes of membrane permeability during an action potential depolarise adjacent areas of membrane sufficiently to initiate further action potentials (Fig. 1.6). In this way an 'explosively' self-propagating change (a spike) can spread along the axon in both directions from the site of initiation. In the physiological situation the site of initiation of the spike is such as to result in unidirectional transmission.

Summarising then, the characteristic properties of the axon of a neuron are excitability and (all-or-none) conductivity.

The myelin sheath, which is a prominent feature of some axons, seems to have the effect of increasing the speed of propagation of the impulse by up to 20 to 25 times. The myelin sheath, an electrical insulator, is not continuous, but is interrupted at intervals of 1·5 to 2 mm. These ring-shaped holes in the myelin sheath, the *nodes of Ranvier*, are the only points at which the axonal membrane is in electrical contact with the extracellular fluid. In the unmyelinated axon the spike is propagated by the current flow associated with the breakdown of the transmembrane potential difference. The current depolarises the neighbouring areas of membrane to a level below the critical potential. In the myelinated axon, however, extracellular currents can enter the cell only at the nodes of Ranvier. Thus, when a spike occurs at one node of Ranvier the adjacent nodes are then depolarised below threshold, so that the spike is propagated by jumping from one node to the next (Fig. 1.6). This jumping ('saltatory') mode of conduction is much more rapid than in an unmyelinated fibre of comparable diameter. In general, conduction velocity increases with diameter in unmyelinated fibres, thus if large numbers of fibres were required to transmit impulses rapidly over long distances, very bulky nerves would be necessary. Myelinated fibres allow a considerable saving in bulkiness in nerves which perform this function.

The terminal branches of an axon may be very fine. Some branches terminate in small ($\sim 1\ \mu m$) structures called synaptic knobs (boutons terminaux, end feet) located on the soma or dendrites of subsequent cells. Other types of axon termination found in the central nervous system include flat plates, a 'basket' which encloses the soma, or 'naked' terminations with no apparent specialised terminal structures. Some types of terminals are found exclusively on dendrites or soma, while other types may be found both on dendrites and soma.

The axon makes functional connections with subsequent neurons at localised sites called *synapses* located on the body or dendrites of the cell. The synapse is a region where adjacent cells are separated by only a very narrow gap. Nevertheless a gap does exist, thus there is not a continuous path for the neural signal and as a consequence the neural message may be extensively modified at each synaptic link.

Some special properties of synapses are as follows:
(1) In contrast with conduction along an axon, transmission across a synapse can only take place in one direction; (2) synapses can exhibit amplification, for example when a cell responds to a single synchronous presynaptic volley of impulses with a train of spikes; (3) synapses can be classified as either inhibitory or excitatory – presynaptic activity at excitatory synapses increases the probability of firing of the postsynaptic cell while presynaptic activity at inhibitory synapses decreases the probability of firing; (4) synapses can modify the temporal pattern of the presynaptic input. Two ways in which this can occur are as follows: Firstly, the maximum frequencies of presynaptic impulses which a cell can follow may be limited not by the length of the refractory period of the axon but by the synaptic terminals. Secondly, a delay of roughly 1 msec occurs during transmission across a synapse. Due to this delay the passage of signals through multisynaptic networks which involve feedback paths may be much easier at some frequencies than at others (Fig. 1.7).

Current notions of the sequence of events associated with signal transmission across a synapse are roughly as follows.

Immediately following the arrival of a spike at an excitatory presynaptic terminal, synaptic vesicles move to the presynaptic membrane where they release an excitatory transmitter substance into the synaptic gap between the presynaptic and postsynaptic membranes. After some synaptic delay, changes

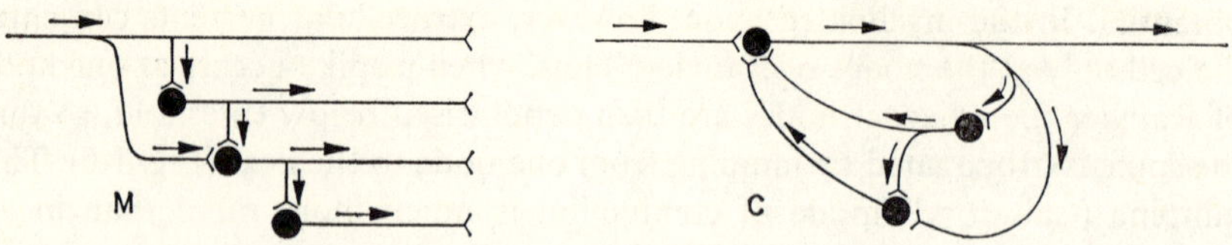

FIGURE 1.7 *Plans of the two fundamental types of neuron circuits. M, Multiple chain; C, closed chain. After L. de No (1938). 'Plans of the two fundamental types of neuron circuits'*, J. Neurophysiol, **1**, 207–44.

occur in the ionic permeabilities of the synaptic membrane. These permeability changes result in a decrease in the electrical potential difference across the membrane (depolarisation). Such a reduction in the postsynaptic transmembrane potential difference is called an 'excitatory postsynaptic potential' (EPSP) (see Fig. 1.8). The EPSP has a synaptic delay of about 0·5 msec and a roughly exponential decay of time constant 4 msec [compare with the shorter and more abrupt time course of an axonal action potential (Fig. 1.8)]. The postsynaptic membrane is restored to its resting condition by the action of a specific enzyme which inactivates the transmitter substance released into the synaptic cleft. The EPSP is a summation of the elementary EPSPs generated synchronously by each individual synapse; temporal summation can also be effective if elementary EPSPs are generated within a few milliseconds of each other (Fig. 1.8). Fig. 1.8 also illustrates that in contrast with the all-or-nothing axonal action potential the EPSP is a graded response.

When activated by incoming presynaptic impulses, inhibitory synapses release packets of a specific inhibitory transmitter substance into the synaptic cleft. When the potential difference across the presynaptic membrane is at a normal level the action of the inhibitory transmitter substance is to produce an increase of this potential difference (hyperpolarisation). This change in transmembrane potential difference is called an 'inhibitory postsynaptic potential' (IPSP) and is in the opposite direction to an EPSP. Whereas an EPSP moves the neuron closer to its firing threshold, the activity of an inhibitory synapse makes firing less likely both by hyperpolarising the postsynaptic membrane (i.e. by generating an IPSP) and possibly also by making the membrane more resistant to depolarisation. The synaptic delay for an IPSP (of about 1·5 msec) is 3 to 4 times longer than the synaptic delay for an EPSP, although the decay time constants (3 and 4 msec respectively) are not dissimilar. The amplitude of an IPSP seldom exceeds 5 mV and is generally smaller than the amplitude of an EPSP.

The EPSPs and IPSPs generated at the many synapses located on the cell body and dendrites spread decrementally across the cell body. If a critical level of depolarisation is reached at some 'trigger site' then an all-or-none spike is initiated on the axon near the cell body. The 'spike' is then propagated along the axon without any decremental loss. It seems clear that it is not only the relative amplitudes of elementary (single synapse) EPSPs and IPSPs which are of systematic importance in determining whether or not a particular cell fires, but also the relative locations of activated synapses from the 'trigger site' of the particular cell. A factor which may introduce variations in the specific spatio-temporal patterns of presynaptic impulses which fire a particular cell is suggested by evidence for the presence on a single neuron of multiple trigger sites some of which might even be located in dendrites. [5 p. 82]

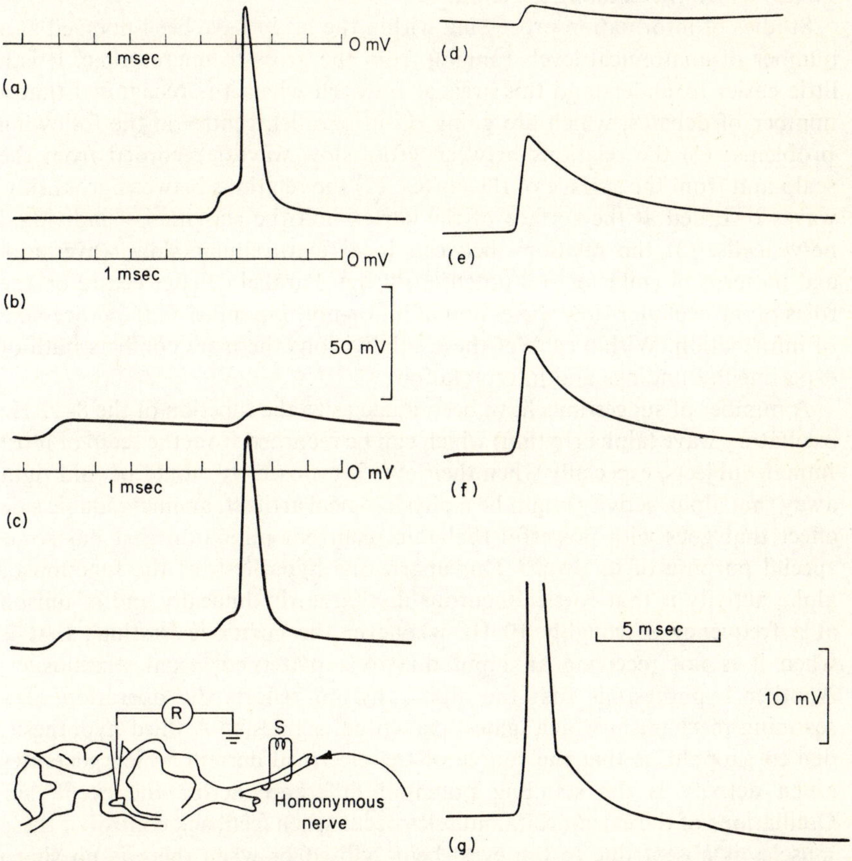

FIGURE 1.8 *Intracellularly recorded responses of motorneurons to afferent volleys of impulses. A, a small depolarisation can be seen immediately before the action potential is initiated; the cell fires when this depolarisation reaches about 10 mV. This prepotential, the excitatory presynaptic potential or EPSP, is believed to reflect the change which is induced in the membrane by the incoming volley and results in the cell firing. B, responses to two incoming volleys both of which fail to fire the cell. C, same as B except that the interval between the incoming volleys is less, so that the second EPSP adds to the 'tail' of the first EPSP and exceeds the critical level of depolarisation (here 13 mV) to fire the cell. D to G, responses of another cell to incoming presynaptic volleys of increasing intensity. In G the EPSP reaches threshold and the cell fires D, E, F, illustrate that amplitude is a continuous function of the strength of the incoming presynaptic volley. From T. C. Ruch, H. D. Patton, J. W. Woodbury and A. L. Towe (Eds.) (1961).* Neurophysiology. *W. B. Saunders Co., Publishers, Philadelphia.*

1.2 General remarks: the activities of single neurons

The previous section gave an outline account of two quite dissimilar forms of electrical activity which have been observed in nerve cells. These are (*a*) graded changes in the potential difference across the limiting membrane, and (*b*) all-or-nothing changes in this potential difference (action potentials or spikes) which travel along the axon.

Studies of information processing within the brain have been pursued at a number of anatomical levels ranging from the gross to microscopic. It is a little easier to understand this area of research when it is recognised that a number of debates, which are going on in parallel, centre on the following problems: (1) the relations between gross slow waves* recorded from the scalp and from the surface of the cortex, (2) the relations between gross slow waves recorded at the surface of the cortex and the activities of individual nerve cells, (3) the relations between local extracellular slow waves and and patterns of spike (action-potential) firing. Parallel debates centre on the roles of intracellular slow waves and of all-or-nothing spikes in the processing of information. Within each of these subdivisions there are conflicts both of experimental findings and interpretation.

A number of suggestions have been made as to the function of the 8–12 Hz oscillatory wave (alpha rhythm) which can be recorded from the scalp of most human subjects, especially when their eyes are closed. It should be said right away that alpha activity might be a physiological artifact, an unavoidable side effect that goes with powerful thalamic recurrent inhibition that has some special purpose of its own.[22] This apart, one hypothesis of the function of alpha activity is that cortical neurons discharge rhythmically and in unison at a frequency of roughly 10 Hz whenever the cortex is 'resting', that is when it is not receiving an input due to a patterned visual stimulus.[9, 10] Another hypothesis is that the alpha rhythm reflects the operation of a scanning mechanism which 'gates' perceptual signals.[845] A third hypothesis, due to Lippold, is that the source of the electrical current which generates alpha activity is the standing potential difference across the eye.[500–502] Oscillations of the extra-orbital muscles occur when feedback control of these muscles is absent due to the eyes' being closed or when there is no sharp image on the retina. These muscles then act as variable shunts for the steady current and so give rise to an alternating electric field on the surface of the scalp. There is, however, some disagreement as to the data which support Lippold's hypothesis. [501, 106a, S43]

Changes in the electrical *resistance* of brain tissue evoked by sensory stimulation have been recorded in the cat.[300, 457] The events responsible for resistance shifts, however, are not identical with those responsible for EPs.[300]

* The slow waves which are recorded from microelectrodes and which can be assumed to reflect the activities of single cells are here referred to simply as 'slow waves'. The term 'gross slow waves' is used to mean slow waves which are recorded with gross electrodes and which reflect the activities of large numbers of cells.

The most characteristic feature of cortical spontaneous activity during barbiturate anaesthesia is the *spindle*. This consists of a sequence of slow waves whose amplitudes gradually increase and then gradually decrease. Andersen and Andersson[22] discussed the physiological basis of the alpha rhythm on the assumption that *barbiturate spindle activity in animals is analogous to the human alpha rhythm*.* They concluded that the thalamus is normally the pacemaker for the cortical alpha rhythm. Their conclusion was based on experiments which involved deafferentation of the cortex, surface or general cooling, the effects of local injection of drugs and the finding that ablation of the cortex did not abolish rhythmic thalamic activity. They speculated that one function of the thalamic recurrent inhibitory mechanism, which (they suggested) underlies alpha activity, may be to transform a single afferent volley originating from a sensory receptor into a train of impulses whose frequency was about 10 Hz and that such a train might be particularly effective in producing cortical excitation. An additional speculation was that rhythmic activity of the thalamocortical network plays an important part in the development of learned responses by keeping information stored in the right place ready to be recalled by the cortex.[22]

1.2.1 *The relation between gross slow waves recorded at the scalp and at the surface of the cortex*

In man Cooper *et al.*[175] compared records from scalp electrodes and from underlying cortical electrodes for both 'spontaneous' EEG and EPs to flash and electrical stimulation. Quite different waveforms were recorded from an occipital scalp electrode (Oz) and from a cortical electrode immediately below. In contrast, there were marked similarities between the waveforms recorded from scalp and cortical electrodes when both were located in the frontal region. Cooper *et al.* confirmed for both EPs and the EEG that scalp records depend not only on the amplitude of cerebral activity in microvolts, but also on the area of cortex involved in synchronous activity. Their records, however, were a superposition of ten traces only so that details of the waveforms would be masked by noise. Heath and Galbraith[366] claimed greater resolution of detail since they summated 100 responses and in addition considered 'early' and 'late' EP components separately. They demonstrated that EPs to flash have different waveforms at cortical electrodes situated in the primary visual cortex and in the temporal cortex. Furthermore, they confirmed that in man EPs to flash recorded over the primary visual area show different waveform at cortical and scalp electrodes. An early component (65 msec peak) was evident in both cortical and scalp recordings in the occipital region, but for later (100 to 300 msec) waves there were latency differences

* Lippold (see above) was careful to restrict his analysis to the 10 Hz oscillatory activity which is often seen in man on closure of the eyes. It has not been conclusively shown that the mechanisms discussed by Lippold and by Andersen and Andersson are one and the same: their hypotheses may not, therefore, be mutually exclusive.

between the EP components recorded at the two electrodes. In explanation of these waveform differences they suggested that activity generated in the temporal cortex spread to the occipital scalp lead whereas the current did not spread to the occipital cortical lead. On the basis of waveform differences recorded from scalp and cortical electrodes in man they concluded that EPs generated in primary and nonprimary cortex are often confounded at a scalp electrode, whatever its location. In particular: (1) activity evoked in sensory specific cortex may spread to scalp electrodes placed over nonspecific cortex, (2) conversely, activity evoked in nonspecific cortex may spread to scalp electrodes placed over sensory specific cortex, (3) similar short-latency components ($\sim$100 msec) are recorded from scalp and cortical electrodes situated over primary cortex and (4) similar longer-latency (100–400 msec) components are recorded from scalp and cortical electrodes situated over nonprimary cortex.

At first sight there appears to be conflict between the findings of Domino *et al.*[233] and Giblin[317] for somatosensory EPs in man and the reports of Cooper *et al.* and Heath and Galbraith for visual EPs described above. Both Domino *et al.* and Giblin found that EPs recorded from an electrode on the dura were of similar waveforms to EPs simultaneously recorded from adjacent scalp electrodes. The only marked difference between the recordings was that the scalp potentials were some twenty times smaller in amplitude. However, these findings may not be inconsistent with Heath and Galbraith's conclusions if it is accepted that *short-latency* components of the somatosensory EP are generated in the primary cortex only, since the records of Domino *et al.* extended over only 125 msec and Giblin's over only 100 msec.

In contrast with the findings of Cooper *et al.* and Heath and Galbraith for flash EPs in man, similarities between waveforms of scalp and epidural EPs recorded over primary cortex have been reported by Vaughan and Gross for rhesus monkey.[821] In contrast with the results of Domino *et al.*, Vaughan and Gross' findings cannot be explained by the omission of long-latency components.

Vaughan and Gross stimulated by spatially-unstructured brief flashes which were presented either aperiodically, or regularly at 1 Hz. Waveforms recorded from electrodes placed over the striate cortex under and on the dura were found to be identical, and were also identical to waveforms recorded from an adjacent scalp electrode. The attenuation between responses recorded from the scalp and over the dura was surprisingly small – roughly 50% for bipolar recordings and 25% for monopolar recordings. Vaughan maintains that this small value of attenuation was not due to the skull and scalp being 'bridged' by a low resistance path round the implanted electrodes,[536 p. 191] and has suggested that other workers' conflicting findings of differences in waveform between EPs recorded at scalp and over dura might be due to inaccuracies in their placements of scalp electrodes over intracerebral electrodes. Vaughan has also claimed that the average EP to photic stimulation (spatially unstructured flash) recorded from the scalp overlying the occipital pole 'reflects in detail the configuration of the evoked cortical response beneath, with little contribution from anterior portions of striate cortex.[815 p. 205] This conclusion conflicts with the findings of a number of other workers[175, 366, 847] and moreover Vaughan's substantiating illustrations have the unsatisfactory feature that the intracerebral and scalp responses being compared are from different subjects.[815 p. 206]

There is the further question of possible interspecies differences between monkey and man. In rhesus monkey the primary visual cortex displays relatively more of its area to the surface of the scalp than in man.[611] As a consequence, EPs generated in primary visual cortex might be less attenuated on the scalp for rhesus monkey than for man, so that scalp and cortical EPs might differ in waveshape more for man than for rhesus monkey. Another point is that the intracranial EP waveforms recorded by Heath and Galbraith (for man) and by Vaughan and Gross (for man and monkey) show marked differences which may be relevant to the conflict between their conclusions. These disparities between EP waveshapes might be due in some measure to differences in recording techniques. Both groups used extracranial references in their monopolar recordings. Vaughan used the skull as an 'indifferent' electrode; Heath and Galbraith used a variety of 'indifferent' placements – left or right ear, both ears, or forehead. There is evidence that the choice of extracranial reference electrode can have a marked effect on the waveforms recorded from intracerebral electrodes, and that the effect can be quite different at an adjacent scalp electrode.[366 Fig. 1]

Whether an electrode lies over or under the dura might also affect the relation between 'cortical' and scalp recordings when the activity of small areas of cortex are involved. Geisler and Gerstein[312] have shown both experimentally and on theoretical grounds that the major part of the 'diffusion' of potential distribution caused by the layers of material overlying the cortex is actually due to dura and cerebrospinal fluid under the dura. Those workers[233, 366, 821] who placed their intracranial electrodes *over* the dura may therefore have eliminated only a part – and the smaller part – of the diffusing effect of overlying structures on the potential distributions generated by small cortical areas. When responses generated in small areas of cortex were involved, evoked potentials recorded from the scalp electrodes and from electrodes on the dura would tend to resemble each other more than recordings from the cortical surface and the scalp.

A number of attempts have been made both to calculate the potential distribution on the scalp which would be produced by hypothetical sources within the skull, and also to relate such theoretical sources to neuroanatomy[324, 413, 488, 816, 826, S1] (see Chapter 2, Sections 2.10.1, 2.10.2, 2.10.3, 2.10.4). These endeavours have met with a number of problems. For example there are mathematical difficulties in calculating the potentials which are produced on the surface of an irregular isotropic volume conductor by an internal generator. Beyond this though there seems to be some doubt as to whether the brain can be regarded as an isotropic volume conductor,[536] or even whether it is reasonable to regard it as a volume conductor at all.[536 p. 536] Morrell and Morrell[555] have argued that scalp EPs are a composite of volume-conducted and neuronally-conducted activities whose relative contributions change with the subject's age.

If the (neurophysiological) current generator of a surface field are assumed to be extended surfaces, then the (theoretical) equivalent source cannot in general be described as an equivalent dipole, but must rather be described by an expansion of multipole terms (e.g. a dipole term plus a quadripole term plus an octapole term, etc.).[57, 99] For current generators which consist of surfaces of simple shapes there are a number of methods for obtaining a good theoretical fit by calculating no more than the dipole, quadripole and octapole terms. These methods cover the cases of media which are homogeneous and isotropic,[99, 314, 315] inhomogeneous but isotropic[592] and inhomogeneous and anisotropic.[695, 696] (Interestingly, the major part of the mathematical groundwork has been carried out for cardiological rather than for EP or EEG purposes.)

In contrast with the case for generators of simple shapes, when the neurophysiological generator is a surface of some complicated shape (e.g. a fissured surface), then the mathematical procedures for calculating a theoretical equivalent source are at best difficult, and at worst unexplored.[52]

Unfortunately there can be little doubt that all the currently-available methods for describing an equivalent source in terms of a multipole expansion are taxing for the non-mathematician. The EP investigator is faced with the problem whether he should expend the time and effort which would be required to familiarise himself with the more daunting of the equivalent-source mathematics. This is a real problem which is not solved by adopting the following working hypothesis which (to this author) seems implicit in some EP reports: that a finding of no serious discrepancy between the predictions of some simple model, and experimental determinations of the potential field at the scalp is a sufficient basis to suggest that the model may have interpretative value. This working hypothesis is seductive: it is also dangerous. For example, particularly when the imprecision of EP measurements is taken into account, the initial success of a single-dipole model surely gives no reason to suppose that some alternative model might not fit the experimental data equally well. The salient point is that this notional alternative model, although perhaps mathematically more inconvenient than the dipole model, might involve an equivalent source whose neurophysiological implications were quite different from the implications of the dipole model. The only certainty among all these 'ifs' is that if no attempt is made to test models other than that which is simplest on mathematical grounds, it will *never* be clear whether the data can support more than one hypothesis as to the spatial configuration of the equivalent generator. This alarming methodological trap can appear in a variety of guises (see Chapter 2, Section 2.1.1).

Wilson and Bayley,[875] and Frank[294] calculated the distribution of potential which would be generated at the surface of a homogeneous isotropically conducting sphere by a volume conduction from a dipole source located within the sphere.[91, 315, 826] This model did not take into account the effects of the different conductivities of the various layers which surround the brain (e.g. cerebrospinal fluid, dura, skull, scalp). Considerable departure from the physiological situation was also made by treating the slow-wave generators as a single equivalent dipole rather than as a volume distribution of dipoles. Geisler and Gerstein in their model subsequently allowed for the effects of different layers, but restricted their treatment to brain activity which could be adequately represented by a single equivalent dipole – that is, dipole-like activity restricted to a small volume of brain tissue. At the same time they pointed out that an adequate (*but not unique*) model to fit observations on EPs generated in the visual and auditory cortex would in fact be a volume distribution of dipoles. Geisler and Gerstein were able to show on theoretical grounds that the effect of a shell whose conductivity is either lower or higher than that of the underlying material is to attenuate and 'spread' the distribution of potential generated by an underlying dipole; the effect is greater for a shell of higher than of lower conductivity. These theoretical predictions of attenuation effects were shown to be physiologically valid by recording auditory evoked potentials in monkey while successively removing the layers which surround the brain. Evoked potential components generated by small areas of cortex were indeed found to be attenuated much more by the highly conducting layers below the surface of the dura than by the (comparatively) poorly conducting skull. Geisler and Gerstein's treatment accounted for the well-known fact that epileptic discharges recorded from the scalp accurately reflect cortical activity when this activity is synchronous over a large area of cortex, whereas when epileptic discharges are very localised no sign of their presence can be detected by visual inspection of scalp recordings.

In conflict with Geisler and Gerstein, Vaughan has claimed that the effect of the layers overlying the cortex is principally to attenuate. The 'spreading' or 'smearing' effect[312] is quantitatively small when it is measured by changes in the position of the half-maximum-amplitude point of the potential distribution.[816 p. 78]

Vaughan extended concentric-sphere modelling[312, 592, 696] from a treatment of a single equivalent dipole to include calculations of fields due to extended, two-dimensional, dipole sheets. Vaughan's calculations accounted for the experimental finding[175] that synchronous activity generated in a small cortical area is much more attenuated at the scalp than is synchronous activity which is generated over a wide area of cortex. His calculations also predicted that the spatial parameter which determined the degree of attenuation caused by the layers surrounding the brain was not the superficial area but the angular subtense (seen from the scalp) of the synchronously active cortex.

SUMMARY

Different laboratories have reported quite different relations between slow waves recorded at the scalp and at the surface of the cortex. To a large extent this conflict of data is due to the effects of the layers of tissue and fluid which overlie the cortex. These layers have been variously claimed to diffuse the distributions of electrical potential generated within the brain,[175, 218, 312] or to attenuate the amplitudes of potentials without diffusion.[816] Attenuation is greater for electrical signals which are generated within a small region of the cortex than for signals generated synchronously over wide areas of cortex. For example in man the attenuation between cortex and scalp may be 2500 times greater for the signals generated within a small area than for signals generated over a wide area.[175] Visually evoked scalp potentials in man for example, contain not only components generated by localised sources within primary cortex but also components generated by extensive areas of nonprimary cortex. Since EPs in primary and nonprimary cortex may have different waveforms, the disparity between the areas of the cortical regions involved in generating primary and nonprimary EP components may lead to differences between the waveforms of the EPs recorded from scalp and cortex. Moreover, electrical activity can predominate at one electrode of a cortical array in one behavioural state, and at another electrode in another state, although scalp recordings show no change.[536 p. 191] In cats at any rate, anaesthesia can have a marked effect on the relation between scalp and cortical-surface EPs. In the unanaesthetised state the auditory EP waveform is similar at scalp and cortical electrodes whereas under anaesthesia the scalp-recorded EPs become very small and the major component of the cortical EP becomes larger.

1.2.2 *Gross cortical slow waves and the electrical characteristics of individual neurons*

Severe difficulties have been encountered by those who have tried to describe in any detail how gross cortical surface slow waves are developed from the electrical activities of individual neurons. As a result the literature is confusing, not only to the newcomer to evoked potential research.[536 p. 198] Among the difficulties in accounting for gross surface slow waves are:

(*a*) The problem of calculating the geometry of the external electric field generated by an individual neuron. This calculation demands a knowledge of the relative contributions made to the surface field by the characteristically different electrical activities of the axons, soma and dendrites of neurons.

(*b*) Problems due to an insufficient knowledge of the neuroanatomical locations of the active neurons,[S3] and an insufficient knowledge of their degree of synchrony. At the present time the sparseness of such knowledge is a potent source of confusion for anyone who attempts to draw general conclusions about the genesis of surface waves from the results of experiments which are lumped together without any regard for differences due to disparate physiological states and preparations. It seems clear from the literature that distinctions should be made between neurophysiological data obtained with deeply anaesthetised and unanaesthetised preparations, between alert and asleep states and between primitive and primate brains.

(*c*) The purely mathematical problems of allowing for the different locations of a large number of active neurons in calculations of the resultant surface field (see Section 1.2.1).

EXPERIMENT AND THEORY

One early hypothesis of the generation of surface slow waves invoked the 'envelope' of the brief-lived (1–2 msec) axon spikes which was the mode of neural activity best understood at the time.[81] In 1936, and indeed for many years, it was possible to uphold the 'axon-spike' hypothesis of cerebral gross slow wave generation even in the face of the findings that the briefest isolated events which (at that time) could be recorded from the cortex were no shorter than 10 msec or so.[9, 10] Hypotheses involving axon spikes as the sub-units of surface slow waves grew less popular, however, in the face of such evidence as Renshaw's[658] demonstrations of lack of any relationship of the slow waves and brief axon spikes recorded from small groups of neurons, and the finding that unitary spike activity could be suppressed while slow-wave activity persisted.[21, 492, 493, 618] Nevertheless there is evidence that spikes can make some contribution to gross surface slow waves.[830, 832]

A second hypothesis firmly excluded both brief (1–2 msec) axon spikes[830] and slow changes in the membrane potential of individual neurons, and postulated that small groups of cortical cells had the special property of generating longer-lived spikes of 10 to 100 msec duration. Surface cortical slow waves were, it was suggested, made up of prolonged spikes, summated over many neurons.[9, 10, 81] Adrian and Matthew's conclusion that slow waves were summation effects and had no counterpart in the activity of individual neurons was based principally on their recordings from closely-spaced electrodes placed on the cortex of anaesthetised rabbit. They reasoned that if slow changes of potential difference between two cortical electrodes were due to a summation of brief waves, then the slow changes would be relatively more in evidence when the distance between the cortical electrodes was large. In contrast, only a succession of brief waves would be observed in the limiting case of electrode separations, so small that only a single neuron could contribute to the record. On the other hand, if surface slow waves were due to correspondingly slow changes in the potentials of individual neurons, then slow waves should still be evident between electrodes at separations so small that only a single neuron could contribute. In fact Adrian and Matthews found an increased amplitude of the brief cortical waves (10–100 msec duration) *relative to* the amplitudes of the slow waves for a small electrode separation. (For small electrode separation a concentric needle electrode of 1 mm diameter was used; these records were compared with monopolar recordings from a 'pointed gelatine electrode'). Adrian and Matthews concluded that the 'brief' (10–100 msec) monophasic spikes which, they proposed, were the sub-units of surface slow waves were themselves the synchronous discharges of a small group of neurons, but that the discharges of each individual neuron had appreciably slower time courses than the 1 and 2 msec discharges of myelinated axons.[10 pp. 448–9] Twenty-eight years after Adrian and Matthews, and with the benefit of modern microelectrode recording techniques, Elul carried out an experiment similar in aim and design to the original Adrian and Matthews experiment.[266] A number of Elul's findings, however, conflicted with the earlier data. He found that extracellular slow waves had only 1% of the amplitude of intracellular records. This suggested that the intracellular slow waves were not generated by an external source, but on the contrary were generated by individual cells. In conflict with Adrian and Matthews, Elul supported a third hypothesis of the generation of gross surface slow waves. This third hypothesis (which dates back to 1931)[8, 94] is that certain cellular potentials are of a sufficiently slow time course that they can lead directly to surface slow waves without the need for temporal summation (i.e. the postulate that surface slow waves reflect the 'envelope' of briefer-lived electrical changes, basic to the first two hypotheses, was rejected).[269, 619] In short, Elul proposed that the gross EEG was not made up of brief potentials, but was a statistical summation of elementary slow waves whose time courses were comparable to that of the gross EEG, and which emanated from cellular-sized generators. However, the slow waves produced by these small generators were found to differ considerably in waveform from the gross EEG. Only *extracellularly recorded* slow waves (made up presumably of a number of individual cellular generators) resembled the gross EEG both in waveform and frequency content. The problem of how individual contributions of individual cellular generators could summate to give the gross EEG is discussed in Section 1.2.3.

Evidence has accumulated[185, 491, 512] to add to that marshalled earlier by Purpura[94, 493, 617] that cortical surface slow waves can be largely accounted for by graded dendritic* postsynaptic potentials, although in some circumstances it seems that highly synchronised axon volleys can be recorded at the cortical surface and may contribute to the earliest component of the visually evoked potential.

Although many authors have reported close correlations between postsynaptic potentials and cortical surface slow waves, it is difficult to form a clear hypothesis of the causal relationships between the two since some authors found surface negative waves to be associated with excitatory PSPs, while in contrast others reported surface negative waves to be associated with inhibitory PSPs. Creutzfeldt's solution to this problem was to suggest that *slow* membrane potential changes are closely in phase with the surface potential, whereas *fast* membrane potential transients may be out of phase with surface waves by angles of up to 180°.[188, 189, 536] The time course of an excitatory PSP may therefore partly determine whether the resulting surface wave is of positive or negative polarity. Creutzfeldt further found that the relations between intracellular activity and surface waves were different for each of three visually identifiable classes of surface wave. Creutzfeldt sug-

* It is worth noting that the surface area of the dendrites may amount to 80–90% of the total superficial area of a cortical cell.

gested that if, as in some studies, all three classes of wave were lumped together, confusion would result.

Creutzfeldt's hypothesis of the generation of the EEG is that it results from volume conduction of the synchronous activity of pyramidal cells. These cells contribute uniformly to the EEG because of their common vertical orientation relative to the surface of the cortex.[189, 5 p. 148] The hypothesis is based on evidence gathered from intracellular recordings of PSPs and EEG waves for sensory motor cortex in cats which were anaesthetised with Nembutal. Creutzfeldt was able to associate different features of the surface EEG with a number of different electrical events in individual neurons (Fig. 1.9). These were: (1) EPSPs which occur in the apical dendrites and which generate a superficial sink; (2) IPSPs and EPSPs which are electrotonically* conducted to the apical dendrites from more deeply located parts of the neuron and which generate a superficial source and a superficial sink respectively; (3) deeply located fast transient activity including (*a*) the discharge of afferent and efferent fibres generating a deep sink and therefore a superficial source, and (*b*) the onset of PSPs–EPSPs leading to a brief superficial source and IPSPs leading to a brief superficial sink.

As examples of items (1) to (3) above, synchronous EPSPs deep in the cortex would appear at the surface as a fast transient positivity, and then later (when they are electrotonically conducted to the dendrites) as a negative wave. Similarly, Creutzfeldt suggests that IPSPs originating deep in the cortex would appear at the surface as a brief negativity followed by a positive wave. Again, synchronous activity in (deeply located) afferent and efferent fibres would rapidly appear at the surface of the cortex in the form of a brief positivity.

It should be emphasised that Creutzfeldt's model of EP generation is based on data obtained from the motor cortex of cat which was stimulated electrically. Two points should be borne in mind: (*a*) most of the cells studied were pyramidal cells which are regularly orientated at right angles to the cortical surface; (*b*) the electrical characteristics of all cells were similar – possibly due to the method of stimulation. For these reasons the extension of Creutzfeldt's model to the *visually* evoked potential may not be entirely straightforward since (i) for visual in contrast to electrical stimulation, the inputs to the cells in the visual cortex may be organised in a variety of ways and may therefore simultaneously produce a variety of response patterns and (ii) the geometry of the cells may not be so regular and simple as that of the pyramidal cells in motor cortex.[536 p. 194] It has been claimed that models of

* 'Electrotonic currents' are formed by the passive spread of charge from more polarised to less (or oppositely) polarised regions of the membrane surface. The effect of electrotonic currents is to eliminate the potential differences established by the active processes associated with neuronal conduction. The tendency for membrane potentials to equalise over the surface of a neuron during passive decay is analogous to the tendency for temperature to equalise over an unequally heated metal plate while it cools: the formal mathematical treatments of the two problems are identical.

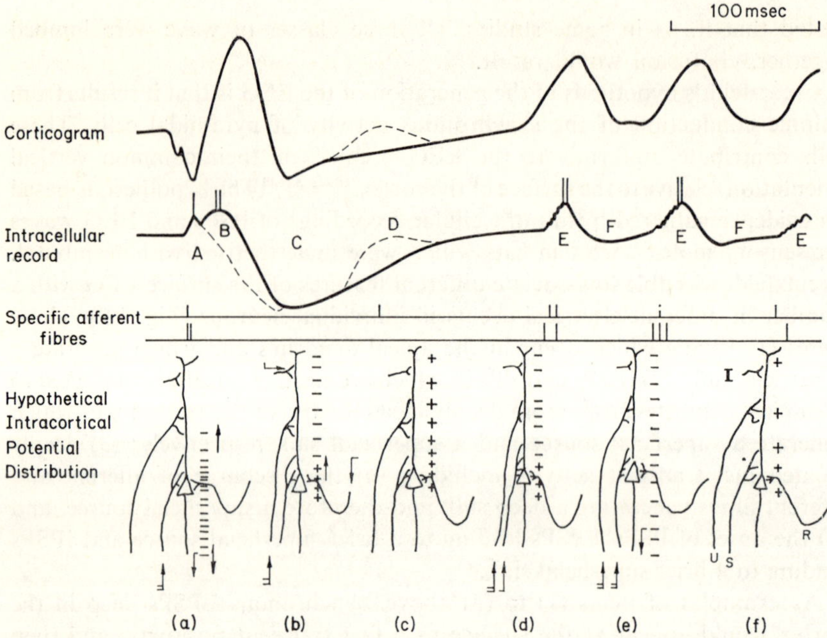

FIGURE 1.9 *Hypothetical transcortical potential distribution during an evoked potential.* (*Tentative model based on data of Creutzfeldt* et al). Top trace: *schematic evoked potential of the sensori-motor cortex after electrical stimulation of the specific thalamic projection nucleus (VPL). Surface positivity downwards.* Second trace: *intracellular record from a pyramidal cell (EPSPs upward, IPSPs downward, action potentials not fully shown.) The broken lines show deviations from the 'typical' potential sequence. The letters refer to the corresponding drawings of the neuron at the bottom.* Traces 3 and 4: *examples of the activity of two afferent fibres.* Bottom: *schematic drawings of a pyramidal cell with its specific (S in* **f**), *non-specific (U) intracortical (I) afferents and the recurrent collateral (R), which comes from a neighbouring cell. The recurrent collateral (R) is considered to be inhibitory, the other afferents excitatory. The arrows with tails indicate the direction and intensity of fibre activity, simple arrows the direction of electrotonic potential spread along the soma-dendritic membrane.* **a**: *highly synchronised afferent volley produces EPSPs in the deeper parts of the neuron and efferent spike activity. Depolarisation spreads upwards along the dendrite and the afferent fibres: surface positivity.* **b**: *activation of non-specific afferents on apical dendrites and fast development of IPSP on the soma due to activity of recurrent collaterals (the IPSP may mask the apical dendritic polarisation if the electrode records from the soma): surface negativity.* **c**: *the polarisation due to the IPSP has involved the whole neuron: surface positivity.* **d**: *the polarisation may be interrupted by non-specific (apical dendritic) depolarisation: surface negativity.* **e**: *loosely synchronised excitatory activity from specific and non-specific afferents produces a depolarisation of the whole soma-dendritic membrane and some efferent, discharges during the after-discharge (and during spontaneous spindle waves): surface negativity.* **f**: *no afferent activation results in return of membrane potential to resting level; recurrent inhibitory activity may produce slight polarisation of the cortical neurons: isoelectric baseline or slight positivity in surface record. From O. D. Creutzfeldt, S. Watanabe and H. D. Lux (1966). Relations between EEG phenomena and potentials of single cortical cells,* Electroenceph. clin. Neurophysiol. **20**, 1–18, 19, 37. *Elsevier Publishing Co., Amsterdam.*

the generation of surface EPs which treat neurons as dipoles orientated at right angles to the surface are in general inadequate since such dipole behaviour can be found only in very specific situations; in particular a dipole model is not an appropriate basis for models of visually evoked potentials.[536 p. 194]

It is a noteworthy feature of Creutzfeldt's hypothesis that a single 'average' neuron is responsible for all the different 'waves' of the surface EP. He does not postulate that different waves reflect the arrival of signals which have traversed different routes, nor does he postulate that different sets of cells or morphologically distinct generators are responsible for different EP waves as has been suggested elsewhere.[21, 115] Creutzfeldt's model has the merit that it embodies an attempt to provide a detailed account of the features of gross slow waves on the basis of rather few facts about the electrical properties of single cells. This approach of course carries with it the dangers of oversimplification. For example, Creutzfeldt's model might need some modification if it were required to include the following points. (*a*) The effect of the distributed capacitance of dendrites can be that a local fast current transient is 'seen' by a distant electrode as a much slower transient;[620, 621] (*b*) extracellular potential differences are due to the extracellular currents generated by neurons. However, the membrane current density at any point on a neuron is not necessarily proportional to the membrane potential at the extracellular surface.[623] In general, therefore, extracellular potential differences cannot be predicted in any simple way from the values of potential at a single site on the neuron's membrane; (*c*) an electrode does not necessarily record a positive potential when it is placed on a portion of the membrane from which current flows into the extracellular volume.[624, S4]

1.2.3 *Statistical relations between gross slow waves and slow waves recorded from single cells*

As described earlier Elul was able to record slow oscillations of the resting potential of implanted cortical neurons and the time courses of these oscillations were comparable with the time course of the gross EEG. These findings led to the hypothesis that the gross EEG is compounded of slow waves generated by individual neurons. If this hypothesis is assumed, then the question of how the contributions of the individual generators are compounded to form the gross EEG merits some attention.

One suggestion is that the EEG is simply the sum of time – locked neuronal activities.[188, 189] Purely visual inspection of the intracellular and gross EEG records appears to lend support to this hypothesis since the frequency of the intracellular and gross EEG waves are superficially similar, and furthermore the frequencies of both change in a similar way when the animal changes from sleep to wakefulness.[269] However when longer sections of record are examined quantitatively for awake cat, the relationships between intracellular waves and the gross EEG turn out to be fleeting.[268] Elul filtered simultaneous records of EEG and intracellular activity into narrow frequency bands. The stability of the relationship between the amplitudes and phases of the records *within a single frequency* band was evaluated. This is the 'coherence' measure[840] and can give an estimate of how closely the two activities are linearly related (when the effect of noise can be neglected). In records lasting 200 to 600 secs coherence between intracellular and gross EEG records *never* exceeded the level by chance alone. Some part of the conflict between Elul's finding and the emphasis laid by other workers on the closeness of the correlation between surface EEG and intracellular waves[189] may be due to the use of unanaesthetised *versus* anaesthetised preparations since there is evidence that (particularly deep) anaesthesia has the effect of increasing the regularity of discharges of cortical neurons.[S5] Additional evidence against a large degree of synchronisation of individual neurons is Elul's finding that twin microelectrodes separated by as little as 30 μm still pick up completely different wave activities.[268]

Elul suggested therefore that the EEG is not produced by linear summation of elementary time-locked (synchronous) slow waves. He proposed a solution for the problems raised by the reported differences between the waveforms of intracellular and gross EEG records and for their lack of long-term coherence.[268] This is that the individual generators are nonlinearly related to each other and that their outputs sum statistically. If these and two other conditions hold then, Elul claimed, it follows from the *central limit theorem* of statistics that the outputs of individual generators will sum to give waves similar to the EEG waves observed in practice.

For any sample of EEG, an amplitude histogram can be computed which, for a sufficiently large number of samples, approximates to the amplitude probability distribution of the EEG sample. Elul pointed out that although the amplitude probability distribution of the gross EEG is approximately Gaussian, the distribution for cortical intracellular records departs appreciably from Gaussian. The central limit theorem of statistics states that a Gaussian amplitude probability distribution may be the result of summing a large number of individual probability distributions *regardless of the nature of these individual distributions.* The conditions required for the theorem to be applicable are: (*a*) the component distributions possess a mean, (*b*) the component distributions possess a finite standard deviation and (*c*) the component distributions are independent. Elul provided experimental evidence that conditions (*a*) and (*b*) can be satisfied in practice. Although independence of the generators would seem to be unlikely [condition (*c*)], Elul[269] argued that the relation between generators is probably nonlinear, is certainly not in general linear, and furthermore, that the central limit theorem would therefore be applicable.

Elul's hypothesis of generation of the gross EEG by combination, according to the central limit theorem, of the contributions of individual cellular generators carries with it some possibilities of the reverse procedure, that is, deduction of cellular events from observations of gross cortical or scalp potentials.[269,5]

Elul's application of the central limit theorem has a corollary which is relevant to the concept of synchronisation of generators. The amplitude of the gross EEG in the extreme case of independence of individual generators will be a function of the square root of the number of generators. In the extreme case of total synchronisation the amplitude of the gross EEG will be a function of the total number of generators. In view of the likely magnitude of the number of generators Elul[269] pointed out that amplitude differences observed between aroused EEG and sleep spindles are far too small (an amplitude change of roughly 10 : 1, which corresponds to the synchronisation of 100 generators). Alternatively, an amplitude change of 10 : 1 could result from a very small change in the synchronisation of a more realistic number of generators, but in any case the amplitude of the intracellular waves themselves are larger during sleep than wakefulness. Either alternative suggests that the concept of 'synchronisation' is of little importance, although some weak interaction between generators during sleep must be postulated since the intracellular waves only double in amplitude while the gross EEG increases tenfold (but see this chapter, Section 1.2).

1.2.4 *Summary and comments*

SLOW WAVES RECORDED FROM THE SCALP AND FROM THE SURFACE OF THE CORTEX

A number of laboratories have reported that evoked potential waveshapes recorded from scalp and cortical surface show marked similarities, although there is some disagreement on the relative amplitudes of the potentials recorded from the two sites. On the other hand there have been some reports of waveshape differences between scalp and cortical slow-wave records. It seems probable that these disparities between the reports of different laboratories are largely due to the attenuating effect exerted by cerebrospinal fluid, skull and other overlying material on the potential fields generated by coherent intracranial sources – especially coherent intracranial sources of small physical dimensions.[175, 506, 847] On the other hand, for slow waves which are generated coherently over a large cortical area, scalp and cortical recordings are similar in waveshape, and not very dissimilar in amplitude.[175, 847]

SLOW WAVES RECORDED BY GROSS ELECTRODES ON SURFACE OF THE CORTEX AND THE ELECTRICAL ACTIVITIES OF INDIVIDUAL NERVE CELLS

Different laboratories report quite different relationships between, on the one hand gross surface slow waves, and on the other hand extracellular slow waves and action potentials. Evidence is accumulating that there is no single fixed relation between spike firing and cortical surface slow waves and that the relation at any particular time is determined by a number of factors such as, for example, whether the surface slow waves in question are evoked potentials or 'spontaneous' EEG, whether the animal is anaesthetised or unanaesthetised, alert or drowsy. The influence of these factors on the relation between cortical-surface slow waves and single-unit activity can probably account for many of the discrepancies between the reports of different investigators.

There is evidence that glial cells can make important contributions to surface slow waves since these cells are electrically coupled to each other by a low resistance pathway and thus behave like a single long conductor.[164] Furthermore, the effect of the glial cell contributions can be that the resultant surface slow waves may have waveforms entirely different from the waveforms of the actively-contributing neurons.[123, 164, 343] The reason for this seems to be that glial cells become depolarised when neighbouring neurons are active, independently of the sign of the neuron's change of potential.[61, 164] So far the evidence on this question of waveform changes due to glial cell contributions relates only to *Necturus* and cat. Nevertheless, it is very clear that the question of glial cell contributions to evoked potentials is of the first importance in the interpretation of EP experiments.

The question whether the investigation of gross surface slow waves is likely to lead to worthwhile knowledge of brain function provokes a variety of responses ranging from the view that the study of surface slow waves can be compared to 'holding an oscilloscope probe 6 feet in diameter up to a computer and pronouncing from the resultant waveform on the underlying structure and function'[603 p. 297] to variants of the feeling that gross slow wave, especially evoked potential, studies provide a 'window' on to the CNS complementary to that afforded by single-cell techniques, and that the relative values of the single-cell and gross-recording methods cannot be assessed in the present primitive state of understanding of brain function.

EXTRACELLULAR SLOW WAVES AND ACTION POTENTIALS

Once again different laboratories have reported different relationships between spike-firing and local slow-wave activity.[230, 291, 292, 425, 612, 831, 832] A considerable part of this conflict seems to be attributable to the different animal states and preparations studied in the various laboratories, and to the use of different electrode diameters which sample different numbers of neurons. Once again, too, evidence is accumulating that there is no fixed relation between spike-firing and local slow-wave activity, but rather that the relation depends on a number of factors including whether or not the animal is anaesthetised,[493] if unanaesthetised whether the animal is alert or drowsy, and whether the slow-wave activity in question is evoked or 'spontaneous'.

The term 'synchronised EEG' has been used with the implication that in this state many neurons are active simultaneously. Conversely, the term 'desynchronised EEG' has been used with the implication that in this state such simultaneous firing does not occur. There is evidence that, although such a clear distinction is not evident at the level of single cells, nevertheless some enhancement of the grouping of spikes does occur during appearances of 'synchronised' gross slow waves[833] (Fig. 1.10).

THE ROLE OF INTRACELLULAR SLOW WAVES IN THE PROCESSING OF INFORMATION

The classical view is that a nerve cell invariably 'fires' when the potential difference across the neural limiting membrane falls to a certain critical value. Although incoming spike trains incident on the synapses of a single nerve cell may be transformed into graded postsynaptic potentials before being 'weighed', their eventual outcome is all-or-none spikes, and on the classical view it is only by all-or-none spikes that neurons can communicate with each other. On this view, intracellular slow waves and spikes reflect the same information processing[291, 292] (Fig. 1.10). If there is an exclusive, mutually causal relation between local slow waves and spike firing the question 'which is the more basic' may have a similar answer to questions about eggs and chickens. The suggestion has even been made that at least in some parts of the nervous system it is the action potentials rather than the slow waves which are best regarded as epiphenomena.[603 p. 290]

There is evidence that some neurons may directly influence each other by means of slow graded changes of potential (for example via dendrite-to-dendrite connections.[622, 625, 632] Furthermore, some workers claim that the potential difference across the neuronal membrane does not unequivocally determine the firing of the cell,[603 p. 299]* and from such data Adey has speculated that slow waves and spikes might reflect separate transforms of information.[603 p. 299] He has further suggested that travelling waves[4, 477] (for which there is some experimental evidence)[555] may play a role in cortical integrative action.

THE ROLE OF ALL-OR-NONE SPIKES IN THE PROCESSING OF INFORMATION

As mentioned above, the classical view is that the only way in which neurons influence each other is by synaptically-transmitted spike activity, and furthermore, that the neuronal correlate of information processing in the CNS is to be found in spike activity. There are two hypotheses of information processing in central regions of the brain. In one view the activity of a small number of cells represents (symbolises) an item of information; the 'labelled' cells 'stand for' the items of information. On the other view an item of information correlates with the activity or *state* of a large population of neurons. The correlation is statistical so that any individual neurons may enter and leave the population with negligible effect on the functioning of the brain.[418, 700, 705, 706, 761, 768, 828, 832, 833 p. 419] In contrast it is generally agreed

* The question has, however, been raised that cells whose intracellular potentials show evidence of variable relationships between membrane potential and firing probability may have sustained damage as a result of electrode penetration.

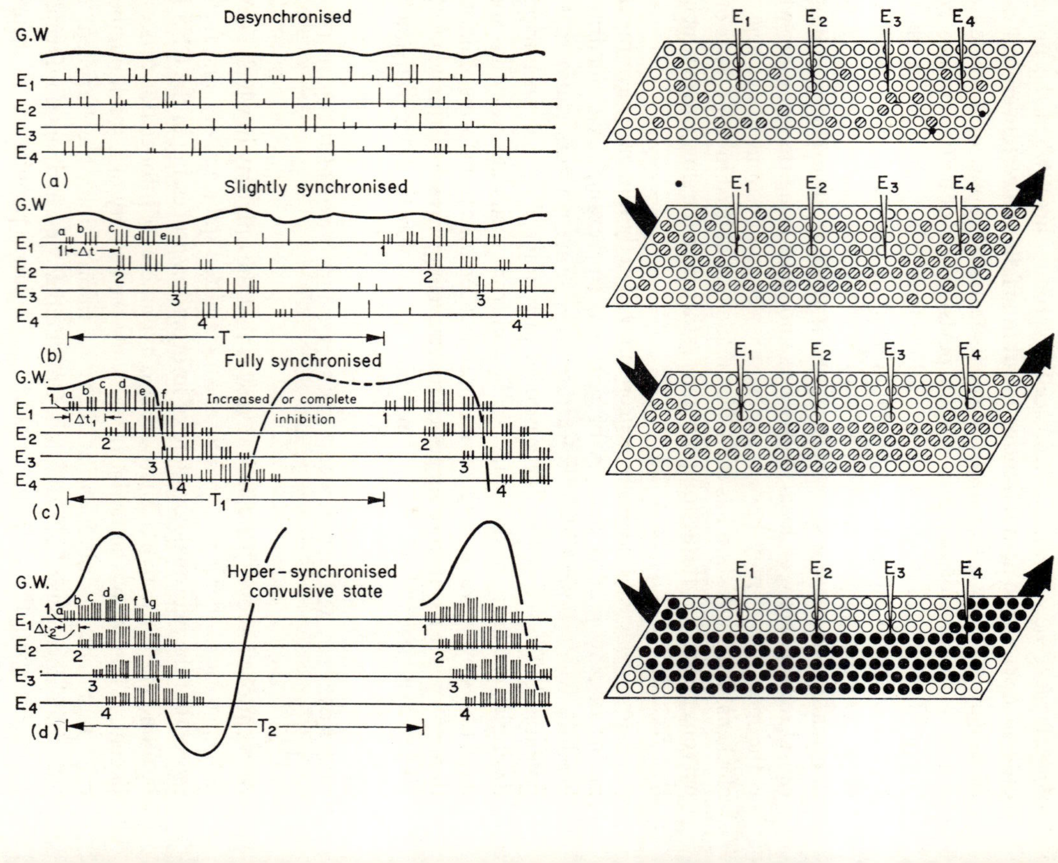
Desynchronised
G.W
E1
E2
E3
E4
(a)
Slightly synchronised
a b c d e
Δt
T
(b)
Fully synchronised
G.W.
Increased or complete inhibition
Δt1
T1
(c)
Hyper-synchronised convulsive state
a b c d e f g
Δt2
T2
(d)

that at more peripheral levels of the CNS the behaviour of neurons are generally much less labile than at central levels, so that an individual neuron may show a close and enduring correlation with some feature of a stimulus.

Analogies between, on the one hand, all-or-none neuronal activity and digital processing and transmission of information, and on the other hand between graded postsynaptic potentials and the analogue processing and transmission of information, have optimistically been pointed out by a number of writers. In this context the possible role of systematic changes in the level of transmembrane potential 'noise' (whether random or periodic) on the transfer characteristics of individual neurons has so far received little attention, although such fluctuations of transmembrane p.d. have been reported to reach up to 35% of the total transmembrane p.d. and may occur in the absence of spike firing.

The promise of the 'information theory' approach to studies of brain function has so far been realised to a disappointing extent. One reason for this lack of success may be a too literal usage of the concept of information theory. Neural pathways are not merely communication channels, since they not only transmit but process information.[603 p. 229] 'The concepts of information theory

FIGURE 1.10 *Relations between neuronal discharge, circulation of neuronal activity and synchronisation of the gross waves, as they appear when recorded simultaneously with four microelectrodes with tips separated by 100 to 150 μm. Left: diagrammatic representation of oscilloscope tracings, showing the progressive changes which take place from the desynchronised to the hypersynchronised state. Right: diagrammatic two-dimensional representation of neuronal fields, showing the neuronal activity corresponding to each successive state.* E_1, E_2, E_3, E_4 *represent the microelectrodes through which oscilloscope tracings* E_1, E_2, E_3, E_4 *(at left) would be obtained; the circles represent neurons in the field of the microelectrodes; the degree of darkness in each circle represents the degree of excitation of that particular neuron; the arrow represents the direction of the circulation of neuronal activity.* a: *oscilloscope: infrequent clustering of the spikes, no circulation of neuronal activity, no synchronisation of the gross waves. Neuronal field: scattered, sporadic neuronal activity, at low level of excitation; no circulation of neuronal activity.* b: *oscilloscope: increased clustering of spikes; occurrence of neuronal activity in regular succession at each one of the tips of the microelectrodes, indicating circulation through the neuronal network; decreased activity in the interval between successive passages of circulating activity through the network; gross waves slightly synchronised. Neuronal field: neuronal activity at higher level of excitation, concentrated mostly in the pathway of circulation (arrow); decreased activity outside this pathway.* c: *oscilloscope: high degree of clustering of spikes; increase in the velocity of circulating activity; activity abolished in an increased interval between successive passages of circulating activity through the network; gross waves fully synchronised. Neuronal field: neuronal activity at high level of excitation in the pathway of circulation; no activity outside the pathway.* d: *oscilloscope: extreme degree of clustering of spikes; high velocity of circulation; further increase in the interval between successive passages of circulating activity through the network; neuronal activity in this interval abolished; hypersynchronised gross waves of high amplitude. Neuronal field: neuronal activity at very high level of excitation concentrated exclusively in an enlarged, multilane pathway of circulation; activity completely abolished outside this pathway. From M. Verzano (1963). 'The Synchronisation of Brain-waves' in* Acta. Neurolog. Latinoamer. *9*, 307.

are at best metaphors (*of questionable aptness*) when applied to the nervous system. . . .' The results of neurophysiological experiments designed within a framework of information theory 'do not imply that the assumptions and methods used by the investigators in their decoding efforts bear any resemblance to processes employed by the nervous system itself'.[551 p. 507]

2

Sensory information processing and evoked potentials

2.1 Introduction

2.1.1 *Correlations between physical and mental events; theoretical models of perception*

How are features of the world variously represented within the brain? What are the physiological processes which underlie sensory perception? This chapter discusses both the contributions already made by EP studies towards the resolution of these questions, and their future role in this area of research.

Correlates between evoked potentials and neural activity have been sought at a number of different levels of information processing. At the lowest level the search has been for EP correlates of such elementary stimulus features as colour or contours. Even at this level, experiments have been bedevilled by artifacts due to processes not immediately related to perception. At a higher level there have been attempts to identify EP correlates of neural processing such as that which underlies the identification of simple geometric shapes. Yet more ambitious studies have attempted to find EP correlates of the high level of information processing which underlies such discriminations as those between different words. Up to the present time the second and third type of study have been hindered by a lack of understanding of EP correlates of even the lowest levels of information processing.

At this point it may be helpful to distinguish between two types of EP experiments. In the first type one measures features of the EP which correlate with an *objective stimulus parameter* (e.g. intensity). In the second type of experiment one measures features of the EP which correlate quantitatively with the *sensation* aroused by the stimulus.

Often the result of the first type of experiment is that, over a small or large range of stimulus variation, some feature of the EP (for example latency) is found to correlate with the chosen stimulus parameter. Given such an experimental result there is an immediate problem in progressing beyond the mere descriptive statement that 'A correlates with B'. It does not necessarily follow that A *causes* B or vice versa. On the contrary, A and B might have no causal relationship whatsoever, but might both be causally determined by C in such a way that A and B are strongly correlated. It follows that, although tempting, it is nevertheless invalid to conclude that an EP feature which correlates with some psychophysical measure (or stimulus measure) *therefore* reflects physiological activity which is directly related to perception. However, if such a correlation is found to hold over a very wide range of stimulus conditions, then there can be greater confidence that the correlation has physiological significance than if the correlation holds only over a narrow range of stimulus conditions. It is easy to see, for example, that quite different functions (for example a power function and a saturation function) may agree fairly well over small ranges, and can only be seen to differ when stimulus parameters are varied widely. The converse, however, cannot be assumed to be true: the failure of a correlation to hold over more than a narrow range of stimulus conditions does not necessarily mean that it has no physiological significance. Uttal[809, 810] illustrated one difficulty in assessing the physiological significance of a correlation between subjective and objective measures when he distinguished between on the one hand a correlate which reflects a physiological 'code' (i.e. neural activity which carries a message which has sensory meaning for the organism) and on the other hand a correlate which reflects neural activity which does not carry a message with sensory significance to the organism (a physiological 'sign').

As mentioned above the aim of the second type of EP experiment is to identify some feature of the EP to a stimulus such that the feature correlates quantitatively with the *sensation* aroused by that stimulus. Examples of this kind of experiment are (*a*) those in which the stimulus intensity at psychophysical threshold and the stimulus intensity required to elicit an EP of some criterion amplitude are both determined for each of a series of stimulus frequencies; the two sets of values of stimulus intensities are then plotted *versus* stimulus frequency on logarithmic paper in order to compare the shapes of the graphs, and (*b*) those in which EP amplitude is compared with subjective estimates of sensory magnitude.[589, 766]

What can one hope to learn from such experiments which compare objective features of EPs with subjective quantities? If the experimenter's working hypothesis amounts to no more than 'it might be interesting to see what happens', then most probably he will learn little unless he is very lucky. In most cases the value of such experiments will largely reflect the quality of the hypothesis that the experiment is designed to test, and this in turn will depend on the experimenter's model or models of the physiological processes which underlie perception, however general these models may be. Von Holst has emphasised that it is just as true in the biological sciences as it is in physics and chemistry that if a hypothesis is to contribute to our understanding of phenomena, the hypothesis should amount to more than a mere generalised description of observations, and should rather predict what will happen under defined conditions: the hypothesis can then be verified or disproved by experiment.[388]

An experimenter's choice of scientific questions and experiments may be dictated by his (possibly unconscious) acceptance of arbitrary models of perception which sometimes masquerade as the natural and logical way of thinking (for example the notion that an internal 'spirit' or 'ghost' looks at brain signals flowing from the sensory receptors).* This point is brought out in MacKay's discussion of the question whether incoming sensory signals should necessarily be expected to be proportional to perceived sensory magnitude (as measured for example by Stevens'[766] method). MacKay showed that this is not the case, since it cannot be taken for granted that the neural substrate of 'intensity perception' lies in the visual pathway.[529, 697] As an illustration of this point, MacKay proposed a model in which stimulus intensity was encoded logarithmically at a peripheral stage. At a more central stage, the organism generated a 'matching response' to the incoming neural signal.[533] MacKay pointed out that an internally-generated matching response to signals from sensory receptors would 'amount logically to an internal representation of the features in the incoming signals to which it is adaptive', and proposed the matching response as the physiological correlate of perception.[527, 532, 533] Here, an important consequence of MacKay's approach is that for a wide range of possible relationships between the stimulus and the peripheral response, the functional relationship between the central *matching response* and the incoming signal could be such as to give the observed power law relation between stimulus intensity and the matching response (and hence between stimulus intensity and sensory magnitude).

Central to MacKay's model of perception is a view of perception as an active 'updating' process in contrast to the position of, for example, Kant[441] who considered perception to be a passive phenomenon. Although MacKay's line of argument can guide the experimenter in his formulation of general

* A related and somewhat intriguing point which was emphasised by Boring[87] is the important influence of scientific fashion in the interpretation of scientific data. As an illustration of this factor, Rosner and Goff[685] cited Matthew's[518] investigation of the effects of mechanical tension on the firing frequency in stretch afferents. In 1931 these data were plotted in log-linear coordinates and gave a close fit to a straight line. This suggested that the relation between tension and firing frequency was logarithmic, in accord with the currently-fashionable Fechner Law. Twenty-six years later it was possible to plot Matthew's data in the now-fashionable log-log coordinates,[685, 767] and find that the points fitted a straight line just as closely as in the original log-linear plot. The same data, then, suggest a power function relation just as strongly as they suggest a logarithmic function. The moral which Rosner and Goff drew from their story for the neurophysiologist was: 'Beware of psychophysicists bearing gifts.' Perhaps, conversely, the psychophysicist would be well advised to beware of the helpful neurophysiologist or EP researcher who can be persuaded to stare into the variability of his 'objective' data until he sees laws emerging from it. On first starting research into evoked potentials it is easy to feel daunted by the neutrality and sheer unhelpfulness of the raw data. Nevertheless, if only to avoid wasting his colleagues' time, minimal caution demands that before publishing an 'experimental demonstration' of some functional relationship, the younger EP research worker should make some effort to find whether his data points fit any other plausible functions, even if the result of his efforts is to blunt the edge of his sharp conclusion.

questions, his model, perhaps because of the generality of its formulation, does not *of itself* point to specific physiological forms which the matching response might take; it would therefore be difficult to disprove the existence of the matching response by experiment, and indeed MacKay has described his model as 'not so much a theory as a programme'.[532] The model outlined above is in essence an attempt to find which questions might most appropriately be asked about the way in which motor output and sensory input are coordinated. MacKay's is a comprehensive model of perception only to the extent that perception can entirely be described in terms of action and readiness for action, in other words only to the extent that passive modes of perception can be excluded.

MacKay's model has implications for the design of evoked potential experiments. For example it suggests that what was learned from an EP experiment would depend on whether the EPs recorded reflected the peripheral neural signal or the more central matching response, or both. More specifically, the EP components which (in MacKay's view) reflected matching activity might be expected to correlate closely with the subject's perception of the stimulus. On the other hand, EPs which reflected the form of peripheral neural signals might be expected to correlate poorly with perception.

MacKay's model of perception leads naturally to the suggestion that EPs reflect activities from many different functional levels, only a limited number of which are accessible to psychophysical investigation. Indeed it is an intriguing possibility that EP methods might allow brain functions to be explored which are inaccessible to perception. By basing experiments on one or other explicit model rather than allowing habits of thought to act as *de facto* models, findings such as poor correlations between perception and some EP feature can perhaps be made to lead to constructive questions about the functional level of activity recorded in the CNS.

Several models of CNS activity are principally concerned with the stability of visual perception against voluntary and involuntary eye movements. These models involve the notion of a 'corollary discharge'[S6] (Fig. 2.1) which is initiated in the motor regions of the brain simultaneously with the motor signals destined to result in motor activity.[388, 786] This corollary discharge is then compared with subsequent incoming messages from the sensory organs which signal *the result of the intended motor activity*.[388] The *difference* between the corollary discharge (which in a sense represents the intended action), and the messages from the sensory organs (which in a sense represent the action in fact achieved) can either influence further action, or can 'ascend to a higher centre and produce a perception'[388] (but 'ascend' in some unspecified manner to some unspecified region).

Both qualitatively, and in terms of information flow, the models of von Holst and MacKay of the mechanisms responsible for perceptual stability are similar in many respects but they differ in the quantitative accuracy demanded of the physiological mechanisms. In von Holst's model the corollary discharge is *subtracted* from the signals flowing inwards from the sensory organs; on the other hand, in MacKay's model the matching response does not cancel the incoming signals but *evaluates* them. The familiar maintenance of stability of the perceived world during voluntary eye movements can be explained along the lines of MacKay's model without requiring the neural evaluation mechanism to operate with any greater accuracy than the accuracy of the eye movements.[533] In contrast the fact of perceptual stability demands, in von Holst's terms, that the cancellation and corollary discharge mechanisms should operate with a very high (according to MacKay an improbably high) accuracy which is of the order of the resolving power of the eye.[533, 87]

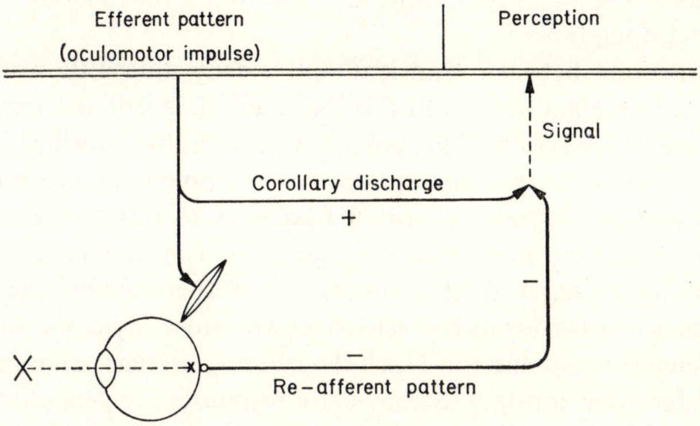

FIGURE 2.1 *Diagram to indicate postulated interaction between afferent, efferent and re-afferent processes in perception. Self-induced motion of the eye (efferent pattern) causes peripheral motor effects and, concurrently, a central discharge back into the appropriate sensory system (corollary discharge) which normally matches (i.e. cancels) the sensations produced by the active movement (re-afferent pattern). Under normal conditions, corollary discharges and re-afferent patterns balance, so that signals from the environment are perceived (e.g. motion of external objects) and distinguished from relative motions due to the perceiver's own movements. When the visual field is inverted, the same feedback becomes positive and maladaptive, causing subjective spinning of the visual field and (in lower species) forced movements of the body. See References 755 and 532. From H.-L. Teuber (1960). 'Perception' in* Handbook of Physiology, *Section 1, Vol. III. American Physiological Society, Washington. (Adapted from von Holst and von Holst and Mittelstaedt.)*[388]

In day-to-day life, information about changes in brightness is generally of less significance to us than is information about the position and velocity of light-dark boundaries (edges) in the visual field. Such 'edge information' tells us where objects are located relative to our bodies, and whether, and in what direction the objects are moving. There is growing evidence, both indirect from single-cell recordings in animals (e.g. References 51, 399, 489), and directly from psychophysical studies in man[23, 50] of the presence in the human visual pathway of neural organisations ('feature filters')[23, 50, 51, 283, 399, 489, 533] which emphasise ('abstract') important *features* of the retinal image such as, for example, the orientation and movement of edges. It seems clear that the auditory system too contains 'feature filters'.[283, 327] If it proves feasible to study the functioning of such neural mechanisms of 'feature emphasis' by the use of EP methods, then EP studies might well assume a valuable role complementary to single unit and psychophysical methods. Evoked potential methods have here the particular advantage over single-cell techniques that they can be recorded from conscious, cooperative human subjects as an everyday procedure. As a result, psychophysical data and the subject's sensory reports can be correlated straightforwardly with objective EP recordings taken at the same time. Electrophysiological studies of feature emphasis in the human visual system are badly needed at the present time, not least to test the reliability of animal-to-human extrapolations.[S56]

The distinctions between transient and steady-state EPs are discussed in Chapter 5. In brief, a transient EP is the result of an isolated abrupt change in some stimulus parameter. This potential is generally described in terms of amplitude *versus time*. In contrast, steady-state potentials are evoked by a stimulus of sufficiently high repetition frequency to result in an overlap of responses such that no individual response cycle can be related to any particular stimulus cycle. A further distinction is that steady-state responses are recorded when the brain has settled down into a 'dynamic steady-state' and is producing a response for which the running averages of amplitude and phase are effectively constant. Steady-state responses are generally described by plots of amplitude (and phase) *versus frequency*.

To anticipate, there is evidence that different features of visual information processing* (both sensory and nonsensory) are reflected by different components of transient EPs and by different frequency regions for steady-state responses respectively. A similar point applies to correlations between features of perception and the EP; both different transient components and different frequency regions of steady-state responses relate in different ways to sensation.

The methodological point that in EP studies the stimulation procedure is at least as important as the methods of data analysis has recently been emphasised by the findings of workers who have used more refined stimuli than the conventional Xenon flash. There is growing evidence that there are a variety of neural organisations within the visual pathways which selectively emphasise restricted features of the visual world such as, for example, contours or motion. The commonly-employed Xenon flash is likely to excite several of these neural organisations inefficiently, simultaneously and to varying degrees. The result is likely to be the creation of further considerable obstacles to the already formidable problem of interpreting a response. It seems probable that one step towards easing the problem of interpreting EPs in physiological terms would be to investigate the effects of changes of stimulus parameters which are chosen, not on the basis of technical con-

* 'Information' here not only covers visual information which enters into the context of perception, but also visual information which does not do so.

venience or ease of physical description, but on the basis of their appropriateness to the already-existing functional organisation of the brain. Specific examples of this approach are the use of spatial structure and of motion as the primary stimulus parameters.

2.2 Evoked potentials and the physical intensity of the stimulus; evoked potentials and sensation

2.2.1 *Introduction*

Almost without exception, EP measurements have been restricted to amplitude and latency in studies of the relationships both between the EP and stimulus intensity, and between the EP and the subjective quantities of brightness, loudness or touch. For this reason alone the question whether there are EP correlates of stimulus intensity, and of subjective brightness and loudness can be by no means regarded as having been decided, since the use of different EP measures might lead to quite different conclusions. Indeed, even within the narrow limits set by amplitude and latency measurements, there are a number of uncertainties remaining. First of all there is the question of which of the various 'amplitudes' is the most appropriate measure of EP amplitude. Technical convenience has sometimes dictated the choice of the peak-to-trough amplitude of a prominent pair of features in the transient EP waveform.[29, 30] However, it seems that different components of the transient EP may behave differently when stimulus intensity is varied,[668] so that a peak-to-trough measure might well confound two differently changing components. It has been claimed that a single wave can be isolated by measuring its peak-to-baseline amplitude,[816] but on the other hand there may be considerable ambiguity in defining the baseline (Chapter 5, Section 4.8). In addition, both of the above amplitude measures are open to the objection that (as for example in the case of motion-evoked potentials) a single EP wave may be a composite of two subpeaks whose amplitudes relate differently to the stimulus.[536, 542] Another source of uncertainty in some visual studies are the relative contributions which 'contrast-specific' and 'unstructured-field' components make to the total EP.* It seems like that the relative importance of these EP components could be markedly affected by such procedural

* EPs can be elicited by changes in the contrast across well-focused sharp edges in a stimulus pattern. These EPs are discussed in Section 2.4 of this chapter and will be referred to as 'contrast specific' EPs. Such EPs differ in a number of ways from the EPs to spatially-unstructured fields (this chapter, Sections 2.3 and 2.4). The differences are most marked for foveally-presented stimulus patterns whose pattern elements are small (roughly 5′ to 20′). The differences between, for example, the EPs to reversals of a 10′ checkerboard pattern and to modulation of the luminance of a spatially-unstructured 10° field could be interpreted in two ways: (*a*) that the scalp potentials specifically evoked by changes of contrast of a spatially-structured field are qualitatively different from the potentials evoked by unstructured fields, or (*b*) that the properties of EPs are a continuous function of the spatial frequency of the stimulus field; the EPs to 10′ checkerboard patterns lie towards one end of the continuum and the EPs to diffuse fields lie at the other end.[120, 38]

details as the sharpness of focus of the edges of the stimulus field, the presence of 'accidental' contours within the stimulus field, and the size of the stimulus field. In many experimental reports such details are not given.

Quite apart from any questions of experimental design, though, the implications of relating EP amplitude to estimations of sensory magnitude are far from straightforward (if not downright incomprehensible). Rosner and Goff,[685] and Sutton[775] have written illuminating reviews of this problem.

Sutton has pointed out that a sensory threshold for any given subject is not unique, but depends on which psychophysical method is used to measure the threshold.[S13] He quoted as an example that when a subject attempts to judge whether a visual stimulus is a single flash or two closely-spaced flashes, a certain forced choice method[589] gives a threshold which is lower by a factor of two than the threshold obtained by the method of constant stimuli[589] Furthermore, the different instructions given by different experimenters and the idiosyncrasies of different subjects may have the result that even the same subject may use quite different threshold criteria in different experiments. The resulting lack of uniqueness of the psychophysical threshold poses problems for the experimenter who asks the question whether 'the' psychophysical threshold is lower, higher or identical with the evoked potential threshold. Furthermore, a physiologically-meaningful definition of 'the' evoked potential threshold has so far proved elusive (see footnote in Chapter 4, Section 4.2.1). If the EP threshold is defined as 'that intensity level at which a recognisable EP waveform can be detected by visual inspection', then, although EP threshold may be clinically useful (Chapter 4, Section 4.2.1), its quantitative value depends on arbitrary factors such as the number of sweeps of the averager, the type of averaging device used, electrode location and the skill of the experimenter in recognising characteristic EP waveforms. An alternative method of determining EP threshold by a graphical extrapolation procedure rests on the assumption that the functional relation between EP amplitude of stimulus strength observed for high EP amplitudes also holds at low EP amplitudes (see footnote in Chapter 4, Section 4.2.1). Sutton[775, 777] has pointed out that the behavioural response in psychophysical trials has often a binary form (i.e. yes – no), while EP amplitude is a continuous (graded) quantity. There are problems in comparing two such mathematically different quantities.[781] A further point relating to the question of whether it makes sense to compare psychophysical and EP thresholds is whether the brain's powers of temporal and spatial integration are related in any simple way to the corresponding capabilities of the experimenter's averaging device.

Clearly a first requirement before comparing EP and psychophysical thresholds is that the psychophysical and evoked potential data should be measured in similar experimental situations, and preferably during the *same* set of trials. The two measures should both be determined while the subject is actively making a judgment, and not, as has often been the case, with the subject attentively discriminating[S28] in the psychophysical experiment but in rather a passive (i.e. undefined) state during electrophysiological recordings.[775, 777] More specifically, it has been shown that differences in late components of the EPs can be produced by changes in a subject's level of attention (see Chapter 3);[239] such effects would be confounded with any effects of stimulus detectability in experiments where the subject's level of attention was different in the psychophysical and electrophysiological trials.[143, 250, 775, 777]

Sutton has drawn attention to the importance of the well-known fact that, at near-threshold levels, identical stimuli can elicit quite different percepts,[775, 777] and went on to question the validity of lumping together the potentials evoked during trials which involved different percepts.[775, 777] A related question is whether potentials evoked in trials which involved different categories of behavioural response (e.g. correct *versus* incorrect guesses) should be lumped together.[775, 777]

A general problem in comparing psychophysical threshold data and electrophysiological measurements is that a given stimulus may often generate not one but several psychophysical cues. For example, a subject might state that his criteria for distinguishing between a double flash and a single flash included subjective impressions that the double flash looked (*a*) double, (*b*) longer or (*c*) a different colour to the single flash, and furthermore that he used different criteria in different trials. If physiological correlates of all these perceptual cues were present in the EP, then confusion might result if individual trials and EPs were not separated into the categories (*a*), (*b*) and (*c*) above. Since it is much easier to instruct a subject to use only one of the psychophysical cues available to him (e.g. doubleness in this case) than to discriminate between different categories of EP, this point indicates that in attempts to compare EP and psychophysical data, the subject's instruction for the psychophysical trials should be as restrictive as possible.

S35

2.2.2 *Visual EPs and the physical intensity of the stimulus: visual evoked potentials and sensation*

One possible complicating factor which has been too often ignored in EP work is the distinction between the absolute change of stimulus *intensity*, and the *percentage change* of intensity during a stimulus cycle.[748] For example, a flash of retinal illuminance* of 500 trolands could be superposed on a 500 troland background giving a 100% change in brightness, and possibly a large EP; the same 500 troland flash superposed on a 10,000 troland background

* In general, not only the physical properties of the stimulus but also the area of the eye pupil determine the light energy incident per unit area on to the retina. This effect of pupillary area is often used to advantage when the pupil is artificially dilated in order to increase the subjective brightness of a stimulus. The illuminating power of the light falling on the retina is measured in *trolands* where one troland is the retinal illuminance produced by viewing a surface of luminance 1 candela per m^2 through an artificial pupil of area 1 mm^2 (see Chapter 5, Section 5.1.1).

would give only a 5% change in brightness and possibly a very small EP. It is easy to see at once how the absolute intensity change is not the sole or even the major determinant of the EP.

As discussed below, the common practice of using only very high percentage changes of brightness can bring with it not only difficulties of interpretation[640] but may also result in the swamping of significant changes in EP features, due to the effect of saturation.[152, 748, 797]

There is some conflict about the way in which the amplitude of the transient EP varies with stimulus intensity. Much of this conflict can probably be attributed to the use of different definitions of EP 'amplitude' and to differences in physical stimuli.

Armington[29, 30] found that as stimulus intensity was increased the amplitude of a peak-to-trough measure of EP amplitude rose at first slowly but then levelled off, and even decreased at the highest intensities.[785] These findings were confirmed by a number of subsequent workers.[152, 228, 666, 815] Shipley *et al.*[735] added that although some components at first grew and then diminished in amplitude as stimulus intensity was progressively increased, the amplitudes of other components increased monotonically to their saturated values.

Kuhnt[472] fitted his amplitude *versus* luminance data by power functions whose exponents for different subjects fell between +0·1 and +0·3. However, inspection of his figures indicates that the data could also be fitted reasonably well by saturation curves.

Most workers have found that the latencies of all components of the transient EP to flashes are decreased when the intensity of the stimuli is increased. Using bright flashes Cobb and Dawson found this to be the case for components within the first 100 msec after the stimulus, and this finding holds generally for components peaking up to 600 msec after the stimulus.[735, 785, 870] On the other hand, Rietveld reported that the latencies of some components were unaffected by stimulus intensity over intensity ranges of 2 to 4 log units.[668] The waveforms of the EPs described by Rietveld and Tordoir, however, differ considerably from the waveforms of the EPs described by Shipley *et al.*[735] and Tepas *et al.*[785] so that some disagreement is to be expected.

There is conflict as to whether any feature of the EP correlates with the subjective magnitude of brightness sensation. The striking claim was made by Vaughan and Hull that the latency of a positive component (100–160 msec latency) and the magnitude of subjectively-estimated brightness are related to stimulus intensity in the same way.[822] At high stimulus intensities this positive EP component tended asymptotically towards a latency (τ) of 108 msec. At lower stimulus intensities its latency (τ) decreased in such a way that a plot of log (τ −108) *versus* log (stimulus intensity) was a straight line of slope −0·33. The relation between (τ −108) and stimulus intensity was therefore a power function of exponent −0·33. Vaughan and Hull associated this finding with Stevens[766] report that the magnitude of brightness sensation was also related to stimulus intensity as a power function of exponent 0·33.* This report of a correlation between EP latency and sensation magnitude would have been even more compelling had both subjective and objective measurements been carried out on the same subjects. To demonstrate a correlation is not of course to demonstrate a causal relation, and in the present instance it is not obvious how the CNS could use latency as a representation of stimulus intensity, since the brain has no time reference[536 p. 233].†[S9]

Keidel,[447] in a similar experiment to that of Vaughan *et al.*, varied light intensity over a wide range between 0·002 and 1400 asb, and found EP amplitude and intensity to be related by a power function of exponent 0·21, in rough agreement with Vaughan's finding. Over a range of 4 log units of intensity Kuhnt fitted his latency data by power functions whose exponents varied from 0·08 to 0·3 depending on the subject.[188]

When the illumination level was reduced to very low levels Vaughan and Hull reported changes in the EP waveform which they described as a sudden increase in latency attributed to scotopic mechanisms. An alternative interpretation suggested by Donchin is that at very low illumination levels stimulus-related EP components are of very small amplitudes so that the response components recorded by Vaughan and Hull to very dim stimuli were only loosely coupled to the stimulus and were in fact related to 'uncertainty resolution' (Chapter 4). On the other hand, Wooten[881] found that EPs recorded at very low illumination levels did have a scotopic spectral sensitivity.

When two equally-intense visual stimuli with adjacent contours are presented in rapid succession, the brightness of the first stimulus appears greatly reduced. This phenomenon is called metacontrast. The initial negative wave of the EPs to diffuse flashes both increase in latency and decrease in amplitude when stimulus intensity is reduced. Schiller and Cordover reported that such EP changes do not occur under metacontrast conditions when brightness is reduced without lowering stimulus intensity.[704]

However, Schiller and Cordover used a parafoveal stimulus. Vaughan and

* Stevens' method of measuring the magnitude of sensations is to instruct the experimental subject to assign a number proportional to the subjective brightness (or weight or loudness, etc.) of the stimulus for stimuli of different intensities, weights, etc.[589, 766, 767] The relation between stimulus intensities and sensory magnitudes are power functions for all sensory modalities so far investigated. Stevens interprets sensory magnitude data as measurements of the inherent operating characteristics of sensory systems, while Warren[852] has suggested that they reflect the subject's prior experience.

† Latency measurements can, whatever their status as candidate codes, reflect *peripheral* processes in the visual pathway. For example De Voe *et al.*[220] showed EP latency to correlate with the Stiles-Crawford effect.

Stiles-Crawford effect: in photopic vision the eye is less sensitive to light which enters near the edge of the pupil than through the centre of the pupil.[768] The accepted explanation is that cones are more sensitive to light incident in a direction parallel to their axes (i.e. light which enters the eye through the centre of the pupil) than light incident at an angle to the cone axes (e.g. light which enters the eye near the edge of the pupil).

Silverstein[827] suggested that Schiller and Cordover's finding of no correlation between subjective brightness and EP amplitude or latency was a consequence of the parafoveal location of their stimulus. Their EPs would then mainly be due to stray light striking the fovea. It turns out that when the visual stimulus is centred on the fovea, a satisfactory correlation between subjective and physiological effects can be observed.[827, s10]

[s11]
2.2.3 *Auditory EPs and the physical intensity of the stimulus; auditory evoked potentials and sensation*

Keidel and Spreng[446, 447, 449, 450, 451] studied the behaviour of auditory EP components whose latencies lay between 130 and 170 msec since these components, they considered, would be linked more closely with stimulus parameters than either earlier or later components. They found that for auditory (and also for vibratory and painful stimulation)[263, 761] the amplitudes of the 130–170 msec EP components were related to the intensity of the stimulus by a power function. Davis and Zerlin[205] also suggested that the plot of the amplitude of the auditory vertex response *versus* intensity is a power function and that its exponent is roughly 0·4. The findings of these objective experiments therefore paralleled Stevens[766] report that the relations between stimulus intensity and subjective estimates of sensory magnitude are power functions for a wide range of stimulus modalities. [Davis and Onishi,[204] however, have commented that even though the amplitude of the vertex potential does rise as stimulus intensity is increased, a number of other properties of the potential, such as its comparatively long recovery time, render it a poor correlate of subjective[s12] loudness (i.e. the potential would reflect a 'sign' rather than a 'code').[809, 810]] Furthermore, the exponents of the power functions reported by Keidel and Spreng for EPs agreed closely with the exponents of the power functions reported by Stevens for subjective sensory magnitude. There does, however, seem to be significant intersubject variability in the exponents of Stevens' power functions, so that correspondence between EP and subjective data has greater force in experiments where both types of measurement are made on individual subjects under identical conditions.

Auditory EPs are further discussed in Chapter 4, Section 4.2.1.

2.2.4 *Somatosensory EPs and the physical intensity of the stimulus; somatosensory evoked potentials and sensation*

In their somatosensory experiments, Franzén and Offenloch used the same subjects for both estimates of sensory magnitude and for EP measurements.[295] They found that power functions described both the plots of stimulus intensity *versus* sensory magnitude and plots of the latencies of the two EP components investigated (positive peaks of latencies 30–40 msec and 43–53 msec). The exponents of power functions for the latencies of the two EP components were *quite different* (mean data for two subjects: exponent 0·56 for subjective estimates, 0·08 for first peak and 0·11 for second peak). Contrasting conclusions emerged from their measurements of EP amplitude. Once again, the relation between stimulus intensity and the EP measure (in this case amplitude) could be described as a power function. However, the exponents of the power functions for EP and subjective data were now in reasonable agreement (exponents: 0·41 for EP and 0·61 for subjective estimates for one subject; 0·47 for EP and 0·58 for subjective estimates for another subject). An additional correlation between the EP amplitude and subjective data was brought out when the results of stimulating two fingers was compared with the results of stimulating one finger only. Two-finger stimulation gave EPs which were larger than single-finger responses by a factor of $\sqrt{2}$; estimates of sensory magnitude were $\sqrt{2}$ times larger for two-finger stimulation than for single-finger stimulation.

Franzén and Offenloch's finding of a close relation between estimations of somatosensory magnitude and EP amplitude appears to conflict with Uttal and Cook's[811] contrary findings. Uttal and Cook claimed that EP amplitude *saturated* in contrast with subjective estimates of sensory magnitude, which continued to rise steadily as the stimulus intensity was increased (cf. similar findings for visual stimuli, Section 2.3.3). However, there were differences between both the stimulation techniques and electrode placements in the two studies. Uttal and Cook stimulated with electrical pulses whereas Franzen and Offenloch used tactile stimulation. The difference between the findings in the two studies might be due to possible differences between the responses of the somesthetic sensory system to tactile stimulation and to 'unphysiological' electric shocks.[578, S40]

Rosner and Goff[685] reported that they had replotted Uttal and Cook's data and found that two of their six published functions did not seem to asymptote, and might even be logarithmic. Rosner and Goff's own experiments showed that the amplitudes of early (up to roughly 80 msec) components of the EP did in fact saturate at high stimulus intensities as previously reported by Uttal and Cook. On the other hand, components of longer latencies did not saturate and, furthermore, the relationship between EP amplitude and stimulus intensity depended on the duration of the shock stimulus. Two-branched curves resulted for both early and later components of the EP when EP amplitudes were plotted *versus* the intensities of 500 μsec shock stimuli. Both branches could be fitted by power functions, but the exponents were lower for high stimulus intensities. Each component of the EP was found to require different power functions. Rosner and Goff claimed that their data were better fitted by dual power functions than by a single power function, even when the single power functions included 'threshold correction' (see below). The transition between the high-intensity and the low-intensity regimes coincided with the stimulus intensity at which an early ipsilateral negative wave first appeared. Rosner and Goff claimed that plots of psychophysical estimates of sensory magnitude *versus* stimulus intensity were also best described by dual power functions, whose transition points also coincided with the first appearance of the early negativity. Rosner and Goff underpinned their theoretical treatment by suggesting that the early ipsilateral negative wave was generated in somatosensory cortex, and was due to signals carried by a group of peripheral fibres which conducted only at high stimulus intensities.

In a later further study, and following an instructive re-analysis of the original Rosner and Goff data,[326] Beck and Rosner[65] came to quite different conclusions. They considered that the most likely reason for the original judgement that the psychophysical and EP data were fitted better by the dual power functions

$$R = a_1 I^{k}{}_{1},\ I \leqslant I_b$$
$$R = a_2 I^{k}{}_{2},\ I \leqslant I_b$$

than by single power functions $R = aI^k$, or by power functions with 'threshold correction' $R = a\,(I - I_0)^k$ was merely that the dual power function had five free parameters (a, a_2, $k_1 k_2$, I_b), whereas the other functions had only two (a, k) or three (a, k, I_0) respectively. In other words, when an experimenter tries to fit his data by a theoretical equation, his task can be progressively eased by adding more and more free parameters to his theoretical equation! In doing so, of course, he runs a severe risk of progressively limiting the generality, the predictive power and the physiological relevance of his equation. Beck and Rosner[65] found that the location of the points of intersection of Rosner and Goff's two power functions did not in fact have the physiological meaning which had originally been postulated. The hypothetical threshold condition for the appearance of the early ipsilateral negativity did not show the anticipated form of dependence on the strengths and durations of stimulus shocks, nor did this wave show the polarity reversal which would be expected of a wave generated in ipsilateral somatosensory cortex.[475] Beck and Rosner considered this early ipsilateral wave to be due to current spread from contralateral cortex, and furthermore that the original data of Rosner and Goff was adequately fitted by equations of the form $R = a\,(I - I_0)^k$. In further support of this judgement they reported that the 'threshold correction', I_0, agreed well with psychophysical measurements of absolute threshold, and that both EP and psychophysical estimates of I_0 obeyed the anticipated strength–duration law. Nevertheless, Beck and Rosner concluded, their re-analysis of the original data upheld Rosner and Goff's claim that EP amplitude and psychophysical estimates of sensory magnitude cannot be described by the same power functions. Their position, therefore, conflicts with that of Keidel and his colleagues.[449, 450, 451, 761]

If the EP correlates of perceived sensory magnitude reported by Franzén and Offenloch and by Vaughan could indeed be interpreted as reflections of the neural representations of sensory magnitude and were not mere epiphenomena, then these EP studies would suggest that the magnitude of visual (brightness) perception and somatosensory perception have qualitatively different neural representations, since in the visual case the latency of the EP was the sensory correlate, while in the somatosensory case the amplitude of the EP was the sensory correlate.

Libet *et al.*[495] reported that somatosensory EPs could be detected at stimulus levels that were below the behavioural threshold. They suggested that their use of subdural rather than epidural or scalp electrodes was the reason for the conflict between their finding and previous reports[222, 233, 782] that psychophysical and EP thresholds coincided for somatosensory stimuli. Sutton[775, 777] has commented (*a*) that the psychophysical procedure adopted by Libet *et al.* would result in high threshold values, since they required their subjects to be *quite certain* that the stimulus had occurred, and (*b*) that since Libet *et al.* defined the subject's psychophysical threshold as the intensity for which less than 50% of the stimuli were reported, their averaged EPs for threshold stimuli included responses which correlated with detected stimuli as well as responses correlated with undetected stimuli. Furthermore, the problem of comparing binary with graded data (mentioned in the introduction to this section) would be acute in the experiments of Libet *et al.*[513]

Clark *et al.*[143] claimed that, for somatosensory stimulation, subanaesthetic concentrations of cyclopropane disrupts correlations between scalp EPs and psychophysical thresholds in such a direction that at the higher concentrations of anaesthetic an easily-detected stimulus failed to elicit an EP. Donchin and Sutton[250] criticised Clark *et al.*'s experiment on several grounds.

They claimed Clark *et al.*'s data were not sufficient to support conclusions about early EP components and were adequate only for those late EP components whose amplitudes have been shown to be sensitive to the subject's state of attention. A second point was, since an effect of cyclopropane on Clark *et al.*'s subjects was to make them feel 'detached from their environment', their consequently low level of attention would in any case be expected to result in attenuated late components of the EP. In contrast with their electrophysiological method which would give attenuated late EP components, Clark *et al.* used a psychophysical procedure (method of descending limits[589]) which would, they pointed out, tend to give sensitive behavioural thresholds.

Sutton's criticisms suggest that the experiments of both Libet *et al.* and Donchin and Clark *et al.* point to the necessity of using closely comparable psychophysical and electrophysiological procedures in experiments whose aim is to compare subjective and objective data.

2.2.5 *EPs and the physical intensities of odorous and taste stimuli; EPs to odorous and taste stimuli and sensation*

Olfactory EPs might be expected to differ from other EPs in ways which are physiologically significant since, in contrast with the somatic, auditory and visual systems, the olfactory system appears to have no thalamic representation and has no known direct projection to the brainstem reticular formation.[19]

Allison and Goff stimulated their subjects with 100–200 msec pulses of odorised air at 6 second intervals. The odorant EPs consisted mainly of a 450–550 msec positive wave and were largest in the vertex region, although they were widely distributed. Their distributions differed from the distributions of somatic or auditory EPs. Different odours gave EPs of different latencies. Allison and Goff[742] considered that contamination of their odorant EPs by responses to stimulation of nasal trigeminal afferents could not be ruled out: later evidence indicated that their olfactory EPs (and probably Finkenzeller's[285] also) were entirely due to trigeminal stimulation.[742]

Electrical stimulation of the tongue can elicit both taste sensations and evoked potentials. Plattig reported that 'if taste sensations were noticed by the subject, stimulus-locked potentials could be gained by averaging the subject's EEG'.[610] Plattig's EPs comprised the following deflections: P_1 (45–80 msec), N_1 (90–155 msec), P_2 (175–195 msec), N_2 (210–245 msec) and P_3 (285–420 msec). The latency of each deflection decreased as stimulus intensity was increased. The amplitudes of N_1 and P_3 were power functions of exponent 0·76 and 0·57 respectively. Plattig did not investigate the relationship between the subjective magnitude of sensation and any feature of the EP. Correlations have been demonstrated, however, between sensory magnitude estimations and summated nerve responses recorded at as peripheral a level as that of the gustatory nerve.[100]

2.3 Visual evoked potentials to spatially-unstructured stimulus fields

2.3.1 *The effects of stimulus field size; spatially-unstructured fields*

The scalp potentials evoked by foveal and extrafoveal stimulation have been compared in a number of ways including (*a*) comparing responses to centrally fixated discs of various sizes, (*b*) comparing the response to a small centrally located stimulus with the response to an extrafoveal annulus and (*c*) comparing responses to small spots of light located in different retinal positions. In all these experiments the relative contributions of contrast-specific components to the total EP was likely to change when either the stimulus field size or shape was varied so that the characteristics of at least two different types of EP components were liable to be confounded.

In Rietveld's experiments a Xenon strobe tube illuminated discs whose angular subtense was varied from 10′ to 8°. An illuminated surround was used in an attempt to reduce the effect of scattered light, although possibly with dubious success due to the very high peak luminance of the short flashes. This high peak luminance would render very difficult the task of reducing the percentage change in brightness due to scattered light to well below the value of 20–50% which may be sufficient to evoke a fully developed response.[152] Rietveld[666, 667, 669] found that the amplitudes of certain negative waves had reached 50% of their maximum for a stimulus field size of about 2° and thereafter increased in amplitude very slowly as field size was increased (waves peaking at 50–70 msec and at roughly 150 msec). From such data on EP amplitude *versus* stimulus area Rietveld calculated the amplitude of the

EP per unit area of retina stimulated for different retinal areas. These calculations indicated that, per unit retinal area, stimulation of the central fovea was overwhelmingly more effective than extrafoveal stimulation. However, Rietveld's calculation is open to the serious objection that, since the contributions of contrast-specific EP components were likely to be relatively most important for the smallest stimuli, then the procedure of dividing the response amplitude by stimulus area is likely to be most invalid for the smallest, centrally located stimuli. Furthermore, there is evidence that the presence of contours enhances the unstructured-field response.[750] It is the responses to these small central stimuli that are most important for Rietveld's conclusion that the central fovea is so much more sensitive than any other region. A second reservation which was in fact pointed out by Rietveld *et al.* is that light scatter is likely to provide the greatest relative contribution to the EP for the smallest stimuli. Both these factors suggest that Rietveld's calculation seriously exaggerates the relative effectiveness of central foveal stimulation.

An additional method used by Rietveld to compare EPs to stimulation of different regions of the retina was to stimulate with annuli of different radii but constant area. He recorded the peak-to-peak amplitude between two prominent features, a negative peak of latency 50–85 msec and a positive peak of latency 100–150 msec. Although his results were not presented quantitatively, it was clear that the response amplitude per unit of retinal area stimulated fell off rapidly as the site of stimulation was moved from 2° to 7° distant from the foveal centre, and that the amplitude of the largest ring response was less than half the amplitude of the response to a centrally fixated disc of the same area. However, as before, the interpretation of these data is complicated by the unknown importance of changes in the contribution of contour-specific EP components. This uncertainty also hinders the interpretation of Rietveld's observation that some components of the EP (a negative wave at 50–85 msec and a positive wave at 100–150 msec) are evoked principally by stimulation of the central 2°, while later waves (170–240 msec) are evoked principally by stimulation of the extrafoveal retina.[667, 668, 669]

In a separate investigation, the amplitude of the steady-state EP to a centrally viewed 2·2° disc was found to be roughly six times greater per unit retinal area than the amplitude of the EP to an annulus of internal diameter 4° and external diameter 11°.[634] Although similar objections to those described above can be made to 'disc and annulus' studies in which repetition frequencies below about 15 Hz have been used, contamination by contrast-specific components is unlikely in studies where repetition frequencies appreciably higher than 15 Hz have been used.[S14] However, in those 'disc and annulus' studies which have used stimulus repetition frequencies near the alpha frequency Spekreijse[750] has pointed out that complications are like due to the varying effect of field structures on the Q factor (i.e. sharpness of frequency selectivity[83]) of alpha activity (and hence on the amplitude of the EP*).

* This point can be seen more clearly by referring to Fig. 2.13.

2.3.2 *Evoked potentials and the modulation depth of the stimuli; analytic and nonanalytic nonlinearities*

The amplitude of the scalp potentials evoked by a change in the luminance of a visual stimulus is determined not only by the *absolute* change in stimulus luminance, but also by the *percentage* change in stimulus luminance. Although it might seem intuitively that the *absolute* change in stimulus luminance would be the most important determinant of evoked potential amplitude, in fact the absolute change may often have much less importance than the *percentage* change in luminance.

The percentage change per cycle in stimulus luminance is often described in terms of *modulation depth*. Fig. 2.2 illustrates how modulation depth is defined in the case of a repetitive sinusoidal modulating waveform.

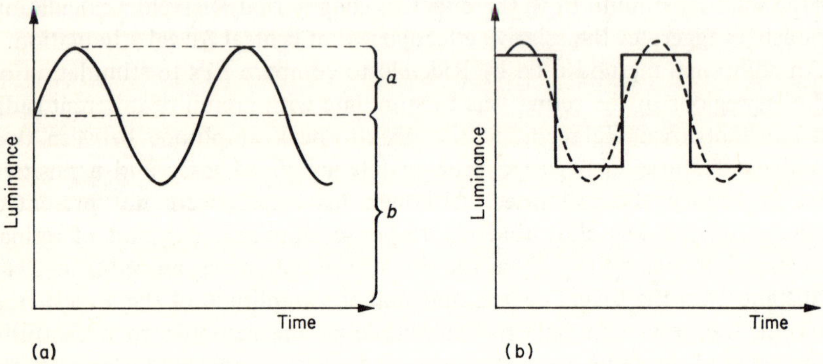

FIGURE 2.2 *A: illustration of the sinusoidal modulation of a stimulus light about a mean level. The modulation depth* m *is defined as* $\left(100\ \frac{a}{b}\right)$ % *B: a long train of square waves of frequency* F *can be represented as the sum of sinusoidal harmonic components of frequencies* F, 3F, 5F, *etc. The fundamental component of a square wave is shown dotted.*

An important feature of light whose luminance is modulated is that the time-average luminance is constant. The mean luminance and percentage change can therefore be varied independently, and furthermore, stimulus repetition frequency can be varied without changing the mean stimulus luminance. In contrast, the result of varying the frequency of brief flashes is that *both* frequency and mean intensity change. An additional point is that with modulated light stimuli 'small signal conditions' (Fig. 2.3 B) can conveniently be used. In Fig. 2.3 the input is the stimulus modulation, and the output is the EP. If a high amplitude stimulus falls on a smoothly-curved part of the characteristic (as at A) the output (which can be graphically synthesised from the characteristic) can be seen to be a very distorted version of the input waveform. However, if the signal amplitude is progressively reduced, then the output waveform becomes less and less distorted (compare outputs in Fig. 2.3 A and B) as the part of the characteristic involved becomes shorter and shorter and therefore approximates more to a straight line. Hence under 'small signal conditions' the system may behave approximately linearly. This type of nonlinearity whose effects can be indefinitely reduced by progressively reducing the amplitude of the signal is called an *analytic* (*'nonessential'*) *nonlinearity.** Fig. 2.3 also illustrates a second type of nonlinearity. When

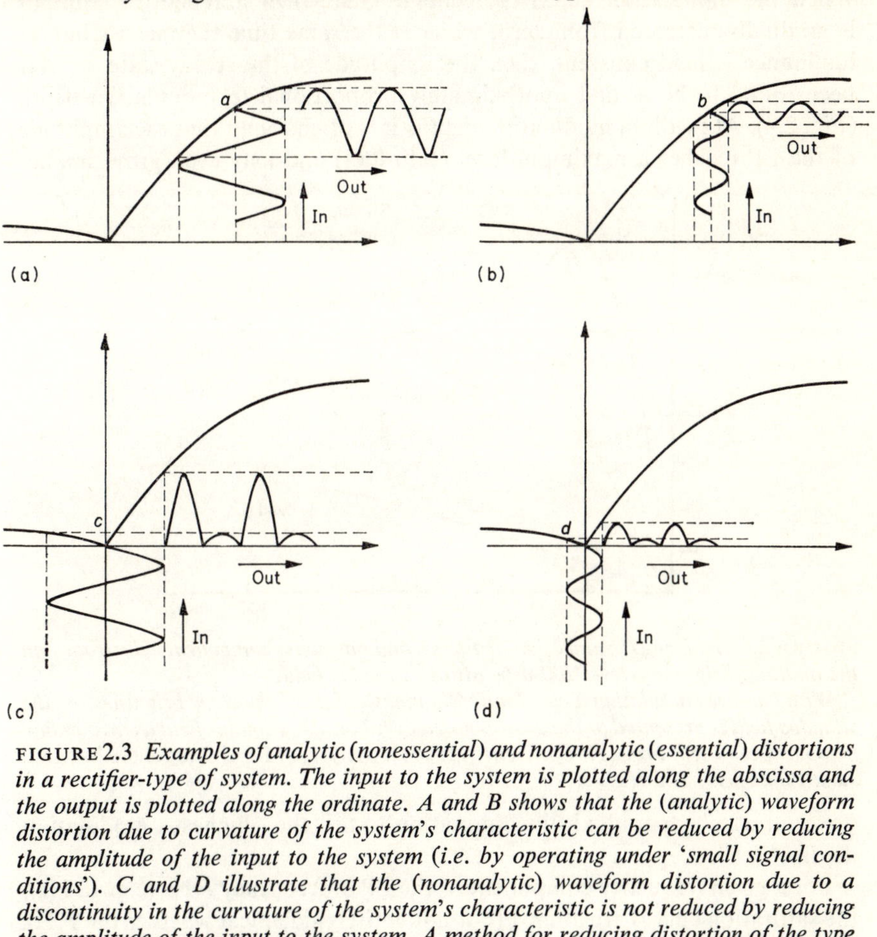

FIGURE 2.3 *Examples of analytic (nonessential) and nonanalytic (essential) distortions in a rectifier-type of system. The input to the system is plotted along the abscissa and the output is plotted along the ordinate. A and B shows that the (analytic) waveform distortion due to curvature of the system's characteristic can be reduced by reducing the amplitude of the input to the system (i.e. by operating under 'small signal conditions'). C and D illustrate that the (nonanalytic) waveform distortion due to a discontinuity in the curvature of the system's characteristic is not reduced by reducing the amplitude of the input to the system. A method for reducing distortion of the type illustrated in B and D is illustrated in Fig. 2.20.*

there is a discontinuity of the characteristic curve or of the slope of the curve in the part of the characteristic traversed by the input (points *c* and *d* in Fig. 2.3 C and D), then the distortion in the output signal cannot be indefinitely reduced by reducing the amplitude of the input signal (compare outputs in Fig. 2.3 C and D). This test enables the two types of nonlinearity to be distinguished, and an identification is of course the essential first step in deciding how to handle a problem in nonlinear analysis.[365, 549] This second

* 'Analytic' here means that the waveform distortion produced by the nonlinearity can be described (analysed) in the form of a series expansion.

type of nonlinearity is called nonanalytic (or 'essential'). Both nonessential and essential nonlinearities have been identified in human EP research.[748, 751]

2.3.3 *Saturation*

When the modulation depth (percentage change) of a repetitive stimulus is gradually increased from zero, while at the same time the mean stimulus luminance is held constant, then the amplitude of the steady-state EP has been found to be at first approximately proportional to modulation depth (Fig. 2.4). At medium modulation depths it is often found that the amplitude of the EP reaches a maximum level (saturates) and may even grow smaller

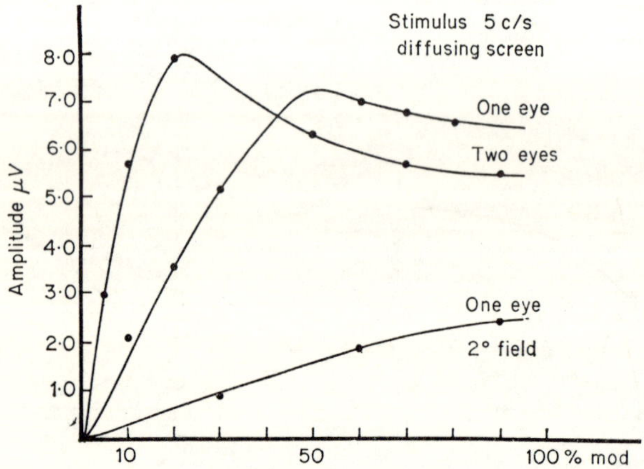

FIGURE 2.4 *Subject D: saturation of the second harmonic component; electrodes on the midline; brightness level 200 asb; diffuse stimulus field.*

With one-eye stimulation a constantly illuminated field of the same brightness as the stimulus field is presented to the unstimulated eye. For a 2° stimulus field a surrounding field has been used. From H. Spekreijse (1966). Analysis of EEG Responses in Man. *Junk Publishers, The Hague.*

('oversaturate' 'paradoxical diminution') at the highest modulation depths.[748, 798]

For a given frequency component of the EP of frequency F Hz (e.g. 10 Hz), the saturation curves are almost (but not entirely) identical whether the F Hz component is evoked by a stimulus of frequency F Hz or $F/2$ Hz. In other words the shape of the saturation characteristic depends almost entirely on the absolute frequency of the EP and not on whether the response is a fundamental or second harmonic.

In Fig. 2.4 the EP to stimulation of one eye alone is compared with the EP to binocular stimulation. For response frequencies near 10 c/sec, the saturated level of the EP to binocular stimulation is similar to the amplitude of the EP to monocular stimulation (Fig. 2.4). One interpretation of this result is that the functional stage at which saturation occurs lies after the signals from the two eyes converge. (This interpretation involves an assumption that the processing of visual signals can be regarded as being serial, and that any centrifugal (central to peripheral) influences can be neglected.) The situation is quite different for components whose frequencies are near 50 Hz (Fig. 2.5). The amplitudes of these 'high-frequency' components to binocular stimulation are considerably greater than their amplitudes to monocular stimulation. With the above proviso, this suggests that the saturation stage for high-frequency EP components is located *before* the signals from the two eyes converge, in contrast with the location of the saturation stage for 10 Hz components.

For components whose frequencies are near 10 Hz, the stimulus modulation depth at which saturation first becomes apparent does not depend on stimulus frequency.[748] Again with the above proviso this finding can be interpreted as an indication that the saturation stage lies *before* the 10 Hz frequency-selective filter stage. Similar arguments apply to components whose frequencies fall in the 45–60 Hz frequency-selective region.

The saturation characteristic depends on both intensity and field size. In the low-frequency region, saturation occurs at lower modulation depths for larger fields than for smaller fields. This suggests that saturation is governed, not directly by the modulation depth of the stimulus, but by the absolute amplitude of the neural signal at the level of the saturation stage. This suggestion is also supported by Spekreijse's data on the ways in which the shape of the saturation characteristic changes as the diameter of the stimulus field is varied. For smaller stimulus fields, saturation occurs at higher modulation depths; the onset of saturation is, however, almost independent of luminance.[750] On the other hand for 'high-frequency' components saturation occurs at roughly the same modulation depths for all field sizes, although it occurs at progressively lower modulation depths as stimulus luminance is increased. This suggests that for 'high-frequency' components saturation

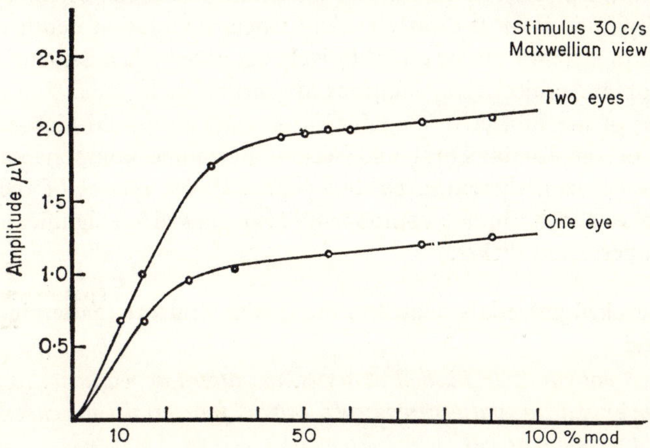

FIGURE 2.5 *Saturation of the fundamental component at high frequencies (subject B). Maxwellian view; stimulus field, 20°; brightness, 10,000 asb; dilated pupil. The unstimulated eye in the one-eye stimulation experiment was covered. From H. Spekreijse (1966).* Analysis of EEG Responses in Man. *Junk Publishers, The Hague.*

occurs not only before the signals from the two eyes converge but prior to the convergence of retinal integration fields.

The shape of the saturation characteristic may also depend on the colour of the stimulus. Regan reported that for 'medium-frequency' EP components of 20 Hz, saturation may be much earlier for yellow stimuli than for red stimuli of the same luminance.[640] In contrast, the saturation curve for high-frequency EP components recorded at the same time and from the same electrodes as the 20 Hz components did not depend on stimulus colour.

According to Spekreijse the amplitudes of the contrast-reversal EPs (Section 2.4.1) to a checkerboard pattern saturate at modulation depths as low as 20%.[748] He found that for a 3·5° target filled with 10′ squares the saturated amplitude of the EP to binocular stimulation was roughly twice the saturated amplitude of the EP to monocular stimulation.[748] Campbell and Maffei[120] used a grating stimulus whose luminance was both spatially and temporally modulated with a sinusoidal waveform (Section 2.4.5). Their measurements were mostly restricted to contrast levels below 0·3 or so, and in this region they found that the amplitude of the EP *versus* log contrast gave a linear plot. In contrast with Spekreijse's checkerboard responses, the ratio between the monocular and binocular EPs could be expressed, not as a constant factor, but in terms of a $\sqrt{2}$ factor between the contrasts of the gratings which gave monocular and binocular EPs of the same amplitudes.[S15]

2.3.4 *Evoked potential amplitude and flicker perception*

Poor correlations have been reported between the amplitude of the steady-state EP and subjective estimates of the amplitude of perceived flicker.[637, 638] As stimulus modulation depth is progressively increased, the subjective magnitude of flicker also progressively increases, but the amplitude of the EP may saturate or even decrease. This dissociation between perceived flicker and EP amplitude is most clearly evident when modulation depth is varied over a wide range, and can be quantitatively described when Stevens' method is used to obtain subjective estimations of sensory magnitude.[766]

Estimates of the subjective magnitudes of supra threshold flicker and the amplitude of the fundamental and second harmonic components of the steady-state EP can, therefore, be dissociated.[648] The phases of the fundamental and second harmonic components also showed no significant correlation with perceived flicker.

2.4 Visual evoked potentials related to the spatial structure (patterning) of the stimulus field

2.4.1 *Evoked potentials to flashed patterns, to pattern-appearance, to pattern-disappearance and to pattern-reversal; evoked potentials to checkerboard patterns and to bar patterns*

It is generally agreed that spatially-structured stimulus fields can evoke potentials whose amplitudes are as large as, or larger than those evoked by spatially-unstructured stimuli, even though the light energy involved may be ten thousand times less.[150, 151] This observation at once raises the question whether the two types of EP reflect the activities of different neural mechanisms. The most direct way of investigating the EPs which are related to the spatial structure of the stimulus is to change the spatial structure of the stimulus *and nothing else*. This may be achieved so as to (*a*) produce a brief presentation of pattern, or (*b*) produce a slow alternation of pattern-appearance, pattern-disappearance or (*c*) result in pattern-reversal at constant mean luminance. There are a number of studies of pattern EPs in which various types of pattern have been flash-presented.[359, 671, 747] This form of presentation is likely to evoke potentials composed of transient responses both to luminance changes and to pattern presentation. These components might summate in a nonlinear rather than a linear manner, and in fact there is evidence that unstructured-field EP components can be enhanced by the presence of spatial structure.[543, 802] In any case the resulting EP is unnecessarily difficult to interpret. Attempts have been made to extract the pattern-specific response by either (*a*) subtracting the EP to a flash-presented unstructured (blank) field from the flash-presented patterned field,[671] or (*b*) subtracting the EP to the defocused pattern from the EP to the focused pattern.[869] Such procedures are in principle unsatisfactory if their object is to examine the pattern-specific response, since it cannot be assumed *a priori* that there is linear summation of the responses to blank-field and to patterned-field stimulation. A more satisfactory procedure is to directly record potentials which are specific to spatial structure by changing the spatial structure of the stimulus *at constant stimulus intensity*.[157, 411, 536, 748] When this has been done and the form of the pattern-specific response is known, then the subtraction procedure can be turned on its head and used as a test for the linearity of summation of pattern-specific and unstructured-field responses. As a matter of fact, it does seem that summation can be roughly linear over a restricted range of variation of stimulus parameters,[411] although nonlinearities may be evident in some circumstances.[802] The force of this point is that linearity of summation is consistent with *independent* operation of the mechanisms underlying pattern-specific and intensity-specific EPs. This question of independence is surely of sufficient importance to merit a detailed quantitative study of the precision to which linearity holds, and the limits over which intensity and spatial contrast may be varied without breakdown of linear summation.

The major (100–120 msec) component[S6] of EPs to the *appearance* of pattern from a previously unstructured illuminated field is opposite in polarity and generally of larger amplitude than the major component of EPs to *disappearance* of pattern[360, 411, 543, 801] (Fig. 2.6).

In most subjects, pattern appearance of a centrally-viewed stimulus field evokes a positive-going major component at the inion, and pattern disappearance evokes a negative-going component[413, 801] (but see this chapter, Section 2.10.2). The amplitude of the disappearance-response seems to be more dependent on the time course of the spatial-contrast change than is the appearance response (Fig. 2.6).[801]

Harter has suggested that the major positive-going wave (155–220 msec latency) which he observed when a pattern of dots was abruptly illuminated reflects mainly photopic mechanisms, whereas the earlier negative wave (90–120 msec) reflects mainly scotopic mechanisms.

The difference in waveform between Jeffreys' and Harter's pattern EPs may be due to a greater intrusion of components due to brightness changes into Harter's records.

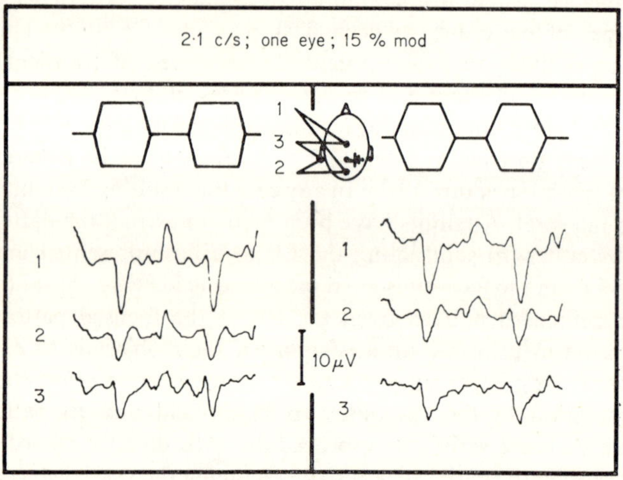

FIGURE 2.6 *Influence of the rate of the brightness change of adjacent checkerboard squares on the responses to appearance and disappearance of a checkerboard pattern. The response to disappearance depends more on the slope (i.e. rate of change) of the contrast change than do the responses to the appearance of the pattern. Decreasing the rate of change of spatial contrast seems only to increase the latency of the 'appearance' response. The downward deflections in the figure are the responses to the appearance of the pattern; the upward deflections are due to disappearance of the patterns. From L. H. van der Tweel, D. Regan and H. Spekreijse (1970). 'Some aspects of potentials evoked by changes in spatial brightness contrast'. 7th International ISCERG Symposium, Istanbul (1969). Published by University of Istanbul Medical Department (1970).*

Potentials evoked by pattern-reversal were described by van der Tweel and Spekreijse[798] and by Spekreijse.[748] The contrast-reversals were generated in the absence of changes of mean luminance by a stimulator whose central feature was a patterned mirror (Chapter 5, Section 5.1.8). At frequencies between (very roughly) 1 and 7 Hz the subjective impression produced by pattern reversal is striking and can perhaps best be described as a haphazard jumping-about of the small squares. This illusion of motion is, however, not necessary to evoke a pattern-specific EP.[801]

There is some evidence that the EPs to pattern reversal are more closely related to the EPs to pattern *disappearance* than the EPs to pattern *appearance*.[415, 803] For example the saturated amplitude of the EP to reversal of a checkerboard pattern (for a pattern of 20% contrast) is roughly twice as great for binocular stimulation as for monocular stimulation.[748] The amplitude of the EP to the *disappearance* of a checkerboard pattern of 20% contrast is much greater for binocular stimulation than for monocular stimulation whereas this is not the case for the EPs to the *appearance* of the pattern.

Spekreijse found that pattern-reversal EPs repeated themselves at the same rate as that of pattern reversals. Indications of the contrast-specificity of these responses and of their distinction from diffuse-field EPs were as follows:[S8] (*a*) the amplitude of the EP was greatly reduced when the retinal image was defocused, (*b*) the EP disappeared when thin black threads were placed so as to obscure the edges between squares, whereas threads located along the middles of the squares had comparatively little effect on the EPs, (*c*) EPs of large amplitude could be evoked by sinusoidal pattern reversal at stimulus frequencies for which the EPs to sinusoidally modulated luminance were insignificantly small (*d*) the amplitude *versus* stimulus frequency curve was quite different for EPs to pattern reversal (flat up to roughly 20–30 reversals per second followed by a rapid reduction in amplitude) and for EPs to diffuse field stimulation (resonant-like peaks near 10, 50 and sometimes 16 Hz) although it should be noted that the relative amplitudes of these peaks depended strongly on the stimulus conditions and varied from subject to subject (see Sections 2.8.2, 2.8.3 and 2.8.4), and (*e*) the topographical distribution was different for the two types of EP. Cobb *et al.*[157] confirmed findings (*a*), (*c*) and (*d*) above by using what was in effect square-wave pattern-reversal generated by a method sharing common features with techniques used by Riggs to study the ERG and later the EP[674, 676] and by Halliday to study the EP[355] (see Section 2.10.2).

There are two lines of argument which lead to the suggestion that the characteristic contrast-specific components of the EPs to pattern stimuli become more and more contaminated by other types of EP when the stimulus check size is increased beyond 20′ or so. These are: (1) defocusing the retinal image produces the greatest attenuation of the pattern EP for check sizes of roughly 10′ to 20′ but for large check sizes defocusing may even increase the amplitude of the EP (Section 2.4.1), and (2) if a grid of fine lines is placed over the boundaries of the checks in a reversing-checkboard pattern, then the EP is abolished only if the check size is smaller than 20′ or so[748] (although no estimate is possible for the intersubject variability of this critical check size as the measurement has as yet been carried out on only a few subjects). On the grounds of argument (2) above it might be expected that the contamination at large check sizes would be due to EP components similar to the second-harmonic components of potentials evoked by spatially-unstructured stimulus fields. An additional effect of increasing check size may be to emphasise parafoveal responses at the expense of foveal responses.[361]

In the absence of a clear definition of the basis on which two components should be judged 'similar' or 'different' it is difficult to answer the question whether transient potentials evoked by patterned stimuli contain components which are qualitatively different from those evoked by spatially-unstructured (blank) stimulus fields.

Spehlman reported that the principal difference between EPs to flash-presented blank-field and flash-presented patterned-field was that a positive wave peaking at 180–250 msec appeared to be much larger in the responses to patterned stimuli (recordings taken from an electrode 3 cm to one side of the inion relative to an ear reference). However, it was possible to say only within rather broad limits that this component was peculiar to pattern stimulation and was genuinely absent in the blank-field EPs. On the other hand, it certainly seems true that when EPs to a blank stimulus field are compared with EPs to a high-contrast patterned stimulus, the *polarity* of a prominent 100 msec wave may be opposite without any apparent change of latency.[359, 540, 671] (Fig. 2.7). Moreover, if the patterned stimulus is progressively defocused this polarity reversal can be seen as a progressive change.[359, 415] For low-contrast patterns the electric fields due to the luminance response and the pattern response respectively might therefore partially cancel at some particular electrode position. As MacKay and Jeffreys pointed out,[543] partial cancellation might result in an *increase* in the amplitude of an EP component if the stimulus strength of one of the effective stimulus para-

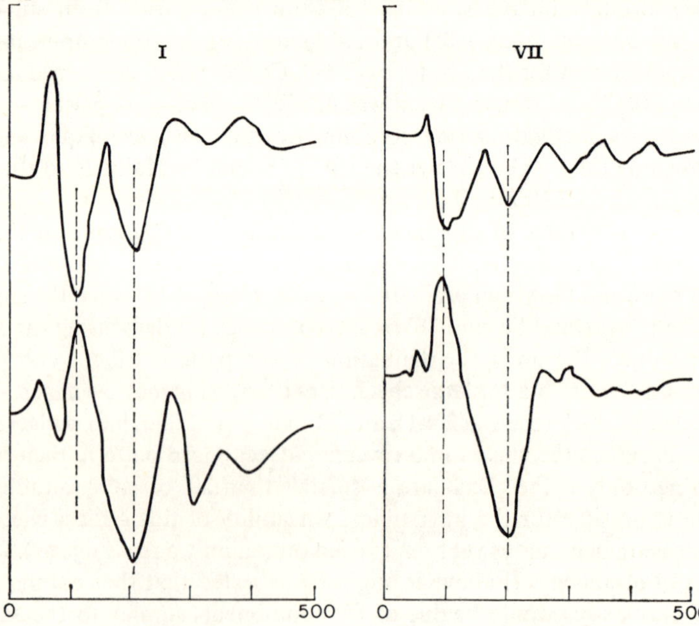

FIGURE 2.7 *Potentials evoked by flash presentation of a blank stimulus field (upper trace) and by flash presentation of a checkerboard pattern (lower trace) for two subjects. The stimulus fields were centrally viewed and were of 9° subtense. The checkerboard squares were of roughly 34′ subtense. Note the polarity inversion for the component of latency roughly 100 msec. From W. J. Rietveld, W. E. Tordoir, J. R. B. Hagenouw, J. A. Lubbers and Th. A. C. Spoor (1967).* Acta Physiol. Pharmacol. Neerl., ***14****, 259–285. North-Holland Publishing Co., Amsterdam.*

meters (here the contrast of a pattern) is *reduced*. They advocated the simultaneous recording of EPs at a number of sites as an aid in detecting such misleading effects.

The polarity of the prominent 100 msec wave can also be reversed merely by changing the retinal location of the patterned stimulus, whereas this is not so for changes of the retinal location of a spatially-unstructured stimulus (Sections 2.10.1 and 2.10.2). There has been some success in attempting to explain these different behaviours of early patterned-field and blank-field components on *geometric* grounds (see Section 2.10.2). Such hypotheses emphasise that the polarity of a scalp-recorded component can be determined *both* by the nature of the electrical events in the cortex and by the orientation (relative to the scalp) of the area of cortex involved. On this basis, the above differences between blank-field and pattern-field EP components might partly be explained, not by assuming that they are generated by cortical events of different time courses, but merely on the basis that they are generated in differently-oriented areas of cortex.

In contrast, there has so far been little progress towards a quantitative or even a qualitative definition of the stimulus parameters which determine the form and the amplitude of the EPs to patterned stimuli. It has been suggested that intersecting contours (corners) play some special role in generating EPs which differ qualitatively from the role played by straight lengths of contour.[536, 671, 750] However, it has not yet been possible to formulate a sharply testable statement of this hypothesis. The appearance and disappearance of pattern have been proposed as EP determinants.[413] An alternative suggestion is that change of the contrast across sharply-focused contrast borders determines the EP.[750, 802] On the face of it, perhaps the most promising way of approaching this problem would be to systematically remove features of the stimulus until some relevant EP feature disappeared; or, conversely, to systematically build up the stimulus pattern until the particular EP feature made its appearance. There is little published material on the results of such experiments; one reason for this speedily becomes clear when the approach is tried in the laboratory. For example, patterns which include corners have been found to evoke considerably larger EPs than striped patterns,[536, 671] even when the total lengths of contrast border are matched,[671] although patterns of dots or visual noise in which there are no corners can evoke clear EPs.[150, 360, 541] Reitveld suggested that intersecting contours (corners) were more effective as stimuli when the corner angle was less, rather than greater, than 90°. If, even by local blurring, the corners of the squares of a checkerboard pattern are now removed, in order to investigate their importance, the pattern looks qualitatively different and the change is difficult to quantify. As a further complication, it is not clear that the EPs to striped patterns and to checkerboard patterns are even qualitatively the same.[803]

On the other hand, coarser judgements as to which stimulus parameters are important may be made by using the above stratagem of altering the pattern. For example, an excellent way to define which components of the EP are related to pattern is to defocus the stimulus.[359, 671, 747] For check sizes below about 20′ the amplitude of both transient and steady-state EPs are very sensitive to accommodation. Flash-presentation of a checkerboard pattern elicits a transient EP component of 90–100 msec latency which is equally sensitive to accommodation for 12′ and 20′ checks and a component of latency 180–200 msec which is more sensitive for 12′ than for 20′ checks. The maximum sensitivity (for the 100 msec component) can be roughly expressed as a 25% amplitude change for a defocusing of 1 dioptre.[359] Steady-state EPs have been reported to show a 50% fall in amplitude when a 0·3 dioptre defocusing of the retinal image is achieved by fixating on a point in front of the plane of the stimulus,[801] although Fig. 2.8 B shows an attenuation of roughly 50% for EPs to 12′ checks when a +1 dioptre lens is placed before the eyes.* After due allowance for refractive errors it seems that in some subjects the result of defocusing may be to *increase* the amplitude of the 180–200 msec component of the transient EP to flash-presentation of large checks (Fig. 2 in Ref. 297). It is interesting that the 6 Hz steady-state EP to pattern alternation may also increase in amplitude when large checks are defocussed (Fig. 2.8 B). This suggests that the steady-state EP may be more closely related to the 180–200 msec transient component to flashed pattern than to the 90–100 msec component. Such a suggestion would be in accord with estimates of 200 msec (at 3 apostilb) and 150 msec (at 3000 apostilb) for the 'apparent latency' of pattern reversal EPs.[748]

MacKay and Jeffreys[543] report that pre-exposure to a static pattern before the transitory presentation of the stimulus pattern attenuates the 'on' response and that the attenuation is greater the more similar the patterns are in form and orientation.

2.4.2 *Regular and irregular patterns*

Little attention has so far been paid to the question whether the pattern EP is fully determined by the mere presence of an adequate number of suitable stimulus contours or whether the *regularity* of the pattern is important. Clynes[150, 151] has described EPs to single dots and to arrays of dots, but does not seem to have compared responses to arrays which are similar in all respects except for a random *versus* regular grouping. Beatty and Uttal[62, 63] claim that even a slight departure from regularity in the grouping of stripes or dots results in a marked decrease in the scalp potentials evoked by the pattern. This interesting claim surely deserves further verification. Beatty and Uttal, however, used only a single bipolar placement, and did not report controls for the effect of the position of the fixation point. It is known that both the amplitude and the topographical distribution of EPs to contoured stimulation depend strongly on the region of retina which is stimulated (see

* Given a depth of field of 0·5 dioptres[117] the net blur produced by placing +1 dioptre lenses before the eyes was probably about 0·5 dioptres, so the EP data may not conflict with that of v.d. Tweel *et al.*

Sections 2.4.4 and 2.10.2). In themselves, either of these effects might result in smaller EPs being recorded to stimulation by patterns containing irregular groupings than to stimulation by regularly grouped patterns, especially when only a single recording site is used as in Uttal and Beatty's studies. In Beatty's[63] investigation, the RMS amplitude of the entire EP waveform was measured, on the grounds that this procedure 'avoids problems of component identification'. The evidence (reviewed in this chapter and in Chapter 3) that different EP components have quite different characteristics suggests that the use of the RMS measure may lead to special difficulties in deriving clear interpretations from experimental data.

The effect of regularity *versus* irregularity of pattern bears on the question whether it might be worthwhile to describe the generation of pattern-EPs in terms of some form of 'regularity detector' (e.g. a travelling wave located at central or peripheral level), or whether pattern-EPs might better be described as (possibly nonlinear) summations of the responses of a number of individual neuronal contour-sensitive elements.

The EPs to regular patterns more complex than checkerboards or stripes might, MacKay has suggested,[536 p. 216] reflect lateral inhibition between 'high-order feature-sensitive elements'.

2.4.3 *The effects of check size*

Rietveld *et al.*[671] found that for flash-presented patterns the baseline-to-peak amplitudes of both a prominent negative component at 100 msec and a positive component at 200–235 msec were maximal for a check size of 20′ (three subjects) or 10′ (one subject). Harter,[359] also using flash-presented patterns, found that the amplitudes of a 200 msec component were larger for 12′ checks than for 20′ or 42′ checks, but in contrast with Rietveld *et al.*,[671] reported that the amplitude of the 100 msec component was relatively insensitive to check sizes.

For pattern-appearance EPs, the amplitude of the prominent 100 msec component is maximal for check sizes of roughly 10′.[415]

Spekreijse reported that steady-state EPs to pattern reversal reach a maximum amplitude for checks of roughly 11′ subtense (one subject).[748 p. 130] In an independent study on a group of 5 subjects, potentials of maximum amplitude were evoked by check sizes which ranged from 11′ to 18′.[649] Regan and Richards[649] found that the power of the scalp responses evoked by six pattern reversals per second was almost entirely concentrated in the 6 Hz frequency component. Fig. 2.8 shows that a log-log plot of the amplitude of the 6 Hz component *versus* check size can be approximated by two straight lines of unity slope. Fig. 2.8 A also illustrates that when the angle of convergence of the eyes was changed by an amount equivalent to a change in the fixation point from 175 to 24 cm, the EP amplitude was not affected for square sizes below 12′, even though the convergence change produced marked changes in the apparent size of external objects.[367] This observation indicates that for squares sizes below 12′ the EP is determined by the physical dimensions of the retinal images of the checks and not by the apparent subjective dimensions of the checks.

There is, of course, an ambiguity in the interpretation of all these studies of the effect of check size, since when check size is increased the number of squares falling on the fovea is decreased, and this may account for part of the observed attenuation of EP amplitude.

Eason *et al.*[259] found that for flash-presentation the check size which gave the greatest EP (90–100 msec wave) was different for upper and lower half-

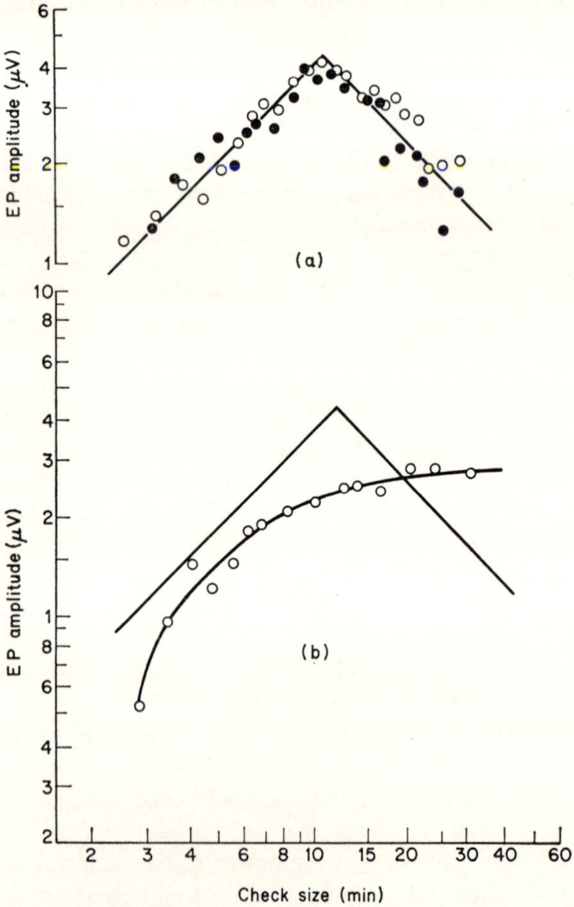

FIGURE 2.8(a) *Amplitude of 6 Hz component of the EP* versus *check size for a 2° checkerboard stimulus, centrally viewed. There were 6 reversals of the luminance contrast of the pattern per second. The circles in (a) show measurements with a stimulus distance of 175 cm; the filled circles are comparable measurements made with the fixation distance effectively reduced to 24 cm by the use of prisms and correcting lenses. The best-fitting lines of 45° slope are shown. In (b) the full line is the same as in (a), but the points are for EPs recorded when the target (at 175 cm) was blurred by placing a +1D lens before the subject's eyes. Potentials measured between an electrode placed 1 cm above the inion and the left mastoid. From D. Regan and W. Richards (1971).* Vision Res., ***11****, 679–684. Pergamon Press, Oxford.*

field stimulation. Checks of 10′ subtense were optimal for the upper field, whereas 40′ checks were optimal for the lower field. Eason *et al.*[259] discounted cortical topography as an explanation of their findings (see Section 2.10.2), and suggested that the difference in optimal check size for upper and lower fields might reflect differences in the sizes of retinal receptive field centres. Such differences, they speculated, would be in accord with the organism's need to detect distant objects in the sky and near-by objects on the ground.[S16]

2.4.4 *The effects of stimulus field size; spatially-structured fields*

Rietveld *et al.*[671] compared the contributions to the EP of foveal and extra-foveal stimulation by means of: (*a*) changing the diameter of a centrally-located black disc in a checkerboard pattern, and (*b*) changing the diameter of a centrally-located checkerboard stimulating field. They subtracted the responses to an unstructured flashed field from the response to flashed patterns and, implicitly assuming a linear addition between blank field and pattern responses, treated the subtracted potential as a 'pure' pattern-specific EP (Fig. 2.9 A). Rietveld concluded that for large stimulus fields, roughly 60% of the EP is due to stimulation of the retina *outside* the central 2°, and roughly 30% is due to stimulation *outside* the central 3° (EP amplitude here refers to a peak-to-peak measure between a prominent negative peak at roughly 100 msec and a prominent positive peak at 200–235 msec). Jeffreys finds that the amplitudes of 80 msec and 120 msec EP components to pattern-appearance are predominantly due to stimulation of the central three or four

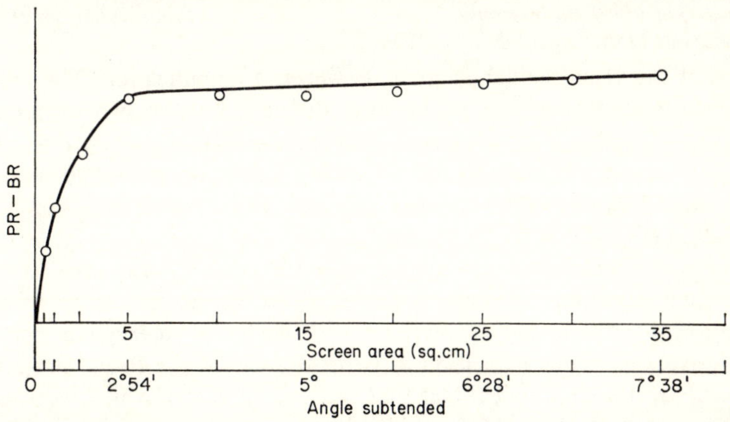

FIGURE 2.9 A *Amplitude of pattern EP* versus *stimulus field size for centrally-viewed target. The figure shows that foveal stimulation is responsible for almost the whole of the response. The peak-to-peak amplitudes of EPs to flash-presented checkerboard patterns were measured between a negative wave of roughly 100 msec latency and a positive wave of 200–235 msec latency. The amplitudes of the pattern EPs were obtained by subtracting the EP to a flash-presented blank field from the EP to a flash-presented checkerboard pattern of roughly 21′ checksize. Potentials measured between an electrode 1·5 cm above the inion and an electrode on one earlobe. The vertex was grounded. From W. J. Rietveld* et al. *(1967).* Acta. Physiol. Pharmacol. Neerl., ***14***, *259–285. North-Holland Publishing Co., Amsterdam.*

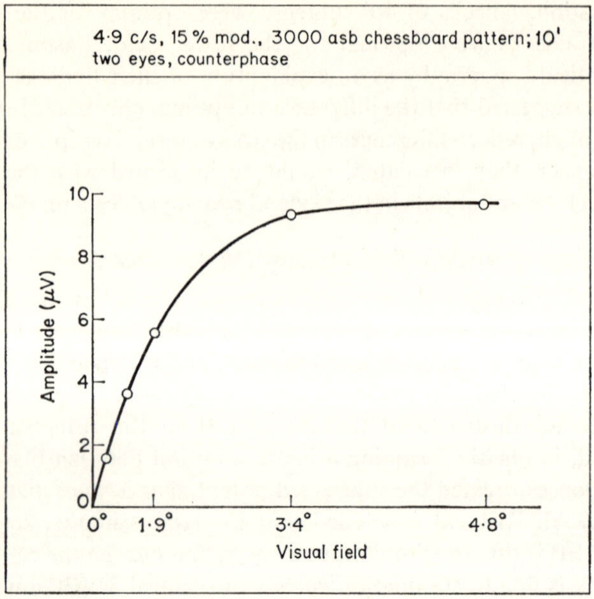

FIGURE 2.9 B *Subject G: natural pupil. Amplitudes of the occipital responses, found by counterphase stimulation with sinusoidally modulated light, as a function of the size of the stimulus field.*

A surrounding field with the same average brightness as the stimulus field has been applied. The modulation depth of the sinusoidal stimulus is 15%, so that saturation effects do not affect the response. From H. S. Spekreijse (1966). Analysis of EEG Responses in Man. *Junk Publishers, The Hague.*

degrees of the visual field.* There is, however, a complication. The relation between EP amplitude and field size is different for the two components attributed by Jeffreys to differences between the spatial orientations of the areas of cortex in which the 80 and 120 msec EP components are generated.[415] Steady-state EPs to pattern-reversal also seem to be mainly due to macular stimulation (Fig. 2.9 B)[157, 748, 58, 16]

The apparently small contribution to the EP made by responses to extra-foveal stimulation has been attributed partly to the larger number of cones per unit area in the foveal as compared with the extrafoveal retina, partly to the relatively generous allocation of cortical area for the foveal projection, and partly to the anatomical fact that the area of cortex which receives the macular projection is more favourably placed in relation to the scalp than the areas which receive projections from other retinal areas.

Vaughan has suggested that the slow rate of increase of EP amplitude

* In contrast, Halliday (personal communication) finds that the amplitudes of the EP components at 80 and 120 msec are not predominantly due to stimulation of the central 3 or 4 degrees of the visual field. Harter's finding may be relevant here that the check size which elicits the largest EPs depends on retinal eccentricity, and in particular that for retinal locations of 7·5° eccentricity, check sizes as large as 60′ may be optimal. Check size is, therefore, an important stimulus parameter when EPs to stimulation of different regions of the refina are compared.

when field size is increased beyond about 3°–4° might be due to mutual cancellation of the responses to stimulation of the upper and lower halves of the peripheral retina. At least for pattern EPs this seems unlikely to be the case, since stimulation of upper and lower half-fields is often found to give EPs of very different amplitudes.[259, 415, 641, 801, S17]

According to Harter[361] the check size which gives the largest pattern EP grows progressively larger as the eccentricity of the stimulus is increased. Harter found that the optimal check sizes depended to some extent both on the subject, and whether waves at 95–100 msec or at 170–220 msec were measured. When the central fovea was stimulated, checks of 7·5′ to 30′ gave the largest responses, whereas for stimuli of eccentricity 4·5° to 7·5° the largest responses were obtained for checks of 30′ to 60′ subtense. Harter[361] suggested that his finding would explain the apparent insensitivity of the extrafoveal retina to check stimulation (Fig. 2.9) when a single, small check size was used. He further suggested that his EP data might reflect the different sizes of retinal receptive field centres in the foveal and extrafoveal regions.

2.4.5 *Evoked potential evidence for orientation detectors*

There is a body of evidence suggesting that in the human visual system there are neurons which are highly selective both to the orientation and to the spatial frequency[S30] of visual stimuli. The direct evidence is mainly psychophysical;[119] relevant single unit studies have been carried out only in non-humans.[607] Recently, however, a linking electrophysiological study has been carried out on human subjects.[120, S56]

Campbell and Maffei were able to give an adequate description of the amplitudes of the EPs generated by 16 reversals per second of a bar pattern merely by measuring the amplitudes of the 16 Hz Fourier component. They reported that, at any rate up to a pattern contrast of 0·3 log units, plots of EP amplitude *versus* log contrast can be fitted by straight lines, much as though Fechner's law were applicable. The way in which the relationship between EP amplitude and stimulus contrast is affected by the retinal locus of stimulation led Campbell and Maffei to suggest that spatial frequencies above 3 cycles/degree or so are handled by the fovea, but the lower spatial frequencies are handled by the parafovea.

A good estimate of subjective psychophysical threshold is given by extrapolating this plot back to zero EP amplitude.[S18] Campbell and Maffei were unable to explore the behaviour of the EP in the immediate region of psychophysical threshold, so that they could do no more than raise the interesting question of whether the EP might follow the frequency-of-seeing curve. A more recent report confirmed their suggestion.[121]

The slopes of the EP amplitude *versus* log contrast plots are insensitive both to the area and to the spatial frequency of the stimulus, and also to whether monocular or binocular stimulation is used.[120] In other words, the EP does not behave as though its amplitude were the sum of the responses of the various areas of cortex activated by the stimulus. Campbell and Maffei[120] suggested that this behaviour might reflect the large size of the receptive fields of hypothetical human cortical cells which were analogous to the complex and hypercomplex cells described by Hubel and Wiesel in cat and monkey.[399]

It is interesting that the slope of the EP amplitude *versus* log contrast graph is doubled when gratings of different orientations are presented simultaneously to the two eyes, as though separate 'orientation channels' were summing. Campbell and Maffei have presented further evidence that such orientation channels are highly selective to orientation (to no more than 15°) and also are unaffected by another spatial frequency which is only one octave removed in spatial frequency.[120]

The characteristics of EPs to bar patterns cannot immediately be related to the characteristics of EPs to checkerboard patterns, as it is not yet clear whether these two types of stimuli excite the same neural populations. One point which should be made, though, is that Campbell and Maffei's bar pattern had a sinusoidal rather than a square-wave luminance profile. This meant that the bars looked a little blurred, even when sharply accommodated. Since it is clear that EPs to checkerboard stimuli are very sensitive to accommodation, it might therefore be asked whether Campbell and Maffei's EPs were contour-specific in the same sense as the checkerboard EPs described earlier. The answer to this question seems to be that there is reason to suppose that grating patterns reversing at 16 Hz should be less sensitive to accommodation than checkerboard patterns. The reason for this is that, in contrast with checkerboard-EPs, EPs to gratings show no peaking as a function of spatial frequency. Instead, the amplitudes of EPs to grating patterns attenuate sharply as spatial frequency is raised (Fig. 4 in Reference 120). The force of this point is that defocusing the retinal image can be regarded as equivalent to attenuating the higher spatial frequencies, so that defocusing would be expected to have comparatively little effect on EPs to grating patterns.[58]

2.4.6 *Evoked potentials to spatial patterns of chromaticity*

Scalp potentials can be evoked by reversing the chromatic contrast in a sharply-accommodated two-colour checkerboard stimulus pattern (Chapter 5, methods Section 5.1.8).[641, 647] Clear EPs of this type can be recorded when the stimulus is made up of 10′–15′ checks and is restricted to a 1·5°–2° foveal field. Under these conditions the resulting EPs would be expected to be least contaminated by components which are (superficially) similar to those evoked by changes in the luminance of a spatially-unstructured stimulus field (see Sections 2.8.2, 2.8.3, 2.8.4). Evoked potentials to 'contours of chromaticity' can be recorded in the absence of any changes of stimulus luminance (Fig. 2.10), and can be of amplitudes equally large as those of the potentials evoked by reversing the luminance contrast in a similar pattern of constant chromaticity (e.g. they can be of comparable amplitudes to the white-light, pattern-reversal EPs described in Section 2.4.1). The characteristics of potentials evoked by reversing the *chromatic* contrast of a checkerboard pattern differ from the characteristics of EPs to changes in the *chromaticity* of a spatially-unstructured (blank) field very much along the lines described in Sections 2.4, 2.3 and 2.8 where differences between the characteristics of the potentials evoked by reversing the *luminance* contrast of a checkerboard pattern and the characteristics of EPs to changes in the *luminance* of a blank field are described. In other words, potentials evoked by pattern-reversal are different from potentials evoked by spatially-unstructured stimulus field, independently of whether it is the luminance or the chromaticity of the stimulus which is the relevant variable.

That chromaticity changes can evoke two different kinds of EPs suggests that the brain may handle information of a chromaticity change in different ways depending on whether the stimulus is (*a*) a change in the chromaticity of a spatially-unstructured field or (*b*) a change in the chromatic contrast across a sharply focused boundary.

There is evidence that the peripheral signals which are generated by changes in chromatic contrast, and which eventually lead to the EP, are restricted to separate colour 'channels', which do not converge until after the stages at which contour-specific signals are generated.[641, 647] This EP evidence is in accord with the psychophysical evidence that contrast sensitivity mechanisms are segregated in separate colour channels.[338] If this hypothesis is valid, and pattern-reversal signals are indeed initiated in parallel colour channels, then it may be possible to use EP methods to measure the spectral sensitivities of individual colour channels under 'physiological' conditions of light adaptation. This would complement the use of 'high-frequency' components of unstructured-field EPs for measuring the photopic spectral sensitivity of the fovea as a whole (see Section 2.9.3).[S18]

2.4.7 *Evoked potentials triggered by eye movements*

The pattern-reversal method has been ingeniously adapted to study both scalp potentials and retinal potentials evoked by eye movements.[33] Armington *et al.* triggered an averaging computer by saccades of an eye which viewed a black and white pattern of bars. The saccadic movement caused an abrupt displacement of the striped retinal image which in turn evoked scalp potentials. It would be expected that EPs of maximum amplitude would result when the angular size of the bars of the pattern were equal to the median angular size of saccades, since then a saccade would cause the whole of those parts of the retina covered by black bars to be illuminated, and vice versa; slightly smaller or larger saccades would reduce the effective retinal stimulation. Armington indeed found that EPs of maximum amplitude were produced by a pattern of bars of subtense 9–13 minutes of arc, which is in fair agreement with the median amplitude of eye saccades.[629]

2.5 Evoked potentials and binocular depth perception

It is known that within the visual pathway of the brains of anaesthetised animals, single units can be recorded which show an optimal response when both eyes are simultaneously stimulated with light.[399] Some binocular units respond, optimally for a specific retinal disparity which is different for

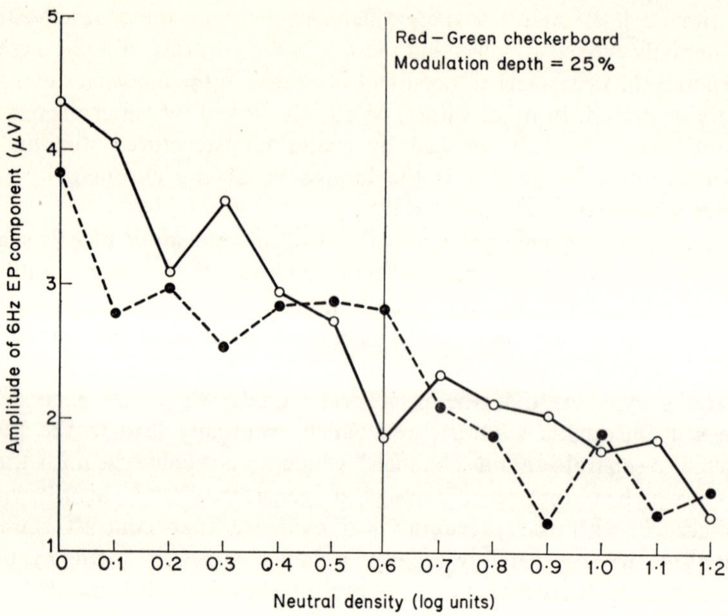

Red – Green checkerboard
Modulation depth = 25%
Amplitude of 6Hz EP component (μV)
Neutral density (log units)

(a)

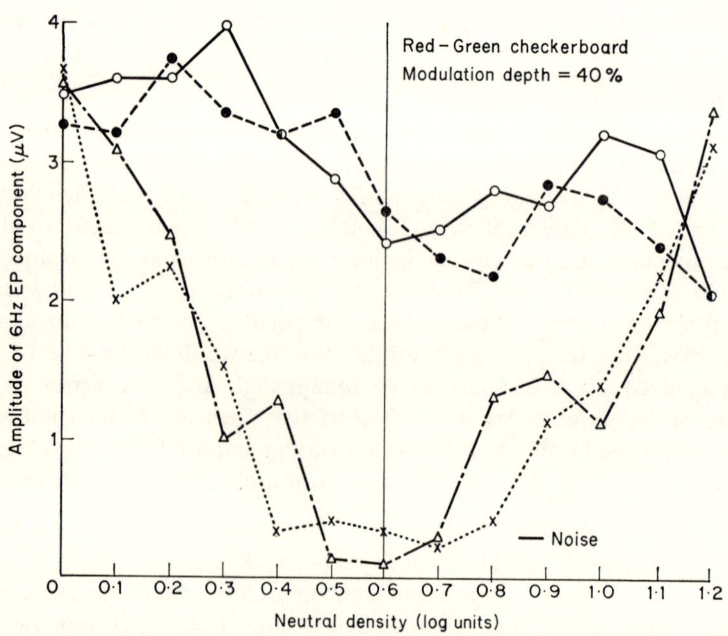

Red – Green checkerboard
Modulation depth = 40%
Amplitude of 6Hz EP component (μV)
Noise
Neutral density (log units)

(b)

different units. The characteristics of such binocular units recorded in animals have been found to be consistent with psychophysically-determined features of binocular depth perception in man.[401, 607] Although it is possible to train monkeys to respond to stereoscopic cues,[89] nevertheless human subjects have the important advantages: (*a*) that it is easy to ensure binocular fusion and (*b*) subjective reports are available. With human subjects electrophysiological recording is, of course, usually restricted to scalp EPs.

Scalp potentials which correlated with changes in perceived depth were first evoked by Regan and Spekreijse[646] who used Julesz patterns.[432] The reference pattern consisted of a random array of small squares. In the comparison patterns a central area was displaced to one side by 2, 4 or 8 pattern elements. Three projectors were used in such a way that the right eye continuously viewed the reference pattern, while the left eye alternately viewed the reference pattern and one of the comparison patterns. This stimulation arrangement ensured that during each stimulus cycle there was no change in the brightness of the fields viewed by either eye, and that the change in patterning was minimal. The rhythmical change of the retinal disparity of the central region of the pattern was an adequate stereoscopic stimulus, and generated the compelling illusion that the central region of the pattern was abruptly moving back and forward in depth. Clear EPs were recorded both to movements out of the plane of the screen and to the return movements (Fig. 2.11 A). When the change of retinal disparity was increased from 10′ through 10′ to 40′, no corresponding increase of EP amplitude was observed, suggesting that saturation might already have occurred for a 10′ disparity. This would not be unexpected, since the psychophysical threshold for stereoscopic vision is much less than 10′.

Changes in binocularly-perceived depth are inevitably accompanied by displacements of the retinal images across one or both retinae. This was a potent source of artifact in Regan and Spekreijse's[646] experiment, since

FIGURE 2.10 *Amplitude of 6 Hz component of the EP to six reversals per second of the chromatic contrast in a 3° red-green checkerboard pattern of 11′ squares plotted* versus *the density of neutral filters in the green beams* (*stimulator shown in Fig. 5.2*). *For filters of 0·6 log units the luminances of the red and green components of the pattern were made equal* (*by flicker photometry at 12 Hz*). *In this situation the net luminance of every point in the stimulus field was constant with time. For 1·2 log units there was chromatic pattern-reversal plus net red luminance pattern-reversal. For 0 log units there was chromatic pattern-reversal plus net green luminance pattern-reversal.* (*a*) *and* (*b*) *show that appreciable EPs are generated when luminance was held constant and there were only changes in chromatic contrast.* (*b*) *also shows a control in which the red filters were replaced by green filters so that colour differences were eliminated, leaving luminance differences only. When luminances were equated* (*at 0·6 on abscissa*) *the EP amplitudes fell to the noise level; contrast this with the situation in* (*b*) *where red-green colour differences were present. Potentials recorded between an electrode 1 cm above the inion and the left mastoid. The right mastoid was grounded. Left eye occluded. Horizontal dashed line shows noise level measured by running Fourier analyser and stimulator at slightly different frequencies* (*6 and 7 Hz respectively*) *without the knowledge of the subject.*

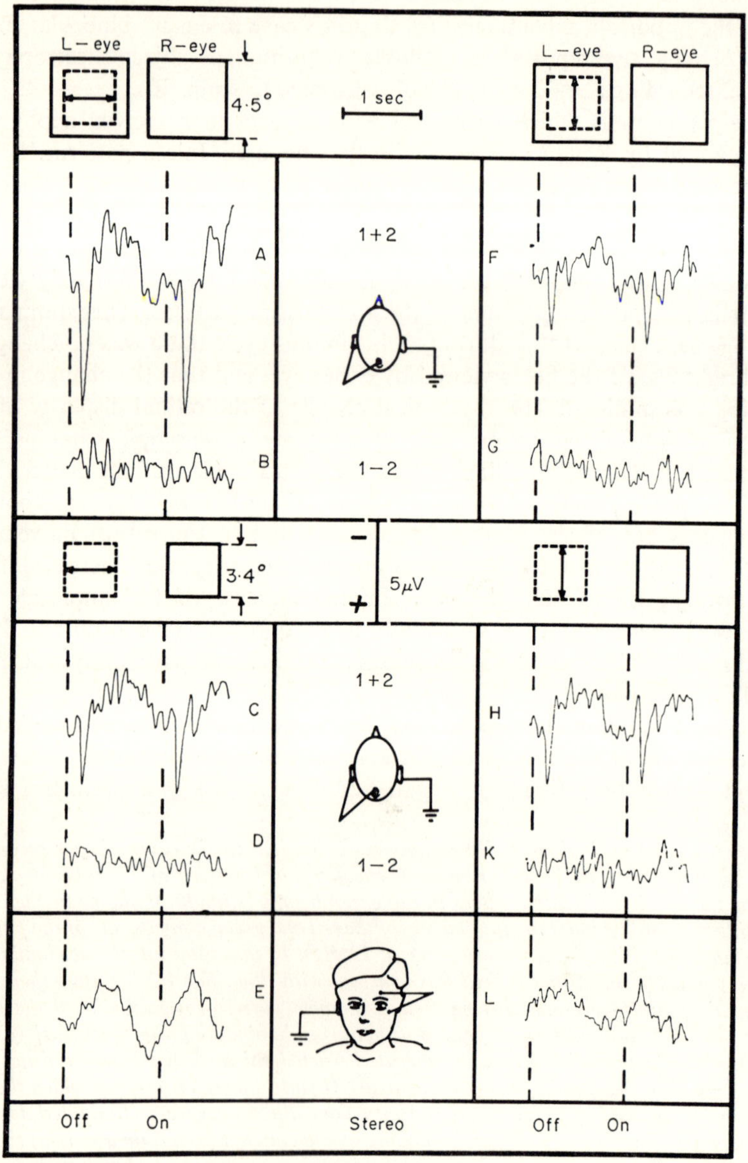
L – eye
R – eye
4·5°
1 sec
L – eye
R – eye
A
1+2
F
B
1–2
G
3·4°
5μV
C
1+2
H
D
1–2
K
E
L
Off
On
Stereo
Off
On

FIGURE 2.11

displacement EPs appeared to have similar waveforms to the 'stereoscopic EPs', and (on rather cursory examination) could not be distinguished on the grounds of topographical distribution. Control experiments for the displacement artifact were carried out by recording EPs to vertical changes of retinal disparity.[646] Vertical disparities, in contrast to horizontal disparities, do not result in depth perception. Vertical displacements were found to evoke potentials which were much smaller than those evoked by comparable horizontal displacements, and which could be negligibly small when the direction of displacement was critically adjusted. This latter adjustment was a problem in Regan and Spekreijse's experiment since the crude design of the optical stimulator was hardly adequate to cope with the unexpectedly exquisite sensitivity of the EP to small retinal disparities. It was confirmed that EPs to retinal image displacements alone were the same for horizontal and vertical displacements, so that Regan and Spekreijse concluded that their EP correlated with the binocular perception of depth. A further difference between EPs to displacement alone and their so-called stereoscopic EP was that monocular stimulation with 20′ and 40′ image displacements gave EPs much smaller than those to the 10′ disparity, whereas 'stereoscopic EPs' for 10′, 20′ and 40′ disparities were not very different.

The reason for the differences between the three displacement EPs might have been that an illusion of apparent sideways movement occurred for

FIGURE 2.11 *Scalp potentials evoked by stereoscopic stimuli and control stimuli. The right eye viewed a static random pattern of small black and white squares. The left eye alternately viewed a pattern identical to that viewed by the right eye, and a pattern in which the central region had been bodily shifted a short distance to one side (dotted line at top of figure). The alternation frequency was 0·45 per sec. In these conditions the central dotted area appeared to jump rhythmically forward out of the plane of the paper and then return. A: potential evoked when retinal disparity of central area changed horizontally and gave rise to a stereoscopic percept (1 and 2 are two separate sessions of 200 counts); B: difference 1–2 showing variability and noise; F: as A except that the retinal disparity now changed vertically and no stereoscopic perception resulted; this is a typical response. It was sometimes possible to align the movement relative to the head so that responses were very small and the response to appearance of depth was near noise level; G: difference between responses to two sets of 200 stimulus repetitions showing variability and noise for a constant stimulus alignment. Lower half of the figure shows responses to displacements of the retinal image similar to the displacements used in the upper half of the figure, but with the stationary border of the field removed by placing black velvet on the screen so that there was no stereoscopic perception; C and H show that similar potentials were evoked by horizontal and vertical displacements of the retinal image; D and K: differences showing variability and noise; E and L: electro-oculograms recorded 4 cm from the centre of the eye showing none of the characteristic brisk responses in A, F, C or H. EEG amplifiers 0·1–200 per sec (−3 dB). Stimulus repetition frequency 0·45 per sec; 2 sec sweep; electrode 3 cm above midline, left earlobe reference. Electrodes 3 or 5 cm to left or right of midline electrode and on vertex showed similar but smaller responses; total angular subtense of stimulus 4·5°; angular subtense of central area 3·4°. Brightness of light areas 0·4 log foot lamberts. From D. Regan and H. Spekreijse (1970). 'Electrophysiological correlate of binocular depth perception in man'*, Nature, **225**, *92–94.*

monocularly-viewed 10′ displacements, but that for 20′ and 40′ displacements there was no illusion of apparent movement.

Julesz[433] has pointed out that Regan and Spekreijse's so-called stereoscopic EPs may have been contaminated by motor potentials related to changes of the angle of convergence of the two eyes. Arguments against this possibility are: (*a*) a fixation point was used which was located in the plane of the screen and (*b*) motor potentials are largest above motor cortex (near the vertex), and are comparatively small near the inion (Chapter 3, Section 3.4), whereas the 'stereoscopic EPs' of Regan and Spekreijse were largest near the inion, and comparatively small near the vertex.

In a quite different stimulus situation to that used by Regan and Spekreijse, Fiorentini and Maffei reported that EPs could be recorded whose amplitudes correlated with binocularly-perceived depth. Grating patterns[703] (see Chapter 5, Section 5.1.6) were presented to the subjects' left and right eyes. When the patterns had equal spatial frequencies the subject saw a single fused pattern in the plane of the stimulating-oscilloscope tube faces. In contrast, when the grating presented to one eye was of higher spatial frequency than the grating presented to the other eye, the subject had the illusion that the grating was tilted in depth (it is helpful here to imagine the views of the left and right eyes when they view a solid grating pattern which is *physically* tilted in depth). The apparent angle of tilt increased as the difference between the spatial frequencies was increased, but only up to a difference of 12% or so.

Fiorentini and Maffei reported that the amplitude of the EP to 16 pattern-reversals per second increased progressively as the apparent angle of tilt of the grating pattern was increased by enlarging the difference between the spatial frequencies of the gratings viewed by the left and right eyes. On the other hand, the EP was unaffected by changes in the spatial frequency difference in circumstances such that the left and right stimuli did not fall on corresponding areas of the retinae so that no illusion of depth was produced. The change in the EP did not seem to be produced by the difference in spatial frequency *per se* (which was presumably far too small),[120] since differences in spatial frequency in excess of 25%, for which the mechanism responsible for the depth illusion broke down, resulted either in no increase in EP amplitude over the 'no depth' condition or even in a decrease in amplitude.

The successful demonstration by Fiorentini and Maffei of a correlation between the *amount* of perceived depth and the amplitude of the EP (in contrast with Regan and Spekreijse's failure to show such a relation) is probably due to the former author's use of smaller retinal disparities. There is a difference between the two experiments which may prove to be of theoretical significance. This is that Regan and Spekreijse endeavoured to record directly characteristic EPs to stimuli which generated changes in perceived depth and nothing else, whereas Maffei and Fiorentini's approach was more indirect in that they reported a correlation between perceived depth and the type of EP which is characteristic of pattern-reversal.

Tsutsui claimed that an occipitally-recorded positive wave of roughly

270 msec latency-to-peak was specific to binocular fusion, since this wave was absent when fusion was broken.[792] In Tsutsui's experiment, however, the breakdown of fusion was accompanied by changes in the retinal locus of stimulation. This might account for the contrary finding of Kawasaki *et al.* that the 270 msec positive wave was not specific to binocular fusion since it could also be evoked by monocular stimulation.

Kawasaki *et al.*[444] found that when similarly-oriented triangular patterns were presented to each eye and the images were fused, then a clear 270 msec wave could be recorded. On the other hand, when the triangles presented to each eye had opposite orientations, the 270 msec wave was attenuated. Kawasaki *et al.* interpreted this attenuation as indicating that the 270 msec wave was suppressed when the two retinal images were not fused. Against the latter interpretation, however, is the fact that an examination of their Fig. 2[444] shows that the amplitude of the 270 msec wave is attenuated by a factor of no more than 1·8 : 1 to 2 : 1. Now the effect of retinal rivalry in the unfused condition would be expected to reduce the amplitude of the EP in the 'fused' condition to roughly the mean amplitude of the EP to monocular stimulation.[157] Kawasaki's Fig. 1 shows that this effect alone would be expected to give an attenuation of roughly 2 : 1.

2.6 Scalp potentials evoked by moving stimuli; lambda waves

2.6.1 *Introduction*

There have been a number of reports that clear scalp potentials can be evoked by moving patterned stimuli[542] or by a single moving spot of light.[43, 44, 49] The question immediately arises whether such potentials reflect the activities of brain mechanisms whose function is to abstract motion information from the total stimulus information flowing into the retina. There is a body of psychophysical evidence for the existence of such a motion-emphasising mechanism in the human visual pathway[50, 318, 528] but there is as yet no compelling evidence that the form of EPs to moving stimuli are indeed determined by these mechanisms. Experimental questions whose resolution may help to provide such evidence are: (*a*) what relationship is there between EPs to moving stimuli and EPs to pattern reversal (see Sections 2.4 and 2.6.2), for example whether the latter EPs are no more than the former EPs in the limiting case of infinitely rapid motion, (*b*) what relationship there is between EPs to moving stimuli and the *lambda waves* evoked by moving the gaze across a patterned target (see below) and (*c*) can EP correlations be found for those subjective after images and visual illusions[50] which constitute the bulk of present evidence for motion-abstracting mechanisms in man?

A number of investigators have studied lambda waves for a quite different purpose than that of investigating the neural mechanisms which underlie motion perception. These workers have seen in the lambda response a possible means of applying crucial tests to certain general models of perception[49] (see Section 2.1.1).

2.6.2 *Evoked potentials to moving stimuli*

Barlow was able to show that an adequate stimulus for scalp potentials was the motion of a spot of light on an oscilloscope screen. MacKay and Rietveld[542] later found that the EP to movement of a single bar was enhanced by the presence of a near-by stationary bar, that is by the presence of a 'landmark' in the subject's visual field. Potentials of much greater amplitude than those evoked by moving a single bar can be produced by reversing the direction of motion of a pattern of visual noise.[542, 543] The amplitude of these EPs is a function of the change of the angular velocity of the stimulus. There is a problem, however, in ensuring that the potentials to motion reversal are not evoked at least in part by the momentary presentation of an unblurred stimulus pattern at the instant that the pattern passes through zero velocity. MacKay and Rietveld's evidence against this possibility was that EPs separately recorded to pattern presentation and motion-reversal EPs were differently affected by the grain size of the pattern.

2.6.3. *Lambda waves*[547] (*see also Section 2.11.2*)

Sharp Λ-like deflection (lambda waves) are triggered by voluntary eye movements especially when the subject is looking at a well-illuminated high-contrast pattern. In some subjects these waves can be of such high amplitudes that they are clearly visible in the raw EEG.[160, 281, 282, 305] Lambda waves are strongly attenuated when the subject views a diffusely-illuminated, spatially-unstructured visual field rather than a patterned field, and furthermore the potentials are totally absent in darkness or when the subject closes his eyes. Lambda waves to stimulation of the upper and lower retinal half-fields show differences of waveform,[132, 601, 657] similar to those observed to pattern presentation and pattern reversal[543] (Section 2.10.2). However, there still seems to be unresolved doubt about the relative roles of sensory mechanisms and oculo-motor mechanisms in the genesis of lambda waves.[49, 569, 659, 711, 819a]

Potentials similar to lambda waves can also result from involuntary tremors of the eye. Armington *et al.*[33] triggered an averaging computer by saccades of an eye which viewed a black and white pattern of bars. The saccadic movement caused an abrupt displacement of the striped retinal image which in turn evoked scalp potentials. It would be expected that EPs of maximum amplitude would result when the angular size of the bars of the pattern were equal to the median angular size of saccades. Armington indeed found that EPs of maximum amplitude were produced by a pattern of bars of subtense 9–13 minutes of arc, which is in fair agreement with the median amplitude of eye saccades.[629]

A familiar feature of everyday experience is that the stability of our visually perceived world is not upset by eye movements. In some models of perception this stability is achieved by blocking incoming visual signals during eye movements, in other words by transient perceptual blanking ('peripheral blocking', see Section 2.11.2). In contrast MacKay's model[533] does not involve the suppression of incoming signals since in his view perception is correlated with an internal *evaluation* of incoming signals (see Section 2.1.1).

Some investigators have seen in the study of lambda waves the possibility of a crucial test of the 'peripheral blocking' hypothesis of perceptual stability. Gastaut and Regis[310] discussed whether lambda waves might reflect the activity of a mechanism for blanking of visual perception during eye movements (see Section 2.11.2). On the other hand, both Scott and Bickford[710] and Barlow and Ciganek[49] concluded that the lambda response is more closely related to movements of visual stimuli across the retina than to any inhibitory mechanisms that might operate during visual scanning.[S20]

Kurtzberg and Vaughan[473] suggested that lambda waves were identical with EPs to pattern movement, although Barlow and Ciganek[49] considered that there were some minor differences in waveform between the two potentials.

For voluntary eye movements, a slow potential change is initiated some 150–200 msec *before* the eyes start to move.[49, 473, 710] Barlow and Ciganek suggested that this potential might be related to the 'readiness potential' of Kornhuber and Deecke (Chapter 3, Section 3.4). Kurtzburg and Vaughan[473] reported a second and later antecedent potential which preceded the onset of eye movement by no more than 25–40 msec. The earlier wave was largest in the frontal region whereas the second wave was maximal over the parietal region.[473] These distributions were compatible with cortical sources in the two areas of the brain where electrical stimulation has been found to produce eye movements in man.[602]

2.7 Rest-motion (R-M) evoked potentials

Clynes has interpreted certain of his EPs as reflecting the hypothetical brain property of specific sensitivity for the transition from a state of rest to a state of change (the R-M, i.e. Rest-Motion Function).[248 pp.363–374] Clynes found that vertex potentials of latency roughly 200 msec were evoked when a stimulus parameter, initially constant, abruptly began to change. For example, when light intensity was modulated by a trapezoidal waveform, vertex potentials were generated at the instant when the trapezoidal modulation caused the light of constant intensity to change its intensity; no vertex potential was initiated by the other corner of the trapezoid when the changing light intensity abruptly became constant. No responses were initiated by sinusoidal or triangular modulating waveforms, nor by a trapezoidal waveform whose flat portion had a duration less than 0·3 sec. Similar vertex potentials were evoked whether the stimulus parameter changed was light intensity, sound intensity or the frequency of a tone. In other words the type of vertex potential recorded by Clynes seems to be evoked specifically by an abrupt transition from an unchanging to a changing stimulus parameter. The response is strongly attenuated if the initial state is one not of rest but of a slow change in the stimulus parameter; interestingly this holds independently of the *direction* of the initial rate of change.

Clynes interpreted his R-M vertex potential in terms of the properties of hypothetical *undirectional rate-sensitive elements*.[152, 248, 548] He had earlier developed the notion of unidirectional rate-sensitivity in modelling a variety of physiological mechanisms. A unidirectional rate-sensitive element is defined as one which (*a*) gives an output signal whose amplitude, but not polarity, is determined by the rate of change of a particular input variable and gives zero output when the variable is constant, and (*b*) responds to an increasing rate of change but not a decreasing rate of change, or vice versa. An example of the experimental findings that Clynes has modelled in terms of unidirectional rate-sensitive evidence is his discovery that the size of the eye pupil shows a momentary increase when the intensity of a stimulus light is abruptly decreased *or when the light intensity is abruptly increased*.[152] An interesting property of systems modelled from unidirectional rate-sensitive elements is that they may be strikingly sensitive to the difference between a state of constancy to a state of change of a specific input parameter. This is because, when the appropriate stimulus parameter is constant, such a system is at an end point. Clynes contrasted the properties of systems based on unidirectional rate-sensitive elements with the properties of systems in which the zero is not an end point, but a point on a continuum between responses of opposite polarities. He claimed that the latter systems are inherently more sensitive to drifting of the zero point and discussed a number of correspondences between the properties of models involving unidirectional rate-sensitive elements and a wide variety of physiological mechanisms. These examples included the mechanisms underlying the scalp potentials evoked by changes in the luminance and chromaticity of visual stimuli and by changes in the intensity and frequency of auditory tones.[248 pp.363–374]

2.8 The effects of stimulus repetition frequency on evoked potentials

2.8.1 *Transient stimulation and steady-state stimulation; time-domain and frequency-domain analyses*

One reason for investigating the way in which EPs are affected by stimulus repetition frequency can most easily be understood by analogy with transient EPs. Transient EPs are elicited by stimuli which are sufficiently widely spaced that the system can be regarded as returning to a state of rest between successive stimuli. To this end, a randomised presentation of stimuli helps to minimise 'locking' of the EEG and may also improve signal-to-noise enhancement[691] (see also Chapter 5, Section 5.4.8). Transient EP waveforms are commonly divided into components of different *latencies* in the hope of associating different components with different functions of the CNS and/or with different locations within the brain. Similarly, one purpose of classifying steady-state EPs into different *frequency* regions is the hope of associating different frequency regions with different brain functions and/or locations within the CNS (see Sections 2.8.1, 2.8.2, 2.8.3 and 2.8.4; see Chapter 4

Section 4.3.3 for a discussion of clinical possibilities of this approach). It is clear that in some circumstances frequency analysis is more convenient and more effective in extracting responses of small amplitude than is temporal (transient) analysis (Chapter 5, Section 5.4.9); there are some grounds for supposing that the two approaches might provide *complementary* information about the CNS.

When the luminance of a spatially-unstructured field is square-wave modulated at a sufficiently slow rate, the (transient) responses to onset and offset of the stimulus have the same polarity, but different waveforms, thresholds and saturation behaviours.[152] The ratio between the amplitudes of onset and offset responses shows marked interindividual variations.[59, 152] When a flash is sufficiently short (less than roughly 25 msec) the resultant EP is not a simple linear sum of the onset and offset responses.[262] For a brief flash the EP resembles an onset response; for a 'flash of darkness' (i.e. a transient reduction of luminance) the EP resembles an offset response.[152]

Transient EPs to infrequently repeated stimuli overlap to an increasing extent as the stimulus repetition frequency is progressively increased. At sufficiently high repetition frequencies, no individual response cycle can be associated with a particular stimulus cycle. When this 'steady-state' regime is established it is no longer appropriate to describe the response in terms of time, that is in terms of the latencies of different components. A more suitable approach is to describe the response in terms of different stimulus repetition frequencies, and for this purpose it has been found useful to analyse the EP waveform into harmonic components (see Chapter 5, Sections 5.4.8 and 5.4.9). A convenient way of presenting these data is to plot the amplitudes and phases of the various harmonic components of the EP *versus* stimulus repetition frequency. It is often more straightforward to interpret the results of experiments in which this steady-state method is used when the stimulus waveform is harmonically simple (for example, sinusoidal). Any harmonic distortions in the response waveform can then be confidently attributed to the CNS. The situation may be confusing when harmonically complex stimuli are used (e.g. repetitive pulses) since, unless the experimenter has prior knowledge of the characteristics of the visual system, it is difficult to say whether harmonic distortions are due to the brain or to the stimulus waveform.

Attempts have been made to predict the amplitude of the EP to flashes whose repetition frequency is higher than 3 flashes/sec solely on the basis of the waveform of the 3 flashes/sec response.[813] This was found to be impossible for any subject tested for frequencies above 11 flashes/sec. In another study a reasonable prediction was possible to a rate of 8 flashes/sec for only two subjects out of ten; little success was obtained for the remaining eight subjects studied.[666] The very limited success obtained in such attempts to predict steady-state responses from transient responses is not surprising in view of the markedly nonlinear behaviour of EPs for stimuli of both low and high modulation depths.[262, 637, 748, 797]

2.8.2 Steady-state EP components of frequency roughly 10 *Hz ('low-frequency' region); analogue model; summation fields*

A visual stimulus whose intensity is sinusoidally modulated at frequency *F* Hz contains no frequency components other than one of *F* Hz. When the luminance of a diffuse visual field is sinusoidally modulated it is found that only very small EPs result for modulation frequencies below about 3 Hz (Fig. 2.12). For many subjects, however, a stimulus frequency which lies

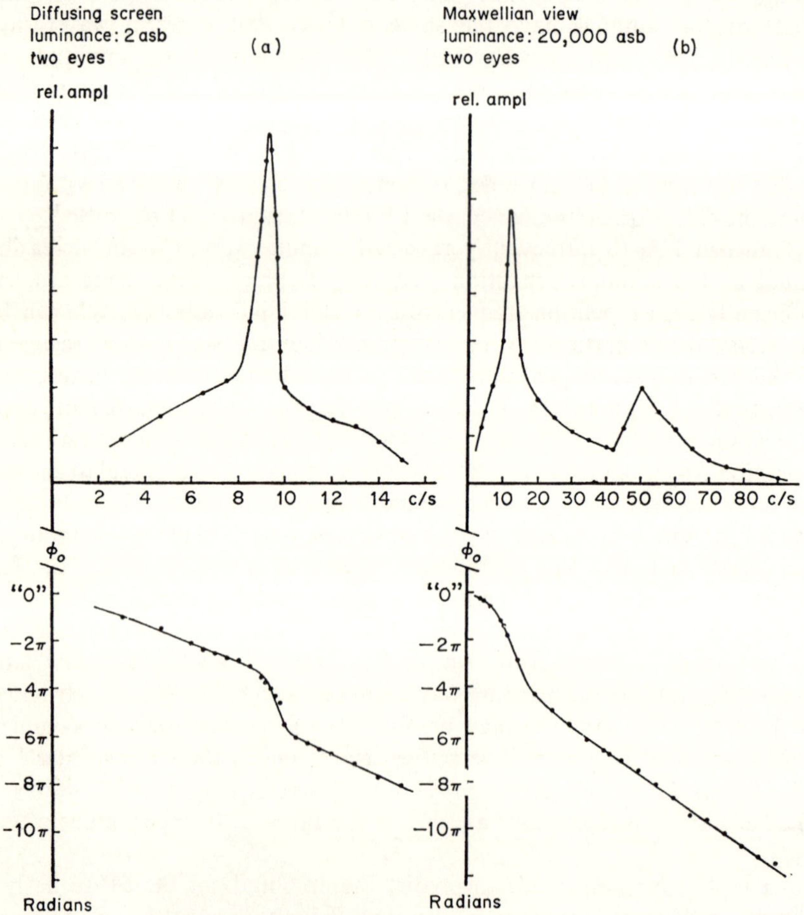

FIGURE 2.12 *Amplitude and phase characteristics for two subjects with sinusoidally modulated light; the frequency scale is linear; amplitudes in relative units.*

(a) *Both the amplitude and phase characteristics of subject A show resonance properties.*

(b) *The amplitude spectrum of subject B shows two preference regions. Neither amplitude, nor phase characteristic shows resonance properties. The phase characteristic shows that the latencies in the low frequency range are longer than in the high frequency range.*

From H. Spekreijse (1966). Analysis of EEG Responses in Man. *Junk Publishers, The Hague.*

within a range centred near 10 Hz evokes a response of large amplitude compared with that at neighbouring frequencies.[550, 634, 748, 753, 797, 843] A number of characteristics of this 10 Hz response are closely related to corresponding characteristics of the spontaneous EEG. The centre frequency of this resonant-like peak in the EP varies from subject to subject, but corresponds closely with the alpha frequency for the subject's spontaneous EEG. In addition the sharpness (Q factor),[83] and amplitude of the EP peak also show close correspondences with the sharpness of tuning and amplitude of spontaneous alpha activity.[748] However, the notion of 'photic driving'[380] in its simplest form is not applicable, since even for stimuli of high modulation depth both alpha activity and the EP can be recorded simultaneously from the same electrode, and they appear to be largely independent and, to a first approximation sum linearly, but this point has not yet been thoroughly investigated.[634, 797]* The large 10 Hz EP component described above can be evoked by a stimulus modulation frequency of 5 Hz as well as one of 10 Hz.[638, 748, 797]

The EPs to the 5 Hz stimulus are almost, but not quite, identical to the responses to the 10 Hz stimulation in amplitudes, sharpness of tuning and centre frequencies. The 'low' frequency 10 Hz components generally show little dependence on stimulus colour although a flattening of the 10 Hz peak has been reported to occur for yellow stimulation.[634, 748]

A plot of the lag of the phase of the EP *versus* stimulus modulation frequency is fairly close to a straight line except at frequencies near the centre frequency of the amplitude peak where there is a well-defined 'step'. (Fig. 2.12.) An estimate of latency can be obtained from the slope of this phase plot (with reservations).* This estimate ranges from 120 to 200 msec depending on intensity and field size.[748, 753, 797]

For a linear filter the phase step and amplitude peak shown in Fig. 2.12 would be expected to be associated in a definite way. Another characteristic of a linear filter is that when a sinusoidal signal is first applied, the amplitude of the response takes some time to build up to the final value, and the rate of

* Let ϕ be the measured phase lag (in degrees) of the fundamental component of the steady-state EP, and f Hz be the stimulus repetition frequency. Let the delay time (latency) of the EP be τ secs. Then:

$$\phi = 360f\tau + A + K$$

where A is a constant and K is a function of f.

$$\frac{\partial \phi}{\partial f} = 360\tau + \frac{\partial K}{\partial f}$$

The 'apparent latency' of the EP is τ' where

$$\tau' = \frac{1}{360}\frac{\partial \phi}{\partial f} = \tau + \frac{1}{360} \cdot \frac{\partial K}{\partial f}.$$

In a frequency region where amplitude changes markedly with stimulus frequency some estimate can be made of $\frac{\partial K}{\partial f}$ on the assumption that the system is a minimum phase-shift system[83] plus a fixed delay (see Reference 506 for a discussion of the plausibility of this assumption). In frequency regions where EP amplitude changes little with frequency, $\tau' = \tau$ if the assumption is made that the system is a linear, minimum phase-shift system plus a fixed delay.[83]

* See pages 236 and 249.

build-up is related to the sharpness of tuning (Q factor[83]) of the amplitude peak. Similarly when a sinewave signal is switched off, the filter continues to oscillate for some time and the rate of decay of response is related to the Q factor. Build up and decay phenomena for the EP have been found to have characteristics which are in accord with those of a linear filter.[748, 795, 797, S21]

The findings described above, and those outlined in Section 2.3.2, led to the suggestion of a simple serial processing model of the form illustrated in Fig. 2.13.[748, 797] It must be emphasised firstly that the model is not unique. It is

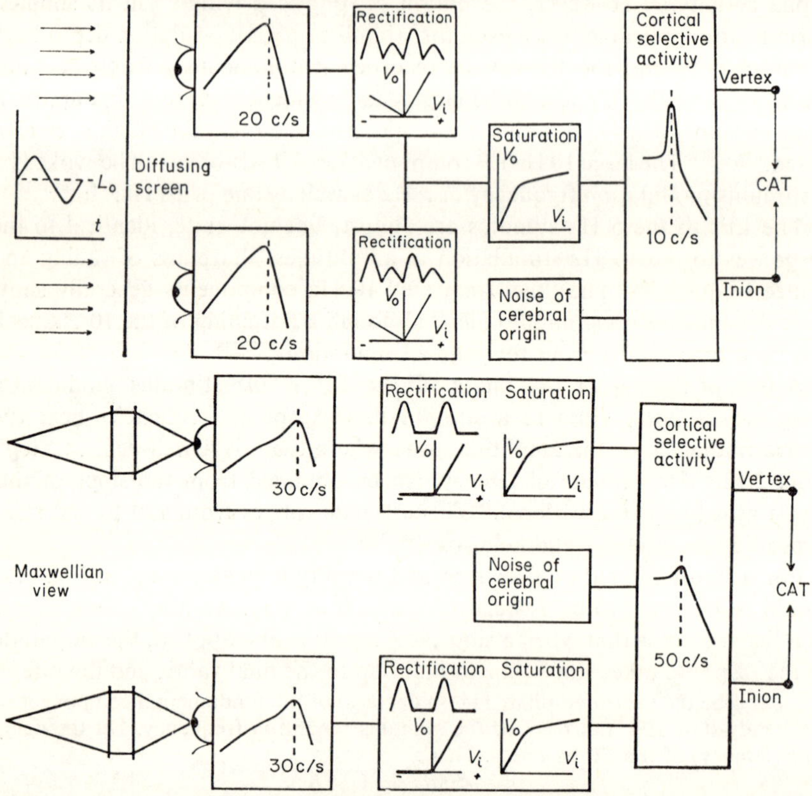

FIGURE 2.13 *Upper half: a simplified model of the retina-cortex system of long latency (i.e. 'low-frequency' region). Lower half: a simplified model of the retina-cortex subsystem of short latency (i.e. 'high-frequency' region). From H. Spekreijse (1966).* Analysis of EEG Responses in Man. *Junk Publishers, The Hague.*

for simplicity intentionally cast in terms of sequential processing and does not invoke feedback[S27] or feedforward elements, nor does it involve any more parallel pathways than are necessitated by the available steady-state data. In order to avoid confusion caused by overlapping of physiological and engineering jargon it is important to remember that the structure of this model, and in fact any other scientific model, can be said to be located in the *minds* of its proposers rather than in the physical world (i.e. in the *brains* of its proposers). In any case it should be emphasised that a model might perform a useful function, even though its component parts could not be uniquely associated with definite physical locations within the brain. However, there is encouraging evidence of correspondencies between peripheral stages of the model and neuroanatomy.[749, 751] The frequency-selective peak near 10 Hz has been modelled by a centrally-located linear filter. The physiological correlate of such a filter is not, however, clear. For example, on the basis of Andersen and Andersson's hypothesis, the physiological correlate of the filter might be the reverberation of signals between cortex and thalamus. On the other hand, Lippold's hypothesis (see Chapter 1, Section 1.2) is that the physiological basis of the 10 Hz resonance is oscillation of the extraocular muscles due to the absence of feedback in circumstances when the visual field lacks spatial structure or when the eyes are closed. The reported absence of a marked 10 Hz resonance when pattern-reversal stimulation is used (Section 2.4.1) would be in accord with this view.

Spekreijse estimated the size of the summation fields for the 'low-frequency' class of EP components in the following way. Pattern-reversal EPs generated by the chessboard mirror method disappear if a fine opaque grid is placed over the boundaries of the squares of the pattern (see Section 2.4.1), showing that the contrast reversal must take place across a sharply focused boundary if pattern EPs are to result. Spekreijse assumed that there is no reason to suppose that the presence of the fine grid would influence EP components which are determined by changes in the luminance of areas of the stimulus (i.e. the 'diffuse field' type of response). Indeed, when the square size exceeds roughly 30′ the amplitude of the EP is little influenced by whether the squares of the pattern are modulated in-phase or in antiphase. However, for a square size of 20′ there is little response when the squares are modulated in antiphase at a frequency set to evoke 'low-frequency' EPs. This finding suggests that the average size of the summation fields for 'low-frequency' EP components is of the order of 25′, although this interpretation may be over simple.[748p.143] Further reservations about the above interpretation are raised by recent findings that the presence of the grid may in fact influence the 'diffuse field' response.[750]

2.8.3 *Steady-state EP components in the range roughly* 45 *to* 60 *Hz* (*'high-frequency' region*)*, analogue model, summation fields*

In many, but not all subjects, the harmonic components of steady-state EPs which fall in the range 45 to 60 Hz ('high-frequency' components) have several features in common with the 10 Hz ('low-frequency' components) described above. A frequency-selective process gives an amplitude peak in this frequency region, which can be evoked as a fundamental component (e.g. by 55·5 Hz stimulus modulation frequency (Fig. 2.14 C)) or as a second harmonic component (e.g. by 24·4 Hz stimulus modulation frequency (Fig. 2.14 A)). This behaviour is similar to that of the 10 Hz class of EPs. Another similarity is that the power *versus* frequency characteristic of the spontaneous EEG contains a peak between 45 and 60 Hz whose frequency

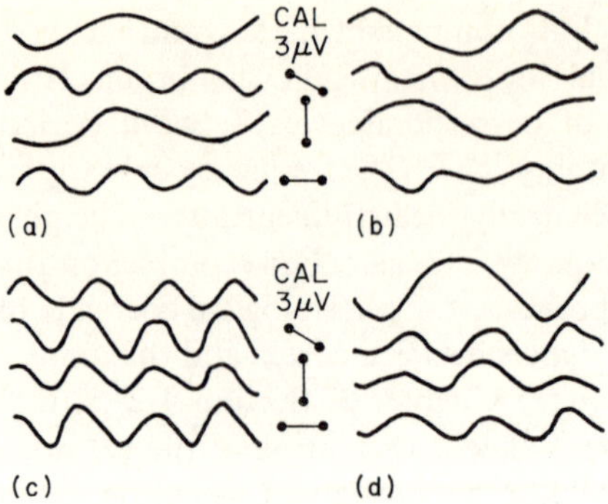

FIGURE 2.14 *Averaged potentials evoked by a red stimulus field of 60° subtense sinusoidally modulated to a depth of 33%. The retinal illumination is about 9300 trolands for* a, b *and* c *and about 930 trolands for* d. *The averaging time was 1 min, the sweep time was 62·5 msec and the number of sweeps was 960 in all cases. The top channel is a calibration of 3 μV peak to peak derived from the stimulus modulation wave. The lines indicate that the second trace was recorded between electrodes 2 and 4, the third trace between 2 and 1 and the fourth trace between 2 and 3 (see Fig. 2.16 for electrode positions).* a: *Stimulus modulation frequency 24·4 c/sec. Subject J.S. Note second harmonic high frequency response in traces 2 and 4.* b: *Same stimulus as for* a *but different subject, F.M.S.* c: *Subject J.S. Stimulus frequency 55·5 c/sec. Note clear responses at fundamental frequency.* d: *Subject J.S. Same stimulus as for a except that it is 10 times less intense. From D. Regan (1968). 'A high frequency mechanism which underlies visual evoked potentials'.* Electroenceph. clin. Neurophysiol., *25, 231–237. Elsevier Publishing Co., Amsterdam.*

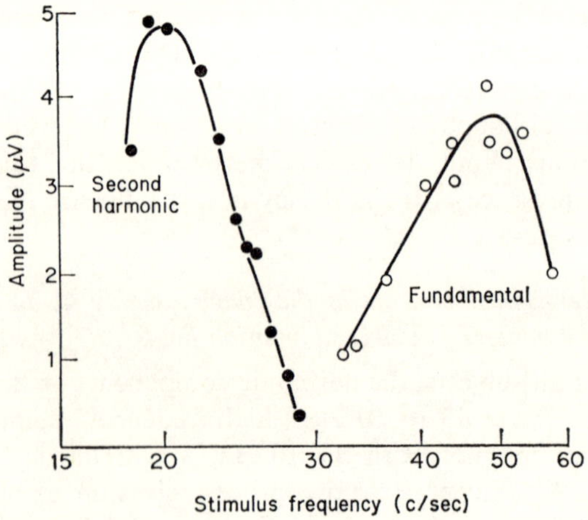

FIGURE 2.15 *Amplitude (in microvolts peak to peak)* versus *stimulus modulation frequency (in cycles per second) for the fundamental and second harmonic components of the steady-state high-frequency evoked potentials. The cross-correlator was used to analyse bipolar recordings made between electrodes 2 and 4 for subject J.S. Same stimulus as for Fig. 2.14a. Note the logarithmic frequency scale. From D. Regan (1968).* Electroenceph. clin. Neurophysiol., **25**, *231–237.*

and sharpness (Q factor) is similar to that of the peak in the amplitude *versus* stimulation frequency characteristic for the steady-state EP. However, the 10 Hz and 45–60 Hz response components are otherwise very different. Independent investigators agree in estimating the apparent latency of the high-frequency responses at roughly 60 msec (Fig. 2.16) (for stimulus brightness of roughly 9000 trolands).[636, 748, 797] The topographical distribution of the HF and LF responses differ (Fig. 2.14),[636, 748] and their relationships with stimulus colour is also quite different (see below). In any case the maximum selectivities (Q factors) of the H.F. peak is generally considerably less than the maximum Q factors of the 10 Hz peak; it is not yet clear whether this is a point of any physiological significance.

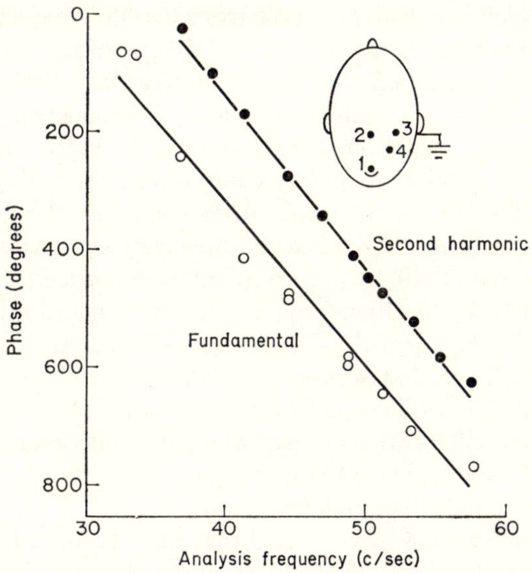

FIGURE 2.16 *Phase (in degrees)* versus *analysis frequency for the fundamental and second harmonic components of the steady-state high-frequency evoked potentials. The cross-correlator was used to analyse bipolar recordings made between electrodes 2 and 4 for subject J.S. Same stimulus as for Fig. 2.14a. Note the linear frequency scale. The zero of phase is arbitrary for both plots. From D. Regan (1968).* Electroenceph. clin. Neurophysiol., *25*, *231–237.*

The *apparent latency* of the second harmonic high-frequency responses evoked by stimuli modulated at 18 to 26 Hz is similar to the *apparent latency* of the fundamental high-frequency responses evoked by stimuli modulated at 45 to 60 Hz (Figs. 2.14, 2.15, 2.16). The maximum (saturated) amplitude of the EP obtained at high modulation depths to binocular stimulation is equal to the sum of the saturated EPs to monocular left and right eye stimulation. These findings above and those described in Section 2.3.2 above are consistent with the model shown in Fig. 2.13 B.

There is some evidence that the amplitude of the HF responses are less affected by stimulus luminance than are the amplitudes of responses in 10–20 Hz range.

Spekreijse has estimated summation fields to be roughly 25′ for 'high-frequency' EP components by using the same method which indicated a size of roughly 15′ for 'low-frequency' components[748] (see Section 2.8.2). This estimate is less open to objection than the estimate for 10 Hz summation fields, since pattern EPs have negligible amplitudes at frequencies as high as 50 Hz.[750]

2.8.4 *Steady-state EP components in the range roughly* 12 *to* 25 *Hz* (*'medium-frequency' range*)

There is some evidence that there are EP components in the range roughly 12 to 25 Hz which are distinguishable from the 'low-frequency' and 'high-frequency' components described above. However, the characteristics of these 'medium-frequency' components are not so well established as are the characteristics of the 'high' and 'low-frequency' components.

'Medium'-frequency EP components seem to be more colour dependent than either 'low' or 'high'-frequency components.[635, 638, 639, 640] Their topographical distribution is different from that of the 'low-frequency' responses.[638] In the subjects studied the frequency selectivity of the steady-state EP is not paralleled by a corresponding frequency selectivity in the spontaneous EEG for 'medium-frequency' components as it is for 'low' and 'high-frequency' components.[638, 748] In order to include such responses in the model of van der Tweel and Spekreijse[748, 797] (Fig. 2.13) it might be necessary to add a parallel channel involving a frequency-selective filter* which differed from the other two filters (*a*) in not performing the function of filtering neural noise to form the spontaneous EEG, and (*b*) whose filter characteristics were sensitive to chromatic adaptation.[638]

A body of evidence has accumulated that there is more than one retino-cortical visual pathway.[402, 403, 859] Whether the different behaviour of the brain to 'low-frequency' and 'high-frequency' stimuli reflect differences between visual pathways is an interesting question which might be approached directly via monkey experiments.

2.8.5 *The effects of stimulus repetition frequency on EPs to pattern-reversal*

EPs to pattern alternation (Section 2.4.1) have amplitude *versus* frequency curves which are quite different from the amplitude *versus* frequency curves for diffuse-field intensity-modulated stimuli of any colour, brightness or field size which has so far been investigated.

Two features which distinguish the amplitude *versus* frequency curve for pattern alternation from the amplitude *versus* frequency curve for blank-field EPs are firstly the much less-pronounced frequency-selective process in the

* The word 'filter' is used here to include *any* physiological mechanism (such as those discussed in Chapter 1, Section 1.2, and Chapter 2, Section 9.4) which can exhibit frequency selectivity.

alpha range or in the 50 Hz range, and secondly the restriction of appreciable steady-state responses to stimuli of rather low frequencies (although steady-state EPs cannot be said to occur for frequencies of pattern-reversal of less than roughly 4 reversals per second, since for these low frequencies each reversal generates a separate response). Stimuli of frequencies greater than roughly 30 reversals per second give pattern-reversal EPs which fall off sharply as frequency increases. In contrast with 10 Hz and 45–60 Hz EP components to luminance modulation, the EPs to pattern-reversal seem to be unrelated to the frequency content of the spontaneous EEG.

2.8.6 *The* (*a*) *subjective and* (*b*) *objective sensitivity versus frequency curves for the visual pathway*

De Lange made an important contribution to our understanding of the perception of flicker when he developed the use of modulated light as a visual stimulus.[217] He was able to distinguish between the effects of the mean luminance ('brightness', see Chapter 5) and the modulation frequency of a stimulus light on the resulting perception of flicker. This distinction was made possible by modulating the light about a constant mean level and then gradually changing the modulation depth at constant frequency (or the frequency at constant modulation depth) until the point was reached at which the subject could just perceive flicker. This point is called the threshold for flicker perception.

De Lange found that the modulation depth at threshold varied with frequency in an instructive way. For example, at 2 Hz the modulation depth which gave just-perceptible flicker might be 1% (A in Fig. 2.17), at 10 Hz it might be 0·5% (i.e. subjective sensitivity was higher than at 2 Hz, B in Fig. 2.17), and then as frequency was increased to 20 Hz (C in Fig. 2.17) and to 60 Hz (D in Fig. 2.17) the subjective sensitivity to flicker fell progressively. Examples of curves of subjective sensitivity (reciprocal of threshold modulation depth) *versus* stimulus modulation frequency are shown in Fig. 2.18. Such curves are called *De Lange curves* and they give a measure of the way in

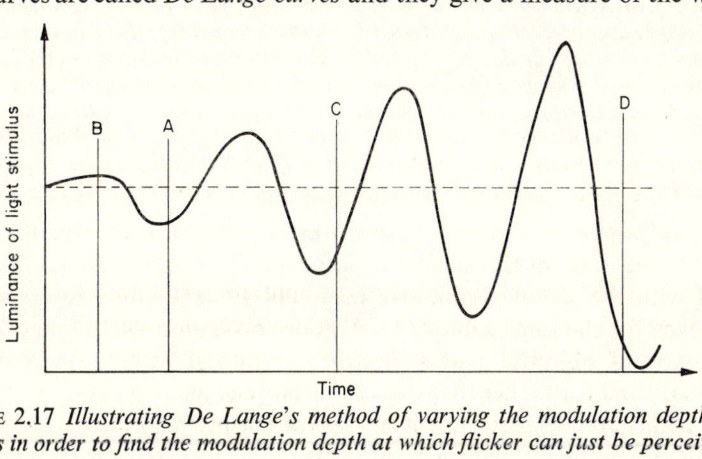

FIGURE 2.17 *Illustrating De Lange's method of varying the modulation depth of a stimulus in order to find the modulation depth at which flicker can just be perceived.*

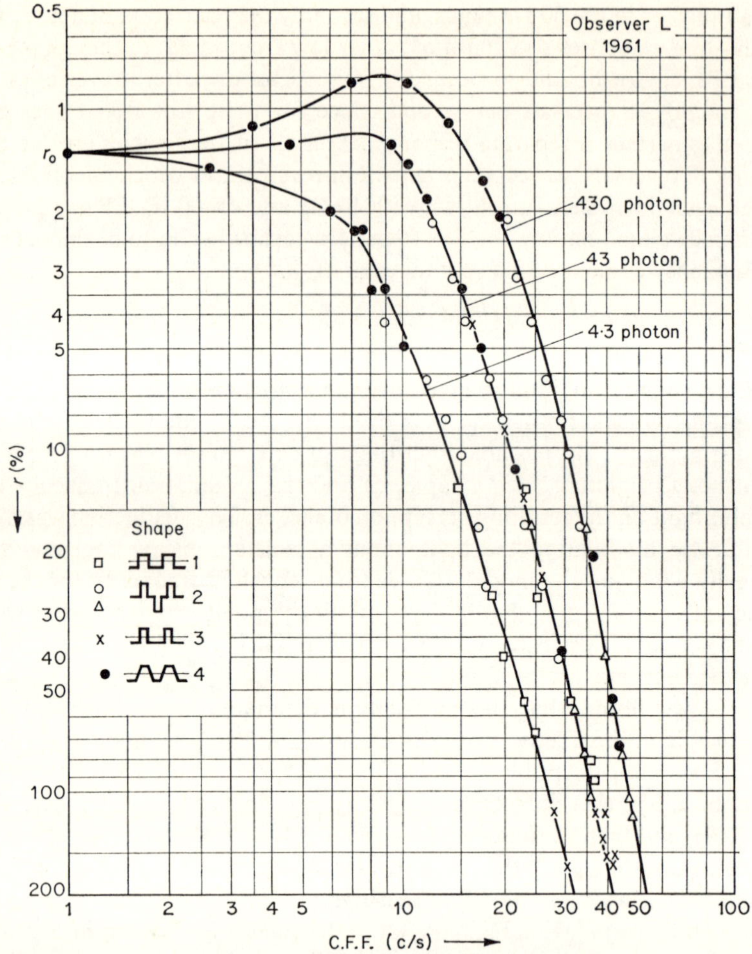

FIGURE 2.18 *Attenuation characteristics for white light of the right-hand system fovea brightness perception; 2° test-field, large surrounding field having the same luminance as the test-field, central fixation. There are four variations in the luminance as shown; 1 and 4 shape of modulation, 2 and 3 mode of interruption. 4 is approximately sinusoidal; ripple-ratio r = fundamental B_1/mean luminance B_a of the stimulus; C.F.F. = critical flicker frequency; r_0 = critical value of the variation at the site of the threshold-mechanism, measured at the input if no attenuation in the system occurs; attenuation $\eta = r_0/r$. From H. De Lange Dzn. (1957). Thesis, Delft.*[217]

which *subjective* sensitivity to flicker varies with stimulus modulation frequency. The *shape* of this subjective curve (in log coordinates) has been compared with the *shape* of objective curves of EP amplitude *versus* stimulus frequency for the same subject.[637, 794] Poor correlations were found between the shape of objective and subjective curves for both lower frequencies (5–25 Hz) and for higher frequencies (45–60 Hz).

At higher frequencies there is a dissociation between the de Lange curve and amplitude *versus* frequency curve for the EP. At frequencies higher than about 13 Hz the de Lange curve falls fairly linearly as shown in Fig. 2.18. It can also be seen in Fig. 2.15 that the amplitude of the EP may be *rising* with increasing frequency under conditions where the subjective sensitivity to flicker is falling with frequency. This dissociation is a stronger observation than the result of comparing the thresholds for perception and the detection threshold for the EP, since EP detection threshold depends markedly on technical factors. Among these factors are the method of signal: noise enhancement, the number of averaging sweeps and electrode position. The dissociation between the shapes of the subjective and objective sensitivity *versus* stimulus curves mean that the attenuation characteristic for the neural pathway which underlies flicker perception is different from the attenuation characteristic of the neural pathway which underlies generation of the steady-state EPs to spatially unstructured stimulus fields. This suggests that the pathway forks at some stage.

The correlation between EP data and the shape of the de Lange curve is, however, less poor when only peripheral EP attenuation is considered.[748] An interesting finding which may be relevant is that single unit spikes recorded from the lateral geniculate body of monkey show attenuation characteristics which are similar in shape to the de Lange curves in man.[750]

The lack of correlation reported above between flicker perception and the amplitudes of steady-state scalp EPs to unstructured fields might seem unsurprising in view of the well-known fact that at cortical level in cat and monkey few cells respond when the eye is stimulated by spatially unstructured fields.[399] However, a large body of classical human psychophysics has been carried out with unstructured patches of light of 2°, 10° or even 55° subtense (for example, the major part of colour theory is based on such experiments).[334] This latter fact indicates that the EP findings described above are not, even with hindsight, self-evident.[S22]

2.8.7 *Evoked potentials, perceived frequency and perceived number*

For low flash or modulation rates (less than 4–7 Hz) the subjective impression of flicker frequency seems to be closely related to the physical stimulus repetition rate. However, for stimulus repetition rates exceeding about 5–7 Hz the subjective impression of flicker frequency grows vague, although it generally seems to be lower than the frequency of the physical stimulus.[460]

In contrast, for any stimulus repetition frequency the EP must necessarily be locked to the stimulus frequency. This follows from the nature of the averaging or analysis process itself. This point raises some doubts whether it is at all reasonable to anticipate correlations between perceived flicker and phase-locked or time-locked EPs.

When an illuminated radial slit is rotated at a suitable speed in darkness an impression may result of a series of bright and dark bands.[526] In order to account for this phenomenon it has been suggested that the response to a transient flash of light is a sequence of impressions of brightness and darkness. In 1942 Talbot and Marshall[511] suggested that the sequence of major positive and negative deflections of the visual EP might correspond to this hypothetical sequence of impressions; they further suggested that the occurrence of such cyclic excitability changes might also be expected to result in disparities between perceived flicker frequency and the physical repetition rate of a stimulus light. Twenty-four years after Talbot and Marshall's paper, evidence was obtained of a close correspondence between the temporal structure of the transient EP and the number of flashes reported by subjects who observe a short burst of flashes.[362, 868] Flashes were presented at a constant rate of 33·3 per second in bursts containing from 1 to 14 flashes. It was found that the number of flashes which the subject reported as having seen was only partially determined by the number of flashes actually delivered. The subjects generally reported from 1 to between 4 and 6 flashes even though from 1 to 14 were presented. If the flash burst did not extend beyond the first phase of the EP waveform, the subject most probably reported one flash; if the flash burst continued up to the second negative peak in the EP he most probably reported two flashes; if the burst continued up to the third negative peak he most probably reported three flashes, and so on (Fig. 2.19).

The likelihood of this correlation being coincidental is reduced by the finding that subject-to-subject variations in the periodicity of the EP waveform were paralleled by corresponding changes in the periodicity of the perceptual effect, and furthermore that variations in EP periodicity caused by changing from red to blue light were also paralleled by corresponding perceptual changes.

A criticism which can be made of the experiments described above is that although a constant stimulus repetition rate of 33·3 flashes per second was used, the result of varying the total number of flashes from 1 to 14 would be to produce marked changes in the frequency distribution of the stimulu energy.[750]

2.8.8 *Linear and nonlinear systems analysis applied to EPs*

Very generally there are two classes of system which may be fully described by their input–output relationships. These are *linear* and *nonlinear* systems. The most important fact about linear systems is that they can all be analysed by using one single method – linear systems analysis.

A system is defined as linear if the superposition principle holds for it. This means that if input x_1 gives output y_1, and input x_2 gives output y_2, then input $(x_1 + x_2)$ gives output $(y_1 + y_2)$. This condition (that each input must be processed as though others were not present) must hold for both amplitude and temporal measures. The steady-state behaviour of *any* linear system is therefore fully described by an amplitude characteristic plus a phase characteristic, and the transient behaviour is fully described by an amplitude *versus* time characteristic. The superposition principle states that the behaviour of a linear system does not depend on the amplitude of the input, so that its output is fully determined by the frequency and phase of the input waveform. If in the steady-state mode a sine wave is applied at the input, then a pure sine wave appears at the output.

All systems for which the superposition principle does not apply are nonlinear. There is no single method of analysis which applies to all nonlinear systems. In some nonlinear systems, operating in the steady-state mode, a sine wave applied to the input does not produce a pure sine wave at the output, but rather a distorted sine wave and this is one unequivocal sign of a nonlinear system.

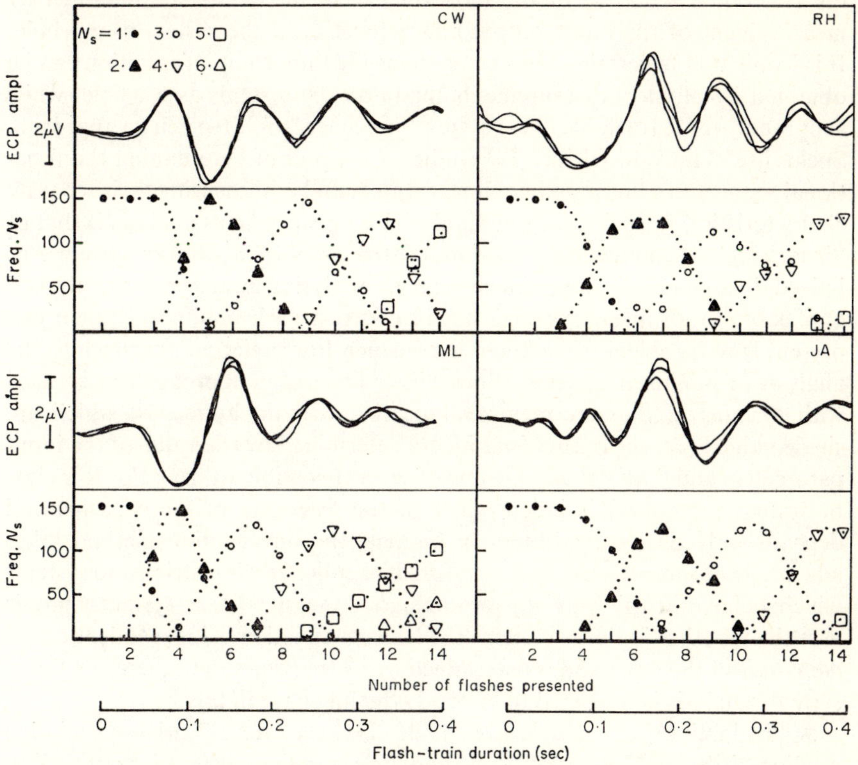

FIGURE 2.19 *Effects of number of flashes presented on evoked cortical potentials (ECP) and perceived number of flashes* (N_s). *Flashes were presented at 33·3 flash/sec. Each of the three superimposed evoked cortical potential traces represents the summation of responses to all flash-trains within a single session (700 flash-trains consisting of 1 to 4 flashes). Negativity downward. Frequency of* N. *reflects the number of times each flash-train was perceived as 1, 2, 3, 4, 5, or 6 flashes, each flash-train being presented 150 times. Due to conduction time-lag, flash-train onset is displaced 35 msec after trace onset. From M. R. Harter and C. T. White (1967). 'Perceived number and evoked cortical potentials'.* Science, ***156***, *406–408. © American Association for the Advancement of Science.*

Since linear systems analysis applies to all linear systems, and is in addition quite straightforward[34], it is the usual practice to restrict the study of physical systems to an operational range where their behaviour is approximately linear (pseudo-linear) by using 'small signals'. The behaviour of some systems, however, is far from linear even when the input signal is very small and then linear analysis is inapplicable.

NONLINEARITIES IN THE VISUAL SYSTEM; LINEARISING; PERIPHERAL ATTENUATION

It is notorious that the analysis of a nonlinear system is more difficult, often much more difficult, than the analysis of a linear or pseudo-linear system. Nevertheless, for a linear system composed of a sequence of linear elements the functional sequence of the individual elements cannot be obtained by measurement of the input–output characteristics of the system as a whole. It is ironic that in certain nonlinear systems the important information can be obtained by physical measurements made on the systems as a whole, while supposedly more tractable linear systems are inaccessible to such an approach. Spekreijse[748] introduced into EP studies a method of determining the functional sequence of linear and nonlinear stages, and of measuring their separate characteristics.[751] Spekreijse's method of nonlinear systems analysis is that of 'linearising'. It applies only to a restricted class of nonlinear systems, as indeed do all methods of nonlinear systems analysis (linear systems analysis is applicable to all linear systems, but in contrast each nonlinear system can present fresh problems since there is no general or preferred approach to the analysis of nonlinear systems). Spekreijse's linearising approach can be used with systems of the zero-memory type (i.e. without hysteresis) which are single valued (i.e. the output is uniquely determined by the value of the input parameters and does not assume one of several possible values). For this class of system the output is independent of the *frequency* of the stimulus and depends only on its amplitude. In essence, the linearisation method takes advantage of this property and therefore its application is restricted to systems which behave in this way. In an analogous manner linear system analysis uses the fact that in linear systems the transfer function is independent of the *amplitude* of the input and is determined by its frequency, and therefore linear systems analysis is restricted to systems which behave in this way.

A distinction was previously made between nonessential ('analytic') nonlinearities and essential ('nonanalytic') nonlinearities (Section 2.3.2). The distortion in the output of the system caused by the former type of nonlinearity can be reduced to any desired extent by reducing the amplitude of the incoming signal, whereas the distorting effect of an essential nonlinearity cannot be reduced in this way. In some circumstances steady-state EPs are found to show a high percentage of second harmonic distortion which cannot be reduced by reducing the modulation depth of the signal. This indicates the presence of an essential nonlinearity (Fig. 2.3).

The principle of linearising is illustrated in Fig. 2.20. The linearising effect of a triangular auxiliary wave on a sinusoidal input is shown for a half-wave linear rectifier. It should be noted that the frequency of the auxiliary triangular wave is here much higher than that of the sinusoidal input signal. When the frequency of the auxiliary wave is close to that of the signal (as is necessary in some physiological applications), a clear output signal will only appear after averaging.

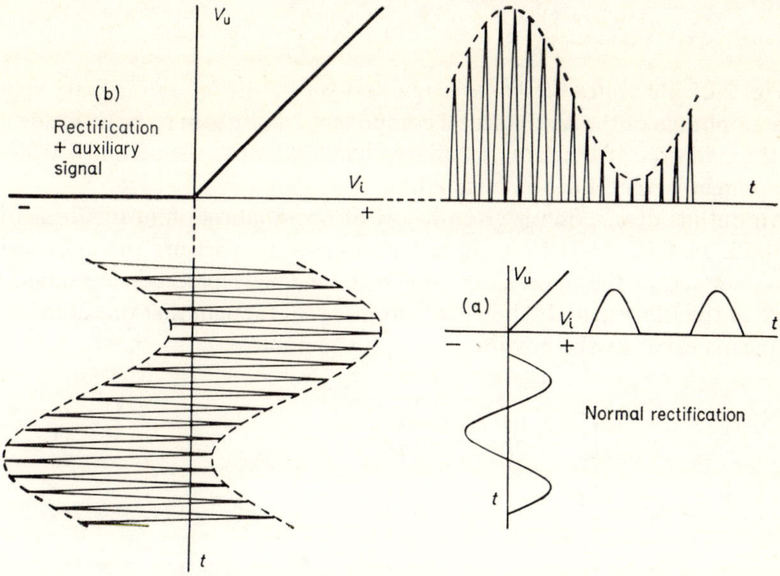

FIGURE 2.20 *The principle of linearising. From L. H. van der Tweel and H. Spekreijse (1969). 'Signal transport and rectification in the human evoked-response system'*, Ann. N.Y. Acad. Sci., ***156***, *678–695.*

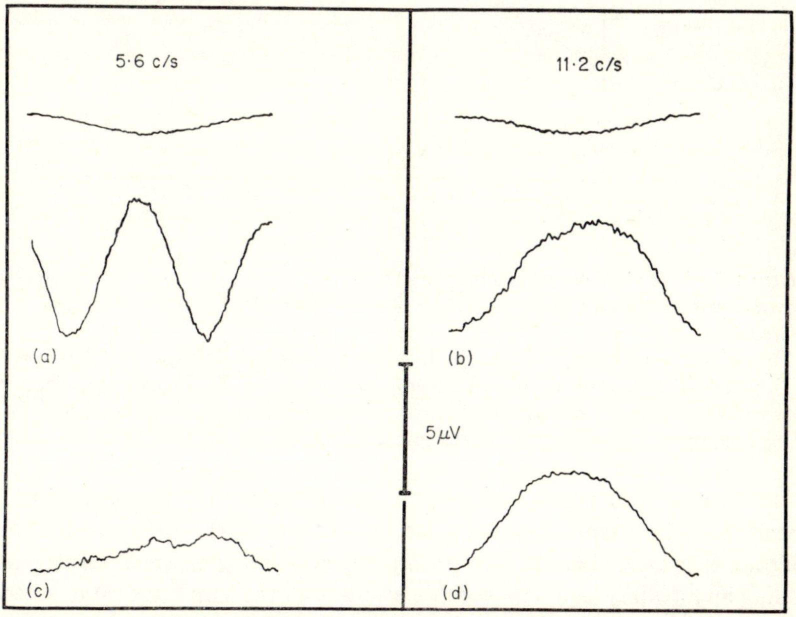

FIGURE 2.21 *Occipital responses recorded with electrodes on the midline for 5·6 cps and 11·2 cps (subject D). Diffuse stimulus field; modulation depth, 10%; natural pupil; brightness, 200 asb; signal-to-noise ratio, $A^2/2\sigma^2 = 0{\cdot}04$. The upper curves represent an averaged photoelectric signal caused by the light. The middle curves show the responses to sinusoidally modulated light (A and B). The bottom curves show the responses to sinusoidally modulated light plus gaussian noise (C and D). From L. H. van der Tweel and H. Spekreijse (1969). 'Signal transport and rectification in the human evoked-response system'*. Ann. N.Y. Acad. Sci., ***156***, *678–695.*

Fig. 2.21 illustrates the linearising effect on the EP of an auxiliary signal. The amplitude of the fundamental component can be seen to be little affected by the addition of the large auxiliary signal, whereas the second harmonic component is very much attenuated.

An outline description is given below of one application of the linearising method. In this application, linearising is used to measure the attenuation characteristic of the linear stage which immediately precedes the nonlinear stage in the EP system. It should be emphasised, though, that this exercise by no means exhausts the possibilities of this method.

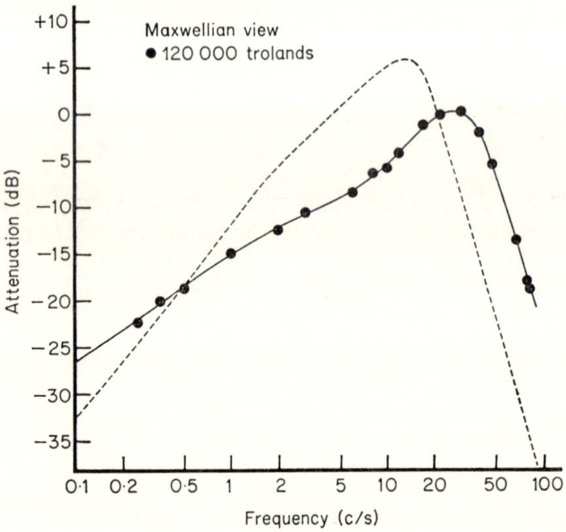

FIGURE 2.22 *Subject B: attenuation characteristic, calculated from the responses recorded with electrodes on the midline. Maxwellian view; 120,000 trolands; pupil dilated.*

The full curve represents the attenuation curve for responses with short latencies.

The dashed curve that for responses with long latencies. The displacement between both curves on the vertical axis is arbitrary. From H. Spekreijse (1966). Analysis of EEG Responses in Man. *Junk Publishers, The Hague.*

If the processes which precede the nonlinearity can be assumed to be linear, then the attenuation characteristic of these processes can be found as follows. It is clear that the reduction in signal distortion which results from adding an auxiliary signal must be determined by the amplitude ratio between the input signal and the auxiliary wave *at a point immediately preceding the nonlinearity.* The case in point is when each of several sinusoidal auxiliary waves of different frequencies produce the same linearising effect on the response to an unvarying sinusoidal input signal. The various auxiliary waves can then be assumed to have equal amplitudes at a point immediately preceding the nonlinearity. In general this result can only be obtained by using auxiliary waves whose amplitudes are made to differ at the point of entry to the visual system. Since the auxiliary waves have equal amplitude by the time they reach the nonlinear stage, the relative amplitudes of the auxiliary signals at the input to the visual system (i.e. at the eye) therefore gives the attenuation characteristic of the stage which *precedes* the nonlinear stage. It turns out that the attenuation for this peripheral stage differs for 'low-frequency' and 'high-frequency' EP components which must therefore be regarded as being separate at even this early stage (Fig. 2.22).[748 p.110]

The possibility of 'dissecting out' a functional sequence of stages of information processing which is offered by Spekreijse's approach must render it a tool of great potential value in both EP and single cell studies. Indeed the method has already been used with promising results in both these areas of research.[748, 749, 751]

2.9 Evoked potentials and colour

2.9.1 *The effect of stimulus colour on the waveforms of transient EPs*

Clynes[146, 149, 150, 153] reported that distinguishably different transient EP waveforms were specific to different stimulus colours. More than one of these colour-specific waveforms could be recorded from any one electrode derivation, so that there was some difficulty in distinguishing between them. However, Clynes designed a computer algorithm to extract the different colour-specific components. The procedure utilised the convenient circumstances that not only did the topographical distributions of the various colour components differ but also their latencies were considerably different[146, 154] (Fig. 2.23). In order to take advantage of topographical differences between different waveforms, Clynes recorded bipolar EPs between electrodes placed 3 cm apart and arranged in a rosette pattern. When red, green and blue stimuli were abruptly switched on, different waveforms were evoked, although these differences were not large[146] (Fig. 2.23). Not only were the topographical distributions of the characteristic waveforms to red, green and blue lights

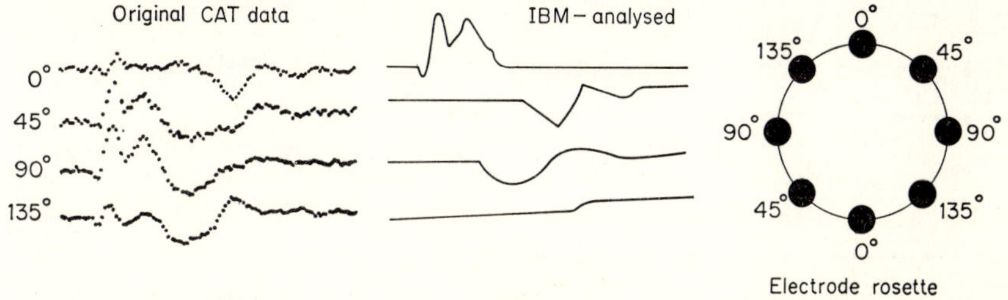

FIGURE 2.23 A: *left side shows evoked potentials recorded simultaneously between opposite electrodes in a rosette pattern. The recorded waveforms are made up from more basic waveforms whose electric fields are differently oriented on the scalp. These basic waveforms can be extracted from the original data by the use of a digital computer (right side of figure). From M. Clynes (1965). Brain space analysis of evoked potential components applied to chromaticity waves. Sixth Internat. Conf. Med. Electron. and Biol., Eng., Tokyo, Japan.*

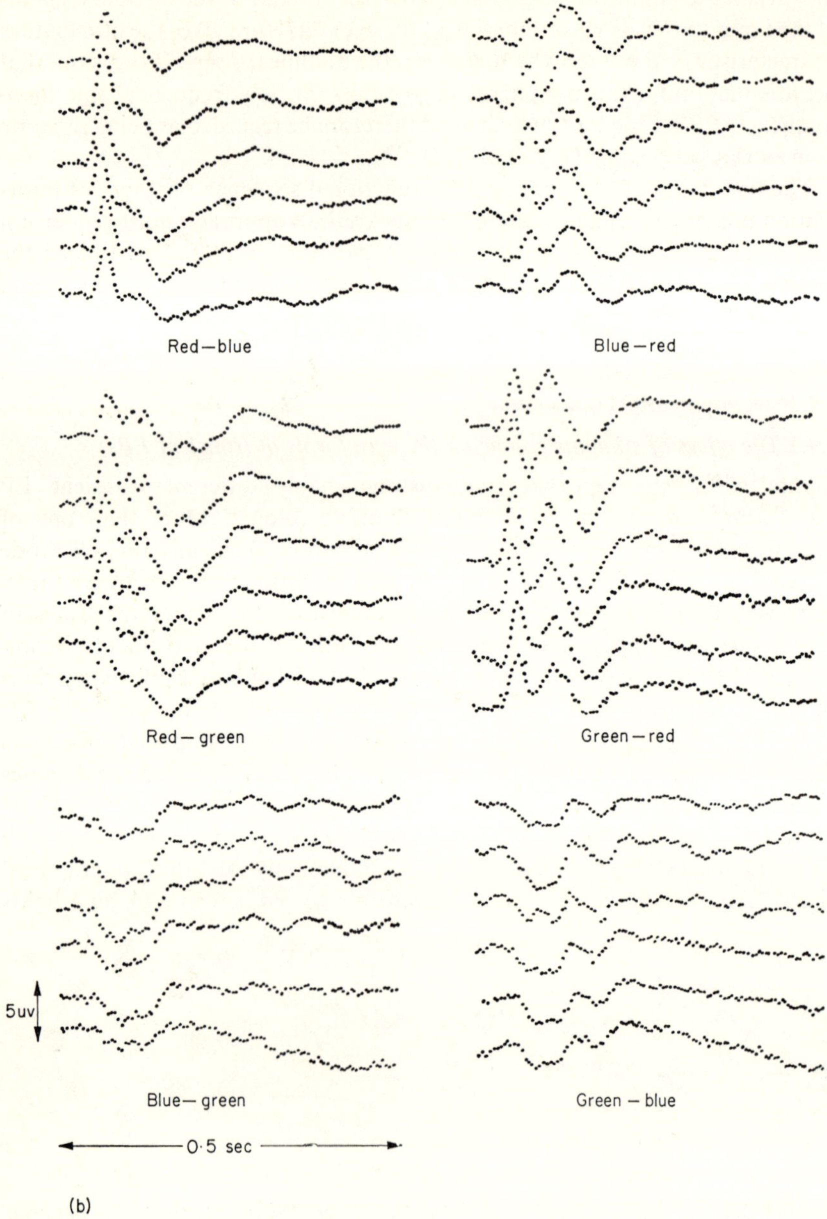

FIGURE 2.23 B: *responses to changes of colour at the same intensity. Red-blue indicates that blue is changed to red. Six pairs of horizontal occipital electrodes were used. Each pair of electrodes was placed 2 cm above the other. Note the characteristic pattern for each colour combination. From M. Clynes and M. Kohn (1967).* Electroenceph. clin. Neurophysiol. Suppl. *1*, **26**, *82–96. Elsevier Publishing Co., Amsterdam.*

different; but also the individual components which made up the specific colour responses differed topographically.[150]

It is difficult to discuss these interesting findings at length since there is little published data on stimulus conditions and control experiments. A rather large field size of roughly 25° subtense[150] was chosen empirically in order to maximise the differences between EPs to differently coloured stimuli.[147] A full description of control experiments designed to distinguish between intensity and colour effects does not yet appear to have been published.

The questions (*a*) whether the shapes of EP waveforms to transient stimulation show colour-specific differences, and (*b*) whether these differences persist over a wide range of stimulus intensities were also investigated by Shipley *et al.*[735] After equating the luminances of the differently coloured stimuli by heterochromatic flicker photometry, Shipley *et al.* varied them over ranges of up to 5 log units.

In an earlier report the less satisfactory procedure was adopted of measuring luminances with respect to a psychophysical absolute threshold.[734] This absolute threshold was measured after 60 seconds dark adaptation. In this report Shipley *et al.* gave no information as to the relative luminances of the differently coloured stimuli. Neither was the relation of the measured absolute thresholds to the (possibly more relevant) chromatic threshold discussed. Shipley *et al.* obtained coloured stimuli by the use of interference filters of roughly 10 nm half-widths and recorded evoked potentials between one electrode on the inion and a second electrode placed 5 to 8 cm in front of the inion along the midline. The stimulus field subtended 11°, and was surrounded by a white adapting field of 27° subtense.

Some of the subjects whose colour vision was normal showed a gradual change in EP waveform as the wavelength of the stimulus was progressively changed from 680 nm (deep red) to 380 nm (far violet). Three distinct EP waveforms could be recognised by purely visual inspection. One waveform was characteristic of the violet–green–yellow range (380 nm–540 nm), one was characteristic of a narrow yellow–orange range (near 590 nm) and one was characteristic of red (near 640 nm). In accord with the finding of Clynes and his colleagues, the 'red' response was the most distinctive, and was marked by a positive peak at roughly 200 msec and a negative peak at roughly 325 msec. Yellow–green responses were marked by two positive peaks near 165 msec and 275 msec separated by a negative peak at roughly 220 msec. Clynes 'green' response is not very similar to that reported by Shipley since it was characterised by a 180 msec peak.[150] At the lowest intensities the earlier components of Shipley's EPs (up to 200 msec) disappeared into background noise, and later components became relatively (and sometimes absolutely) more marked. This finding agrees with Vaughan's report.[822] Both are open to Donchin's[536] comment that this late wave may be related less to stimulus parameters than to the resolution by the stimulus of the subjects' uncertainty.

Ciganek and Ingvar[139] found that the latencies of all EP components to equal-energy monochromatic flashes varied little with stimulus wavelength at high intensities, but for low-stimulus intensities showed a minimum latency in the middle of the spectrum. They reported that the waveform of their EPs depended on wavelength, but did not thoroughly investigate the effect of stimulus intensity on their wavelength-dependent changes of EP waveform.

There are some reservations which must be made which arise from the

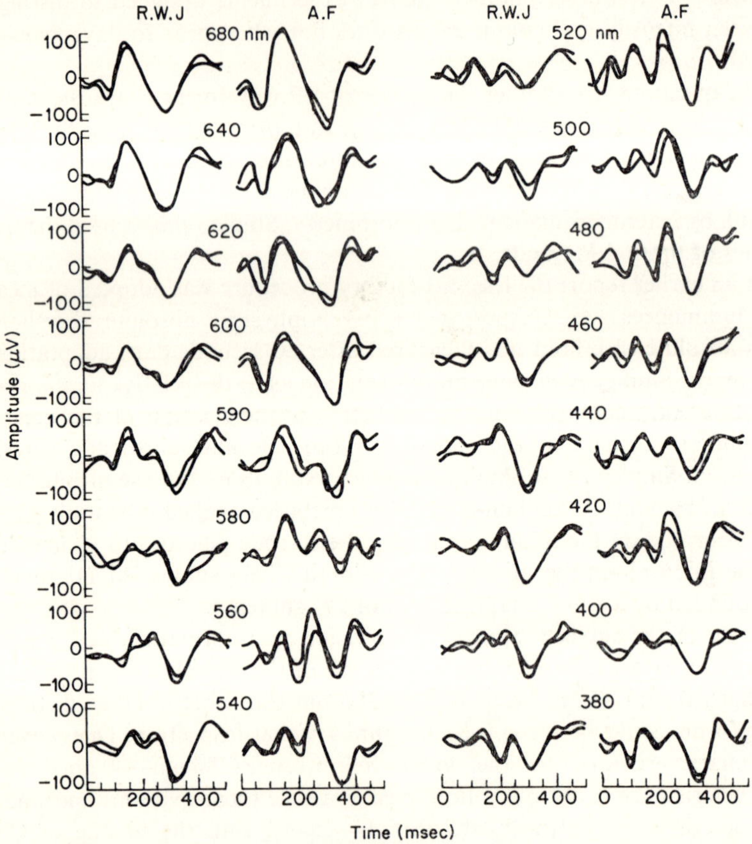

FIGURE 2.24 *The EPs for 16 colours at matched intensities for two colour-normal observers* (*R.W.J. and A.F.*). *From T. Shipley, R. W. Jones and A. Fry* (*1966*). Vision Res., *6*, *657–667*. *Pergamon Press, Oxford.*

rather large stimulus fields used by Shipley *et al.* (11°), by Ciganek and Ingvar[139] and (it seems in most experiments) by Clynes and his colleagues (roughly 25°). Such large stimulus fields as these fall on a markedly inhomogeneous retinal area which includes not only foveal cones, but also extrafoveal cones and rods, all of which have differing spectral sensitivities. The question of whether any conclusions about the neural processing of colour information can be drawn from the colour-dependent EP effects described above would be clarified by confirmatory studies in which stimulation was restricted to the fovea. What evidence that there is available on foveal stimulation is not encouraging. Siegfried[738] found no colour-dependent waveform effects.

Although the colour-dependent effects illustrated in Fig. 2.24 are clear even to visual inspection, the differences between the waveforms are nevertheless difficult to describe quantitatively. This is a problem which at the present time seriously limits the hypothesis-testing power of many EP studies. Such a limitation amounts to a serious weakness since a lack of quantitative precision hampers attempts to establish clear links with previous studies, and to generate predictions which are vulnerable to sharp experimental tests. In such circumstances, when experimental conclusions are entirely restricted to qualitative description, any resulting predictions are likely to be framed in such vague terms that their *disproof* is unlikely.

Clynes *et al.*[149, 150] reported that scalp potentials could be evoked by abruptly changing the colour of the stimulus without changing its subjective brightness, and that the waveforms of these responses depended on both the initial and the final colours. These responses were reported to be more clearly colour dependent than responses to switching on a light from initial darkness, though this is not surprising, since initial colour adaptation would be expected to enhance colour differentiation. However, in spite of their apparently simpler waveforms, such EPs might be expected to be more difficult to interpret than either the responses to switching on a coloured light from initial darkness or the responses to changing the brightness of a light of constant colour. One reason for this is as follows: EPs to an abrupt change in stimulus colour might, in the absence of evidence to the contrary, be assumed to be made up of responses to (*a*) a decrease of the luminance of the first colour (off response), (*b*) an increase in the luminance of the second colour (on response) and (*c*) a response to a change in the *wavelength* of the stimulus. If the spectral sensitivity of the EPs differed from the psychophysical spectral sensitivity, then subjective brightness equality would be an ineffective control. Clynes *et al.* do not seem to have published details of the results of control experiments in which the relative luminances of members of colour pairs were varied. An additional opportunity for intensity effects to masquerade as colour effects is offered if there are any colour-dependent differences between the latencies of components of the potentials evoked by changes in the luminances of lights of different colours (as seems the case in psychophysics).[838] Such latency differences might allow 'on' and 'off' intensity responses to superpose in ways which depend on the initial and final colours. In fact, misleading responses of this nature have been reported in the related situation when EPs are recorded to rapidly alternating colours. For such EPs, colour-dependent saturation characteristics conspire to produce luminance-dependent EP components which closely mimic EP components specific to chromaticity changes[640] (see Section 2.9.3).

Shipley described his EP colour correlates as reflecting neural 'colour coding'. However, it has not yet been convincingly established that *any* EP signals do in fact reflect neural events which have significance for the organism, and more specifically it has not yet been demonstrated that EP colour correlates reflect a neural representation of colour that relates causally with the perception of colour. This last point gains force from Shipley's finding that some colour-normal subjects showed no discernible EP colour correlates. On the other hand, colour-defective subjects did shows a diminished degree of EP colour effects and the failure to find colour effects in some normals might be due to problems of electrode placement.[733]

A possible source of artifact in many colour studies is due to uncontrolled spatial structure in the visual stimulus. Depending on the spatial structure of the stimulus, EP components related to spatial contrast are likely to contribute to the EP to a greater or lesser extent. The amplitude of contrast-specific EPs depend markedly on the sharpness of visual accommodation.[359, 748, 801]

2.9.2 *Spectral sensitivity: transient EPs*

It is generally agreed that there is an intensity region over which the amplitude of any particular EP component rises monotonically as the intensity of light flashes is progressively increased. As stimulus intensity is further raised, the amplitude of any EP component often reaches a maximum (saturates) or even falls off (Fig. 2.25). If measurements are restricted to the pre-saturation region a spectral sensitivity curve for the EP can be measured by the criterion response method* (Fig. 2.25). When this procedure is used some arbitrary criterion EP amplitude is chosen, and the light flux required to evoke the criterion response is then determined for a series of colours throughout the spectrum. Armington measured spectral sensitivity by this method[29] and found that this 'objective' curve agreed fairly well with the psychophysical CIE curve (Fig. 2.26). The peak-to-peak measure of amplitude, used by Armington has the advantage of clarity but the disadvantage that it may lump together components which behave differently (see Section 2.9.3)· Shipley *et al.*[735] reported evidence that the peak-to-trough measure may be of dubious validity, since different EP components reach their maximum at different stimulus intensities. Also, it is difficult to be sure that the disparity between the psychophysical spectral sensitivity curves for Armington's subjects and the CIE curve was not important when compared with EP variability. Cavonius[124] used a similar peak-to-peak measure but for repetitive rather than transient stimulation (4 Hz) and obtained a similar spectral sensitivity to Armington's curve. It is worth noting that at frequencies appreciably higher than those used by Cavonius some caution is necessary when using repetitive stimulation. For example, at repetition frequencies close to 10 Hz a yellow stimulus may give EPs of considerably smaller amplitude than do red or blue stimuli of equal luminances.[635, 748] In the 'medium frequency', range, spectral sensitivity may not be a useful concept.[640]

* The criterion response method is to record EPs to different colours over a range of stimulus luminances. A 'criterion response', e.g. 5 μV is then chosen, and the stimulus luminance is calculated which, for each colour, produces the criterion response. The reciprocals of this range of luminances, when plotted *versus* stimulus wavelength give the relative spectral sensitivity curve.

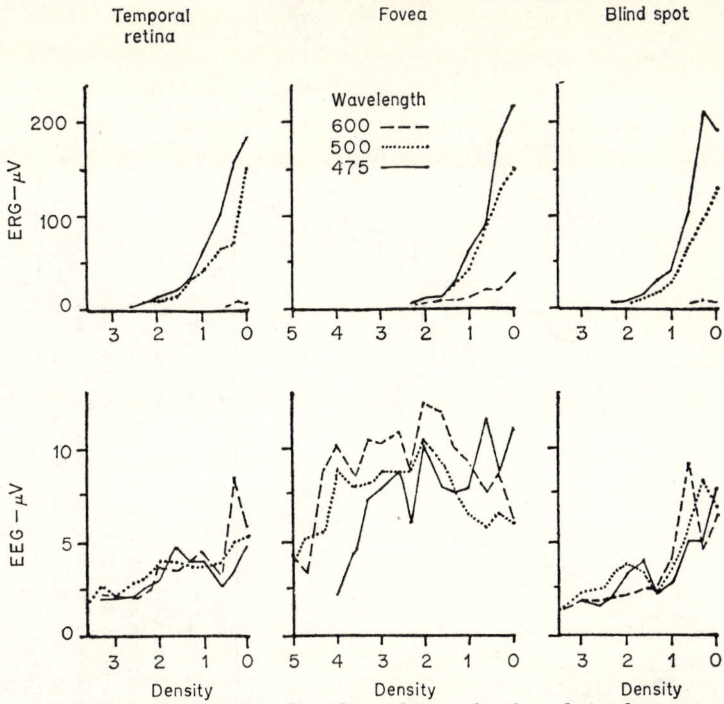

FIGURE 2.25 *Luminance curves describing the amplitudes of simultaneous electroretinograms (above) and electroencephalograms (below). The height of response has been plotted versus the density of filtering in the test beam for three wavelengths. Each point is the average of two responses only. The left column shows data for the temporal retina, the middle for the fovea and the right for the blind spot. Subject J.C.A. From J. C. Armington (1964). 'Spectral sensitivity of simultaneous electroretinograms and occipital responses', in* Clinical Electroretinography, *Ed. H. M. Burian and J. H. Jacobson. Pergamon Press,* Vision Res., *Suppl. 1, 225–233.*

2.9.3 *Heterochromatic flicker photometry*

Heterochromatic flicker photometry is one classical psychophysical method of measuring the spectral sensitivity of the eye.[334, 839, 882] One variant of this procedure has been adapted to give an EP measure of spectral sensitivity, so that in a single subject the psychophysical spectral sensitivity can be compared with EP data. The psychophysical procedure is as follows: The subject views a stimulus field which consists of two superimposed patches of light. One light is coloured and the other is a standard white which is left unaltered throughout the procedure. The white and coloured beams are alternated at a sufficiently high frequency that the colours fuse subjectively but the alternation frequency is not so high that brightness flicker disappears. The luminance of the coloured beam is then altered until the subject reports that flicker is a minimum. At this point, perceived flicker will increase if the coloured beam is made brighter or dimmer; and at the point of minimum flicker the luminances of the white and coloured stimuli are equal (by definition).

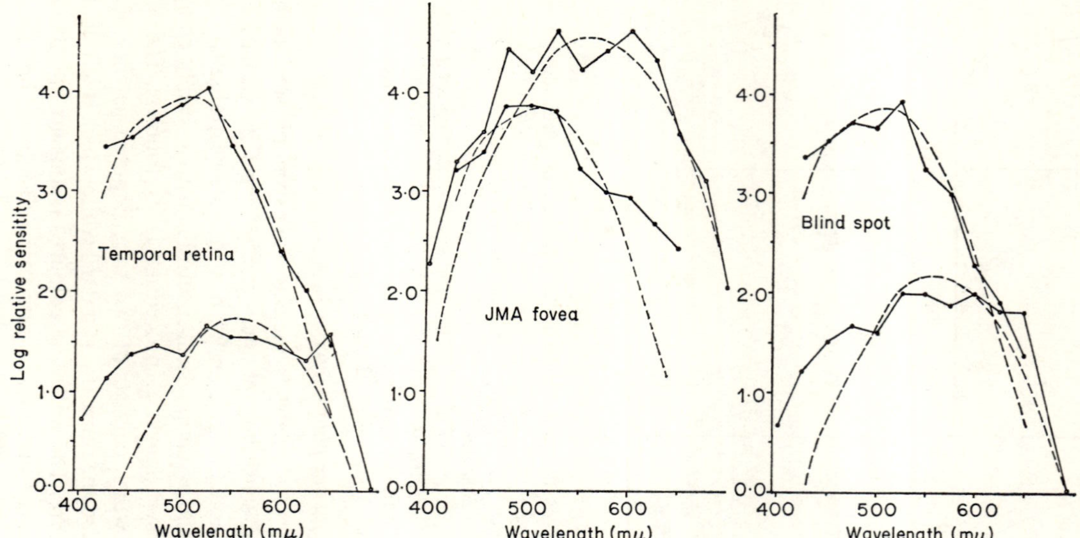

FIGURE 2.26 *A comparison of the spectral curves of the occipital response and the ERG for the three stimulus locations. Open circles connected by straight lines are the data for the occipital response; closed circles are used for ERG data. The photopic CIE curve has been drawn with dashed lines through the occipital data. The scotopic CIE curve has been drawn through the data for the ERG. Subject J.M.A., 5 μV criterion. From J. C. Armington (1964), in* Clinical Electroetinography, *Ed. H. M. Burian and J. H. Jacobson, Pergamon Press,* Vision Res., *Suppl.* **1**, *225–233.*

Siegfried *et al.*[739] carried out psychophysical heterochromatic flicker photometry by abruptly alternating either a red *versus* a white light or a green *versus* a white light in a 3·6° stimulus field which had a white 31° adapting surround. They found that EP amplitude (peak-to-trough) fell to a minimum near the point of minimum subjective flicker; although this was clearer in one than in the other of their two subjects. In contrast, Regan,[640] who repeated this experiment, found a minimum in EP amplitude which coincided with the point of minimum subjective flicker for only one electrode position (out of four) in only one (out of eight) subjects. This suggests that the correlation reported by Siegfried *et al.* between peak-to-peak EP amplitude and the point of minimum subjective flicker is uncommon in the experimental conditions they used.

Putting this in a different way, large EPs can be recorded in many subjects by alternating lights of equal luminances but different colours. The question arises whether these clear responses recorded when lights of equal luminance are alternated can be regarded as reflecting neural activities (central to the photoreceptors) which underlie subjective hue perception and hue discrimination. To anticipate, it seems that in one frequency region EPs may reflect photoreceptor characteristics; in another frequency region EPs may represent photoreceptor properties and in addition some further neural activity, but there are as yet no grounds for associating this further activity with the mechanisms underlying hue perception.[S29]

It is first necessary to distinguish between harmonic components of the EP in the 8–30 Hz region and harmonic components in the 40–60 Hz region. Both types of component can be evoked at the same time in the heterochromatic photometry situation, one as a fundamental component and the other as a second harmonic component. Since it turns out that the two components behave quite differently, the peak-to-peak measure of amplitude, which confounds them, is misleading in this context.

In general, a phase difference of near 180° between the stimulus beams results in minimum subjective flicker (i.e. when one beam grows dimmer the other beam simultaneously grows correspondingly brighter). However, the phase difference between the beams which gave a minimum amplitude of the 8–30 Hz component differs markedly from the 180° condition (for example by 120° for a red–yellow pair).[S29] It is possible to show that *in itself* this phase shift can be sufficient to obliterate any minimum in EP amplitude when the beams are adjusted to produce minimum subjective flicker (Fig. 2.27). There is, however, a further complication. Even when the phase of the stimulus beams were adjusted to give a minimum in EP amplitude, this resulting minimum did not occur at the same stimulus modulation depths which gave minimum subjective flicker (Fig. 2.27 D). The reason for this was that the shapes of the saturation curves for the EP depended on stimulus colour. When the red beam was left unmodulated, and the modulation depth of the yellow beam was progressively increased from zero the EP was found to saturate or even decrease in amplitude at the highest modulation depths. In contrast, when the

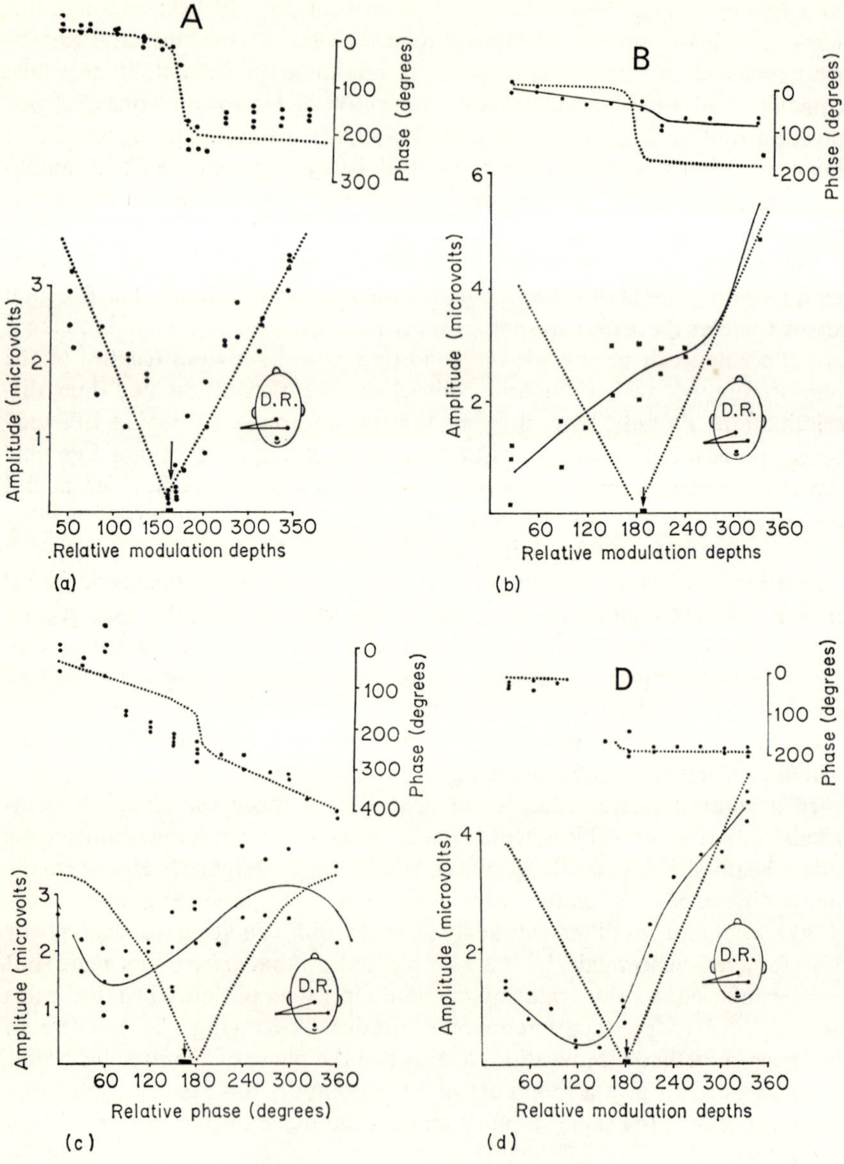

A
Phase (degrees)
0
100
200
300
Amplitude (microvolts)
3
2
1
D.R.
50 100 150 200 250 300 350
.Relative modulation depths
(a)
B
Phase (degrees)
0
100
200
Amplitude (microvolts)
6
4
2
D.R.
60 120 180 240 300 360
Relative modulation depths
(b)
Phase (degrees)
0
100
200
300
400
Amplitude (microvolts)
3
2
1
D.R.
60 120 180 240 300 360
Relative phase (degrees)
(c)
D
Phase (degrees)
0
100
200
Amplitude (microvolts)
4
2
D.R.
60 120 180 240 300 360
Relative modulation depths
(d)

FIGURE 2.27

yellow beam was left unmodulated and the modulation depth of the red beam was progressively increased from zero, the amplitude of the EP showed only a mild tendency to saturate. The result of this was that the relative amplitudes (of the 10–30 Hz components of the EPs) to red and yellow modulation depended on the arbitrary choice of stimulus modulation depth. The difference between the points of minimum EP amplitude and minimum subjective flicker in Fig. 2.27 D can therefore be manipulated by appropriate choices of stimulus intensities and modulation depths. All this indicates that for the 10–30 Hz frequency components, flicker perception and the amplitude of the EP are quite dissociated. This could explain Regan's finding that in most cases peak-to-peak EP amplitude did not correlate with the point of minimum subjective flicker in the heterochromatic photometry situation of Siegfried *et al.*

FIGURE 2.27 *The amplitudes and phases of the fundamental component of the steady-state evoked potential are plotted in A, B, C and D.*

A: Two beams of the same colour (red, 640 nm) were modulated in antiphase and their relative modulation depths varied. Dotted line is output of photocell. Circles are EP amplitudes. The arrow indicates the mean point of zero subjective flicker, and the horizontal black line gives the range of four settings.

B: Similar experiment to A but now different colours (yellow 589 nm and red) were alternated in antiphase. Dotted line is photocell output and full line is EP. Maximum yellow and zero red modulation at 30 on abscissa, maximum red and zero yellow modulation at 330. There is no minimum in EP amplitude which coincides with the point of minimum subjective flicker (arrow).

C: Amplitudes and phases of the fundamental component of the EP versus the relative phases of the red and yellow beams. The relative modulation depths of the beams were held constant at the setting for minimum subjective flicker (B). Dotted line is output of photocell, full line and circles show fundamental component of EP. Arrow and horizontal bar indicate mean and range of 14 settings on point of minimum subjective flicker. Relative phase for minimum EP is roughly 80° from the relative phase for minimum subjective flicker. Note: 180° on scale means beams in antiphase.

D: Experiment B repeated, but now with the relative phases of beams not in antiphase as in B, but set to give minimum amplitude for the fundamental EP (see C). A minimum now occurs in EP amplitude, whereas in B there was no minimum. Arrow and horizontal bar gives mean and range of 4 settings on point of minimum subjective flicker; the point of minimum EP amplitude is displaced from the point of minimum subjective flicker. In addition, an abrupt phase change of roughly 180° occurs near the point of minimum EP amplitude (contrast with B). Dotted line gives photocell output for B; for easier comparison the photocell curve for the phase has been shifted along the abscissa by an amount corresponding to the displacement of the EPs minimum amplitude from the point at which the photocell has a minimum output.

Note. Modulation depth scale, i.e. $\frac{m_1}{m_1 + m_2}$ *is linear* (m_1, m_2 = *modulation depths of beams (1) and (2) respectively. Stimulus modulation frequency = 16 c/sec. The maximum modulation depth of either beam is 30% (at 30 or 330 on abscissa). 10° field of 1800 td with 30° white surround of 540 td. Electrode (1) 1 cm in front of inion, electrode (2) 7 cm in front of electrode (1), electrode (3) to right of midline and 7 cm from electrodes (1) and (2). Electrode behind right ear grounded. Noise level roughly 0·1–0·2 μV. From D. Regan (1970). 'Evoked potential and psychophysical correlates of changes in stimulus colour and intensity'*, Vision Res., ***10**, 163–178. Pergamon Press, Oxford.*

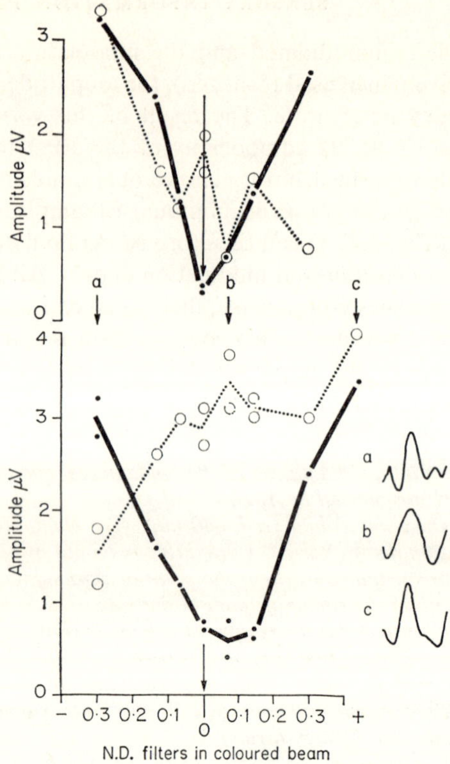

FIGURE 2.28 *Comparison of psychophysical and objective heterochromatic flicker-photometry data. A standard white light was alternated at 24 cps in antiphase with a coloured light whose luminance was adjusted by the subject until he saw minimum flicker (zero on the abscissa). The luminance of the coloured light was then altered in increments of 0.07 log units. The EEG was processed by an on-line Fourier analyser and the amplitudes of the fundamental and second-harmonic components of the evoked potential were plotted* vs. *the luminance of the coloured beam for 580 nm (upper half of the figure) and 460 nm (lower half). The position of the minimum of the second-harmonic component (filled circles, full lines) agreed with the point of minimum subjective flicker, to within the smallest increment of luminance used (0·07 log units, 18%). In contrast, the fundamental component of the evoked potential did not generally have a minimum at all (open circles, dotted lines). The peak-to-peak amplitude of the evoked-potential waveform obtained with an averaging computer gave no reliable indication of the point of minimum subjective flicker (averaged waveforms shown for points,* **a**, **b**, **c**, *in lower half of the figure). The stimulus field size was 15°, with a 30° white surround whose luminance was equal to the luminance of the standard white component of the central stimulus field. The retinal illuminance produced by the standard white component was 100 td. Both beams were sine-wave modulated to depths of 100%. Subject J. S. Bipolar recordings between an electrode 1 cm above the inion and a second electrode on the midline 7 cm ahead of the first electrode. Half-widths of interference filters were roughly 10 nm. Amplifier bandwidth 1·0–75 cps (−3 dB). Fourier analysis carried out during 1 min of stimulation, starting roughly 20 sec after onset of stimulation. An averaging computer was run simultaneously with the Fourier analyser; 800 sweeps, 62-msec sweep time, 100 points. From D. Regan (1970). 'An objective method of measuring the relative spectral luminosity curve in man'*, J. Opt. Soc. Amer., ***60***, *856–859.*

The story is quite different for frequency components of the EP in the 'high-frequency' 40–60 Hz range. In a heterochromatic photometry situation the amplitude of the high-frequency EP component falls to a sharp minimum at the point of minimum subjective flicker (Fig. 2.28). It can be seen in Fig. 2.28 how, in contrast with the behaviour of 'high-frequency' components, the EP components whose frequency falls into the 8–30 Hz range show no such minimum. By measuring the energy fluxes of the white and coloured beams for coloured beams throughout the spectrum, Regan measured the relative

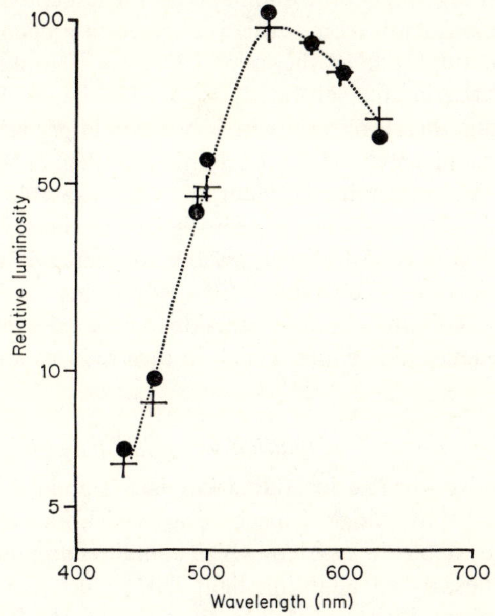

FIGURE 2.29 *Crosses: relative luminosities measured by psychophysical heterochromatic flicker photometry. Full circles: spectral sensitivity determined by method described (by measuring the luminance that gave the minimum amplitude of the second-harmonic component of the evoked scalp potential for each coloured beam). The psychophysical and objective determinations agreed to within the smallest luminance increment used (0·07 log units, 18%). The dotted curve was drawn smoothly through the psychophysical data points. Subject J.S. From D. Regan (1970). 'An objective method of measuring the relative spectral luminosity curve in man'*, J. Opt. Soc. Amer., ***60**, 856–859.*

sensitivities of the eye for a range of stimulus wavelengths through the spectrum. This EP method gave a relative spectral sensitivity curve which agreed with the psychophysical data to within 0·1 log unit, that is, to within the variability of the psychophysical data (Fig. 2.29). The method is considerably more precise than the criterion response method* of measuring relative spectral sensitivity[29, 31, 124] for the following reasons: The stimulus-to-stimulus variability of the amplitudes of transient EPs may amount to a considerable fraction of the difference in EP amplitude produced by stimuli

* See footnote on p. 96.

whose luminances vary by as much as 10,000 : 1. The values of radiant light flux which give an EP of constant criterion amplitude are therefore susceptible to serious variability.[29, 31] On the other hand, in the heterochromatic photometry situation there is a unique value for the luminance of the test colour which gives zero effective stimulation (i.e. zero modulation depth) for the 40–60 Hz components of the steady-state EP. There is a very large relative increase in the effective stimulus for the 40–60 Hz components when the luminance of the test colour is changed by 0·1–0·2 log units. For example, a change of only 0·2 log units in the luminance of the test colour can change the stimulus modulation depth from 0 to 15–25%. Such a change may be sufficient to raise the amplitude of the second harmonic component of the EP from zero to its maximum (saturated) value. The heterochromatic photometry EP technique therefore results in very much larger relative changes in EP amplitude for a given change of EP luminance than is the case when the luminance of a single stimulus is changed as for example in the criterion response method. The heterochromatic flicker method is therefore less sensitive to EP variability. Additional reasons for increased precision are the more effective rejection of unwanted EP components by Fourier analysis than by averaging. This gives both a reduction in residual noise and a shortening of the experimental procedure, which in turn reduces long-term changes in the EP.

2.9.4 *The effects of chromatic adaptation on evoked potentials*

The use of selective chromatic adaptation is a standard method of distinguishing between physiological mechanisms which have different spectral sensitivities. For example, in a system which contains components of differing spectral sensitivities, a red adapting light will reduce the sensitivity of a predominantly red-sensitive component more than that of a predominantly blue-sensitive component. Blue adapting light will have the opposite effect.

Red and blue adapting lights of identical luminances have different effects on both the amplitudes and phases of EPs to repetitive stimulation[104, 638] This suggests that the EP contains components of different spectral sensitivities. It seems unlikely that phase shifts as large as those reported would be due to amplitude changes, so that it is probable that there are differences between the temporal properties of the different colour components of the EP. There is also evidence that the different colour components have different topographical distributions,[638] and may therefore arise from populations of neurons which differ in spatial distribution or orientation.

The reported effects of chromatic adaptation on EP amplitude show some discrepancies. Regan found that one effect of blue adapting light on the EP to a red stimulus which was intensity-modulated at 10 Hz was to slightly increase its amplitude; in contrast, for 16 Hz modulation, the EP amplitude was markedly decreased by this procedure. On the other hand, Burkhardt and Riggs found that for red light flickered at 17·5 Hz (effectively the same as 16 Hz) the effect of blue adapting light was to *increase* the amplitude of the

EP. However, both reports stressed the considerable inter-individual variability of the amplitude changes, even for subjects whose colour vision was judged to be normal by certain standard methods of subjective testing. This inter-individual variability, taken together with differences in electrode placements, might account for the discrepancies between the two reports.

It seems to be agreed then that chromatic adaptation can exert a colour-selective effect on the EP. However, the stimulus fields used by both Riggs and Burkhardt and by Regan were sufficiently large to cover an inhomogeneous retinal population comprising both rods and cones so that the EP changes cannot be unequivocally interpreted as correlates of the neural representation of colour information.

2.9.5 *Wavelength discrimination*

To those who are fortunate enough to possess it the most striking characteristic of colour vision is the rich variety of hue sensations. This variety reflects the exquisite sensitivity of the human visual system to differences of stimulus wavelength (differences as small as 0·4 nm can be distinguished in the yellow and blue-green). On such semi-scientific grounds alone one would expect that a large proportion of researches into colour vision would have been studies of different aspects of wavelength discrimination. For reasons which elude the author this is not the case, not even in psychophysics. In EP research, only Riggs and Sternheim have so far made a systematic study of wavelength discrimination.

Riggs and Sternheim[676] stimulated the eye with a two-colour pattern of stripes. Each stripe was 1° 30′ wide, and the stimulus field subtended 19° 36′. The subject set the luminances of the stripes to be subjectively equal. Scalp potentials evoked by rhythmically reversing the chromaticities of adjacent stripes were recorded from a bipolar pair of electrodes located on the midline 2 and 10·5 cm above the inion. Riggs and Sternheim found the amplitudes of these EPs to increase as the wavelength differences between adjacent stripes was increased. They reported that the wavelength difference between stripes which was necessary to evoke potentials of a fixed criterion amplitude was minimal in the blue–green and yellow parts of the spectrum and that it was in those spectral regions that their subject's psychophysical sensitivity to wavelength difference was also greatest.

An important claim made by Riggs and Sternheim was that the scalp EP is more sensitive to wavelength differences than is the ERG. They suggested that this difference in sensitivity was a consequence of the functioning of mechanisms which, in effect, operated upon visual signals as they travelled along the visual pathway in such a way as to 'sharpen up' the capacity to resolve different stimulus wavelengths.

Riggs and Sternheim's 1969 report raises a number of difficulties. These are mostly concerned with the concept of the 'enhancement of wavelength-discrimination signals'.[676] Riggs and Sternheim's salient finding was that when the wavelength difference ($\Delta\lambda$) between adjacent stripes was large, the amplitude of both the ERG and EP tended towards limiting values. In their experiments it turned out that these limiting amplitudes were roughly 5 μV for both the ERG and EP. Riggs and Sternheim pointed out[673, 676] that this form of nonlinear behaviour meant that a scaling factor could not explain their finding that for values below the limiting amplitudes for the EP and ERG, a given criterion amplitude was evoked by a smaller value of $\Delta\lambda$ for the EP than was required for the ERG. In other words although arbitrary factors such as electrode placement might change the *absolute* amplitudes of ERG and EP, such factors would not be able to account for the large *proportional* differences in $\Delta\lambda$ sensitivity at the two levels.*[673] A relevant point here is that the EP is known to show clear saturation behaviour[748] (Chapter 2, Section 3.3) whereas the ERG does not show such behaviour. This fact would predict that, for sufficiently high modulation depths (such as the 100% depth used by Riggs and Sternheim), the effect of progressively increasing $\Delta\lambda$ would be that the amplitude of the EP would reach its maximum (saturated) value for moderate value of $\Delta\lambda$, while the amplitude of the ERG would rise progressively as $\Delta\lambda$ was increased. The effect of saturation would, therefore, be that for small values of $\Delta\lambda$ the *proportional* sensitivity to $\Delta\lambda$ of the EP would be larger than the *proportional* sensitivity of the ERG to $\Delta\lambda$ – exactly as Riggs and Sternheim reported. Riggs and Sternheim's main finding is therefore explicable on the grounds of the known saturation behaviour of EPs, without necessarily invoking any possible colour discriminating mechanisms and whether or not the assumption is made that the 'red', 'green' and 'blue' signals are separate.

The pattern EPs which were described in Section 2.4 specific to spatially-abrupt, sharply-accommodated spatial transients (i.e. contour or contrast boundaries) of luminance or chromaticity. Such EPs are typified by the EPs to a foveally-viewed stimulus field of no more than 2° subtense which is filled by a pattern of checks whose side lengths are less than 12′ or so which, if repetitively presented, are presented at some frequency which is not a sub-harmonic of the subject's alpha frequency. It seems (to the present author) that, for the reasons (*a*) to (*d*) listed below, the EPs described by Riggs and Sternheim were unlikely to be principally of the type described above. Furthermore, although for the reasons (*a*) and (*c*) listed below, there seems to be a possibility that Riggs and Sternheim's EPs might include substantial contributions similar to those of unstructured-field EPs, the possibility cannot be excluded that Riggs and Sternheim's EPs include a third type of component whose properties are different from both unstructured-field components and from the contrast-specific components described in Section 2.4. Riggs and Sternheim themselves state that their stimulus 'minimised edge effects and

* Riggs and Sternheim found that their stimulator evoked EPs of appreciable amplitudes even when $\Delta\lambda$ was zero and adjacent stripes were of equal luminances. Whether this artifact was constant for all values of $\Delta\lambda$ is not clear, so that it is difficult to estimate its possible effect on Riggs and Sternheim's data (e.g. their Fig. 2 in reference 676).

stimulus artifacts but maximised spatial effects that depend on wavelength alone'.[673]

The arguments that Riggs and Sternheim's EPs were not principally of the same type as those described in Section 2.4 are as follows: (*a*) the large (19° 36′) field size would emphasise the unstructured-field type of EP at the expense of the foveally-elicited pattern EP (Sections 2.3.1 and 2.4.4), (*b*) the wide (1° 30′) stripes would have the same effect, for different reasons (Section 2.4.3), (*c*) one of the stimulus frequencies used (5·5 Hz) might be liable to evoke appreciable second harmonic EP components of the unstructured-field type (Section 2.8.2) and (*d*) Riggs and Sternheim reported that their EPs could be recorded more clearly when a rather wide (45′) black grid was placed in front of the edges of the stripes, whereas contour-specific EPs have been reported to be *abolished* by placing even a narrow occluding grid over the edges of the pattern elements.[748, S23]

2.9.6 *Evoked potentials and colour: summary*

There have been a number of EP studies directed to the general question of how colour is neurally represented and processed within the brain. Two aims of these studies have been to determine what part the relative timing of neural signals might play in the encoding of colour information, and what the importance might be of differences in spatial distributions of signals evoked by different colours. The picture which has emerged so far is complex; EP research seems not only to have failed to provide satisfactory answers to the original questions, but also to have generated additional problems. In all probability these failures are only partly due to weaknesses in experimental design and controls. A probable major factor is that EPs to coloured stimuli reflect neural activities not directly related to colour perception (e.g. rod *versus* cone effects).

Before discussing the effects of stimulus colour on EPs an essential requirement is to demonstrate that these EP effects are indeed specific to stimulus colour, and are not in reality either luminance effects or photopic-scotopic phenomena masquerading as colour correlates. The confounding of intensity-dependent and colour-dependent effects is a notorious pitfall in colour research generally. In psychophysical colour studies it is recognised to be of the first importance to clarify this point by appropriate control experiments. For this purpose it is *not* sufficient to investigate differences between EPs to stimuli of different colours whose brightnesses have previously been adjusted to be subjectively equal. In order to verify that an EP feature is specific to either a particular (physical) spectral region or to a particular (subjective) perceived hue it is essential to extend observations over a range of intensities which is sufficiently wide to exclude any possibility that the observed correlation might be an intensity effect. This equal-brightness control is inadequate because without direct experimental evidence it cannot be assumed that the spectral sensitivity measured by use of a particular EP feature is necessarily the same spectral sensitivity as measured by a psychophysical method.

Discrepancies between spectral sensitivities could arise from a number of factors such as: (*a*) The relative weightings appropriate to stimulation of central *versus* peripheral retinal areas (and to photopic *versus* scotopic processes) may differ for psychophysical and EP responses (this point applies with especial force to studies using stimulus fields appreciably larger than 2° or so); (*b*) Some components of the EP may be associated less with the physical parameters of the stimulus than with the presence or absence of the stimulus (one example of this is the resolution of uncertainty by the stimulus) (see Section 2.2.2); (*c*) The EP may reflect neural activities connected with a variety of functions of the CNS, and some of those may be nonlinearly related or may not even be causally connected with perceptual events.

Most studies of the effect of stimulus colour on EPs have so far been restricted to looking for differences between certain features of the transient potential evoked by changes in the intensities of differently coloured stimuli. The EP features studied have seldom extended beyond the amplitudes and latencies of different EP components. Good correlations have been reported between spectral sensitivities measured using an EP *latency* criterion and spectral sensitivities measured psychophysically. However, as mentioned earlier the view has been urged that latency correlates are unlikely to lead to worthwhile physiological insights of perceptual mechanisms. On the other hand, studies of the relations between stimulus colour and the *amplitudes* of transient EPs are beset not only by variability and by ambiguities in defining the 'amplitude' of a transient EP component (see Chapter 5, Section 5.4.8), but also by laborious recording procedures. Nevertheless, a fair correlation between at least one amplitude measure and psychophysical determinations of spectral sensitivity seems established,[29] although this agreement holds over only a restricted range of intensities.

A promising early report[146] has been followed by remarkably little work on the intriguing colour correlate of *topographical distribution*, although appropriate and powerful techniques developed by Rémond[651, 655] and by Clynes[146] have been available for some time.

The familiar psychophysical procedure of heterochromatic flicker photometry has been adapted to include EP recording so as to give objective measurements of spectral sensitivity. The resulting spectral sensitivity curves have then been compared with psychophysical spectral sensitivity curves for the same subject. For reasons detailed above (Section 2.9.3) the peak-to-peak amplitudes of the steady-state EPs in the 10–25 Hz range seem to be of little value as objective measures of spectral sensitivity. However, EP components in the 45–60 Hz range of frequencies can be used to give a spectral sensitivity curve which agrees well with the psychophysical curve, even though these 'high-frequency' components may be only a minor feature of the EPs.

Quite apart from the fact that practically all the electrical energy of all neuronally-generated scalp EPs seems to be immediately supplied by cortical cells, there is evidence, both direct and circumstantial, that the *forms and properties* of scalp potentials to sensory stimuli are partially determined by neuronal populations other than those which actually generate the EP. For example, EPs to spatially structured stimuli may largely reflect activities of groups of cells located as centrally as the visual cortex (see Section 2.4.5), while EPs to some spatially unstructured stimuli seem to be determined by activities of groups of cells located as peripherally as the photoreceptors (see Section 2.9.3). Contrast-specific ('pattern') EPs have been demonstrated both for contours of luminance (brightness) contrast, and contours of chromatic contrast; these findings raise the possibility of relating subjective data of colour perception to the activities of functionally different populations of neurons, and thus classifying potentials evoked by changes of luminance and colour, not only by means of analysis methods, but also by the use of different types of stimuli.

Two questions whose investigation might be fruitful but which have so far received little attention are: (*a*) whether there are EP features whose time course parallels the time course of colour perception described for example, by Pieron,[608] and (*b*) whether EP recording can give clues to the different aspects of neural information processing which underlie the sensations of hue, saturation and brightness.[S29]

2.10 Evoked potentials and the neuroanatomy of sensory pathways

2.10.1 *Stimulation of localised retinal areas, the topographical distribution of visual EPs and EP generator sites: unstructured stimulus fields*

Differences between the topographical distributions of EP components have been utilised in attempts to associate particular EP components with particular areas of cerebral cortex. For flash-evoked potentials there is evidence that early components arise in the primary visual cortex, whereas a later wave arises in the parietal cortex. There has been some conflict of opinion as to whether early components of the pattern-specific EP arise mainly in a region outside the primary cortex. It has been suggested that monocular stimulation of the left and right half-fields can evoke scalp potentials which arise predominantly in the left and right hemispheres, but some doubt remains about the possible roles of interhemispheric signals. A start has been made on using EP methods to investigate differences between the dominant and non-dominant hemispheres but little progress has so far been made in this difficult endeavour.

A number of workers have illuminated different retinal areas with small spots of light in attempts to compare responses to stimulation of the fovea and extrafovea. The resulting data, however, are often difficult to interpret due to (*a*) uncertainties as to the relative contributions to the EP made by potentials evoked by changes in luminance and by potentials evoked by the boundary of the stimulus field and (*b*) uncertainty as to whether these two types of response might interact.[543, 803] There is evidence that the two types of potential may have different distributions, and furthermore that the contrast-specific components may be affected by the different acuities of fovea and retinal periphery. The interpretation of potentials evoked by small spots of light may additionally be complicated by the effects of scattered light. This is likely to be of particular importance when Xenon flashes of very high peak luminance are used.

Copenhaver and Perry[178] found that the amplitude of the EP to a 2·5° light spot which was flashed four times per second was reduced by 60% when the spot was shifted from the central fovea to a position 2·5° from the fovea. The amplitudes of the EP changed very little when the eccentricity of the spot was subsequently increased from 2·5° to 30°. However, as a consequence of the high peak luminance of the Xenon flashes which were used in this study, light scatter may have been relatively more important for the more peripherally located stimuli. This might have exaggerated the effectiveness of these peripheral stimuli. In contrast, De Voe *et al.*[220] found that a 1° stimulus spot located at 5° eccentricity evoked a response which was so small as to be inappreciable when compared with a response evoked by the same spot centrally fixated. This finding also conflicts with reports of Eason and White[256, 257] and Ohba.[580] The former stimulated the eye with 1° flashes superimposed on a steady background whose luminance was 1 log unit less than the luminance of the flashes; Ohba's stimulation conditions were roughly similar. In the temporal retina the response amplitude changed by only 50% when the 1° spot was moved from the foveal centre to 50° eccentricity[256, 257] or to 20°–30° eccentricity.[580] This surprising result was supported by control experiments in which stimulation of the blind spot was found to evoke responses of much smaller amplitude than stimulation of neighbouring regions. Ohba found that not only did the amplitudes of the individual waves of a 90–250 msec complex attenuate as the stimulus spot was moved from the fovea into the periphery, but that in addition the latency of all components progressively increased by up to 20–30 msec. There was in addition a change in waveform which, Ohba considered, did not prevent identification of the various EP components. Ohba's latency findings conflict with those of Eason, Oden and White[257] who reported that latency fell to a minimum at 10°–20° from the fovea and on the basis of this finding speculated that EP latency and the total number of photoreceptors per unit retinal area might be related.[257, 577]

Vaughan[816] pointed out that Eason, Oden and White's results are not consistent with the well-established finding that EPs to centrally-viewed disc stimuli are predominantly due to foveal stimulation, independent of the size of the disc. Vaughan further speculated that the conflict could be resolved if, for large disc stimuli, there was cancellation between the EP components to stimulation of upper and lower half-fields of the peripheral retina. This speculation is of course open to an experimental test.

The different topographical distributions and waveforms of EPs to stimulation of different retinal areas have been cited in support of hypotheses of the sites of origin of EP components. Rietveld *et al.*[670] found that stimulation of the two upper quadrants of the visual field gave similar EPs as did stimulation of the two lower quadrants. In contrast, quite different EPs resulted from stimulation of an upper and a lower quadrant (or an upper and lower half-fields). These differences could be described in terms of shifts of the latencies of different components, but Rietveld *et al.* did not describe reversals in polarity nor were they able to associate their data with cortical topography (Halliday and Wilson (personal communication) independently came to similar conclusions in the early 1960's). As MacKay and Jeffreys[543] pointed out, the finding of Rietveld *et al.* does show that simple graphs of total response against foveal area with central fixation mean little. Vaughan[816] claimed that the topographical distribution of EPs to flash stimulation of upper and lower retinal half-fields was consistent with two generator sites for the EP. One site was located in the primary visual cortex and a secondary site was located in parietal cortex (Fig. 2.30).[S17, 24]

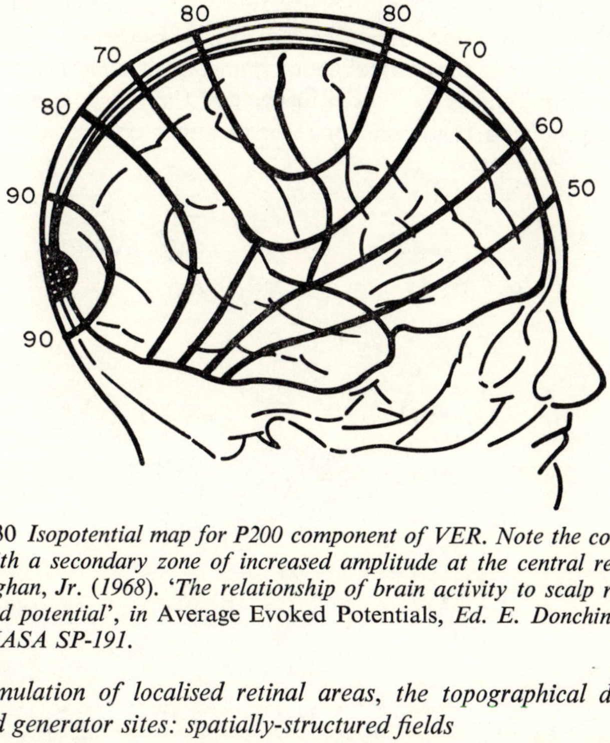

FIGURE 2.30 *Isopotential map for P200 component of VER. Note the complexity of the field with a secondary zone of increased amplitude at the central region. From H. G. Vaughan, Jr. (1968). 'The relationship of brain activity to scalp recording of event-related potential',* in Average Evoked Potentials, *Ed. E. Donchin and D. B. Lindsley. NASA SP-191.*

2.10.2 *Stimulation of localised retinal areas, the topographical distribution of EPs and generator sites: spatially-structured fields*

Jeffreys reported that the EP to presentation of a checkerboard pattern from a previously uniformly illuminated field in either an upper or a lower retinal half-field had a triphasic waveform. The second peak, which is the most prominent,[415] has a latency of roughly 120 msec. All three components show a polarity reversal when stimulation is changed from upper to lower half-field (Fig. 2.31; Reference 536 p. 213).

There has been some controversy over the probable neuroanatomical locations of the generators of the three components. Halliday and Michael[355] were unable to accept Jeffreys'[536] suggestion that all three components of the pattern EP are generated within the calcarine fissure and argued that there was strong evidence to indicate that vertical foveal octants were represented mainly *outside* the calcarine sulcus, while horizontal octants were represented mainly *inside* the calcarine sulcus.[97, 387] Consequently, the hypothetical dipole layers driven by the octants adjoining the vertical meridian would be roughly parallel to each other, so that no polarity reversal would be expected for these octants. Halliday and Michael[355] went on to report that for pattern-reversal the octants adjoining the vertical meridian did in fact show a clear polarity reversal for the 100–120 msec component. Jeffreys[413] subsequently found that this was also the case for EPs to pattern appearance.

This still leaves the problem of explaining both the longitudinal changes of topographical distribution and the changes of EP waveform when the site of retinal stimulation is changed.[355, 412, 413, 800, 801] Halliday and Michael[355] suggested that, since striate cortex does not seem to be the site of generation of the EP to pattern, then the cortical region immediately underneath the zone of greatest EP amplitude (5 to 7·5 cm in front of the inion) might be a likely site. They speculated that polarity reversal might be a consequence of a

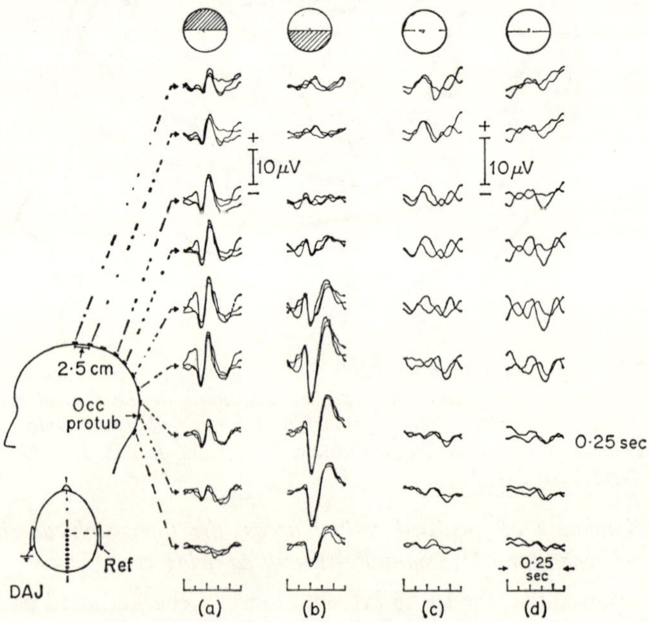

FIGURE 2.31 *Monopolar EPs recorded from midline row of electrodes to the brief (25 msec) presentation of pattern (14′ hollow squares of 3·5′ line thickness) into* (a) *the upper half and* (b) *the lower half of the continuously illuminated* (6°) *stimulus field. The responses obtained to upper and lower field presentations of the same pattern when defocused (+3D lenses) are shown in* (c) *and* (d) *respectively. Modified from D. A. Jeffreys (1971). 'Cortical source locations of pattern-related VEPs (visual-evoked potentials) recorded from the human scalp', in* Nature, **229**, *502–504. Macmillan (Journals) Ltd.*

neural organisation such that upper and lower retinal half-fields projected into layers of different depths in this region of cortex.

In later studies Jeffreys described the transverse and longitudinal distributions of the scalp potentials evoked by the appearance of pattern from a previously illuminated but unstructured field.[413] In conflict with Halliday and Michael's report for pattern reversal EPs, Jeffreys found that the waveforms, amplitudes and topographical distributions of the EPs to stimulation of upper and lower half-fields by pattern-appearance were quite different from the waveforms, amplitudes and distributions of the potentials evoked by changes in the luminance of spatially-unstructured stimulus fields (Fig. 2.31). The EP to full-field stimulation by pattern appearance appeared to be roughly similar to the sum of the EPs to separate stimulation of upper and lower half-fields.[413]

Jeffreys reported that the longitudinal topographical distributions of an early 80 msec EP component were similar for stimulation of upper and lower half-fields (though with polarity reversal, see Fig. 2.31). When the stimulus field was restricted to 30° and 45° sectors it became clear that the 80 msec component of the midline (upper-field) VEP could be evoked much more effectively by stimulating the parts of the retina which adjoined the horizontal meridian than by stimulating the parts which adjoined the vertical meridian.[415] On these grounds Jeffreys suggested the 80 msec component was generated in the striate cortex lying within and immediately adjacent to the calcarine fissure. Jeffreys reported that the topographical distribution of the later 110–120 msec peak was quite different from the distribution of the 80 msec peak. The upper field distribution could be modelled as that due to a single equivalent dipole located in extrastriate cortex on the under surface of the occipital lobe, and the lower-field distribution could be modelled by a single equivalent dipole located in extrastriate cortex on the upper convexity of the occipital lobe. Jeffreys explained certain intersubject variations of EP distribution in terms of intersubject variability in the neuroanatomical location of the calcarine fissure.[413*, S16, 17†]

It is difficult to compare the conflicting data and conclusions of Jeffreys and of Halliday and Michael, since their stimulation and recording procedures were dissimilar. Jeffreys' stimulus was the abrupt appearance of pattern in an illuminated but previously unstructured field of 6° total subtense. The pattern elements were hollow 14′ squares of 3·5′ line thickness. He measured the amplitudes of the various EP components from a baseline. In contrast, Halliday and Michael used a 14°–18° field of 50′ checks to stimulate the retina with pattern-reversal, and measured the peak-to-peak amplitude

* Later work by Halliday and Michael (personal communication) showed that the ear reference used in their 1970 paper was not indifferent, and that when allowance was made for this, then the 100–120 msec component of the EP to pattern-reversal did seem to be generated in the upper and lower surfaces of the hemispheres. However, they found that their responses were of opposite polarities to those described by Jeffreys and suggested that the discrepancy might be due to differences in the activities of the 'indifferent' electrodes used by Jeffreys and by themselves.

† For a discussion of dipole and multipole models see Section 1.2.1 and for a simplified 'focusing' analogy supplementary footnote No. 1.

between a 100 msec wave and the wave immediately following. No systematic study has yet been published of the relation between EPs to pattern-appearance and EPs to pattern-reversal, though the evidence that is available does suggest that EPs to pattern-reversal are more akin to the EPs to pattern-disappearance than to the EPs to pattern-appearance recorded by Jeffreys.[801] Furthermore, there is evidence that Halliday and Michael's use of large checks and of a large field size might have introduced EP components into their recordings which are dissimilar to those evoked by the smaller check sizes used by Jeffreys (see Section 2.4), and (*b*) have emphasised the contribution of the extrafoveal retina.[649, S8, 16]

2.10.3 *Topography of somatosensory evoked potentials: sensory pathways and EP generator sites*

A detailed knowledge of the neural pathways involved in the somatosensory scalp EP is necessary before the power of the EP recording technique can be fully realised in both fundamental research and in clinical applications (see Chapter 4, Section 4.2.2). There now seems to be an encouraging degree of agreement as to the neural mechanisms which give rise both to short-latency and to long-latency components of the somatosensory EP.

In the adult, the early components of the EP are remarkably constant from subject-to-subject, both in polarity and scalp localisation[225] (Fig. 2.32). The topographical distributions of 'short' latency (here, less than roughly 80 msec) EP components correspond to the cerebral somatosensory projection.[211, 214, 225, 317, 321, 382, 410, 454, 816] The latency of the earliest component (18–20 msec peak) is practically accounted for by the conduction time of the afferent volley to the cortex.[590]

The initial activity is a triphasic complex which Goff, Rosner and Allison designated as component I.[321] The third positive phase peaks at 25 ± 4 msec.[321] In the numbering system of Goff *et al.*, component 2 is a positive deflection with a latency of some 31 ± 6 msecs and component 3 is a positive deflection whose latency is 48 ± 8 msec.[321] (Debecker and Desmedt's[221] system is to number third component of Goff *et al.* as component 2, and so on).* A later negative-positive component (65 ± 14 msec and 85 ± 20 msec) is component 4 in the Goff *et al.* system and component 5 is a later negative-positive complex (135 ± 25 msec and 220 ± 45 msec).[321]

There are therefore three quite distinct positive components of the early response, but all three are not always apparent in any particular recording. In recordings which show only two of the three sub-peaks, the early positive wave may split up either into the 25 and 31 msec components or into the 31 and 48 msec components (A. M. Halliday, personal communication). The absence of the first positive sub-peak can easily lead to confusion.

For stimuli whose intensities are higher than twice threshold intensity, the latencies of the early components of the somatosensory EP (Nos. 1, 2 and 3) are constant [in marked contrast with the behaviour of visual EPs (Section 2.2.2)]. In contrast to these early components of the EP (Nos. 1, 2 and usually

* The numbering system of Goff, Rosner and Allison is used in this text.

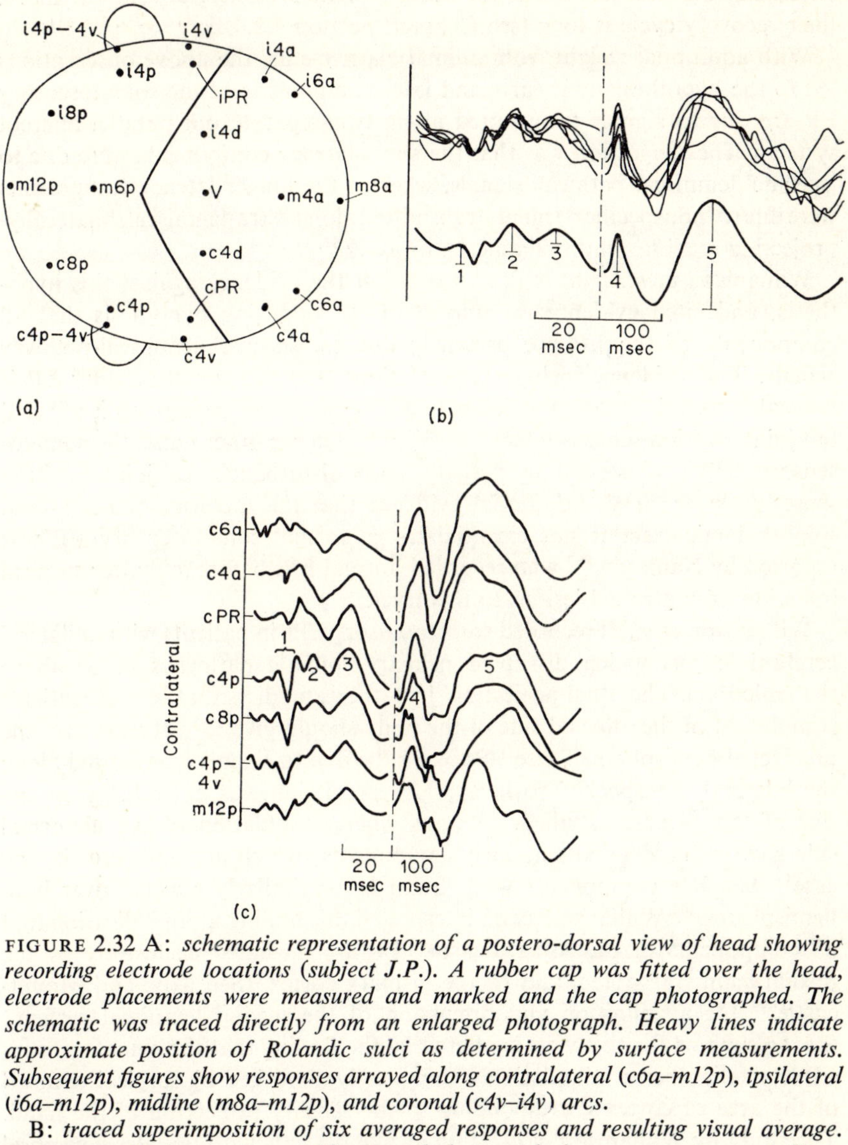

FIGURE 2.32 A: *schematic representation of a postero-dorsal view of head showing recording electrode locations (subject J.P.). A rubber cap was fitted over the head, electrode placements were measured and marked and the cap photographed. The schematic was traced directly from an enlarged photograph. Heavy lines indicate approximate position of Rolandic sulci as determined by surface measurements. Subsequent figures show responses arrayed along contralateral (c6a–m12p), ipsilateral (i6a–m12p), midline (m8a–m12p), and coronal (c4v–i4v) arcs.*

B: *traced superimposition of six averaged responses and resulting visual average. Tracings made from ×5 magnification of photographed responses. Arrows indicate amplitude measurements on the components. In this and all succeeding figures, upward deflection indicates positively at recording electrode.*

C: *Distribution of averaged evoked responses. Subject T.S. Left median nerve stimulation. Subject was right-handed. Electrode locations correspond to those indicated in Part* A. *From W. R. Goff, B. S. Rosner and T. Allison (1962). 'Distribution of cerebral somatosensory-evoked responses in normal man',* Electroenceph. clin. Neurophysiol., ***14**, 697–713.*

3), later components have a bilateral scalp distribution. Again in contrast to the early components (1 and 2), the later components (3, 4, 5) are markedly affected by barbiturates and by the state of alertness or sleep and, furthermore, their recovery cycle is long (see Chapter, Section 4.2.4).[2, 16, 17, 321, 322, 811]

With additional weight from animal experiments, the above observations led to the hypothesis that early and later components of the somatosensory EP are due to signals transmitted along two separate but parallel afferent systems. The suggestion was that the short-latency components were due to 'specific' lemniscal pathway signals, whereas the longer latency components were due to 'nonspecific'* signals transmitted along extra-lemniscal, bilaterally-projecting reticular and thalamic pathways.[2, 71, 811, 874]

Williamson *et al.*[874] have drawn together the evidence against this hypothesis, and cited evidence in support of the opposing hypothesis that all components of the EP are primarily due to 'specific' lemniscal-pathway signals. This evidence includes observations that the somatosensory EP is normal in disease states in which pain and temperature perception is affected but joint position sense is intact.[350, 352, 475, 476] On the other hand, the somatosensory EP is abnormal in patients with disturbances of joint position sense.[317, 352, 475, 565, 566] Additional evidence that the integrity of the lateral spinothalamic tract is not essential for a normal somatosensory EP was reported by Namerow[567] who recorded normal EPs before and after surgical infliction of controlled lesions to this tract.

Williamson *et al.*[874] recorded somatosensory EPs in patients with unilateral cerebral lesions which disrupted primary somatic pathways at or above thalamic level. The 'dual projection' hypothesis predicts that in such patients stimulation of the affected side of the body should give EPs at least over the unaffected hemisphere. These EPs would be due to signals transmitted along the bilateral 'nonspecific' pathway. This prediction was not fulfilled in any one of the 14 cases studied. In cases where stimulation of the abnormal side gave reduced or absent early components (which are unilateral in any case), then late components were found to be similarly affected over both hemispheres.[494] Williamson *et al.* interpreted this finding as an indication that *all* components of the somatosensory EP are mediated exclusively by the medial lemniscal system and by the primary cortex. (See Rose and Mountcastle[683] for a definition and discussion of the medial lemniscal system.) Strong support for this view is offered by the finding that the somatosensory EP to median nerve stimulation is completely abolished by surgical removal of the area of cortex corresponding to the sensory projection of the hand. The study by Williamson *et al.*[874] on awake patients with unilateral cerebral lesions has been replicated on sleeping patients.[326] Williamson *et al.* also claimed that the somatosensory 'K complex' seen during synchronised sleep appears also to be mediated exclusively by the primary lemniscal somatosensory system.

* For a discussion of the notion of 'specific' *versus* 'nonspecific' EP components, see Chapter 5, Section 5.4.8.

Goff[326] states that 'all we can conclude on the basis of our evidence and the evidence cited (in Reference 874) is that late potentials are not mediated by a *parallel projecting* non-specific system. However, late potentials could reflect activity arising from this system activated serially by input from corticofugal fibres arising in the primary area or its immediate association areas. Once activated in this manner through primary cortex, the non-specific system could then project activity to the cortex in the diffuse manner observed. Our evidence does not permit us to distinguish between this possibility and the possibility that late components arise in some other area such as commissural structures'.

2.10.4 *Topography of auditory EPs and generator sites**

Fig. 2.33 shows an isopotential map of the amplitude of a (roughly) 100–200 msec biphasic component of the auditory EP. The locations of the iso-potentials were obtained by extrapolation from recordings at 19 electrode sites (common chin reference). Vaughan claims that, above a line defined by the plane of the Sylvian fissure, responses are opposite in polarity to those recorded below the line.[824] The observed topographical distribution for the 100–200 msec component fits a theoretical distribution calculated from the assumption that the sources are dipole sheets whose dipole orientations are parallel to the scalp and whose locations are in primary auditory cortex. Vaughan has stated that this model applies only when the subject is not making use of the sensory information presented to him.[536 p.202] In spite of this restriction, Vaughan also claims to have succeeded in modelling the distribution of a positive wave, peaking at roughly 300 msec, in terms of equivalent dipole sheets located in parietal association cortex.[816] Other workers however, have claimed that auditory scalp EPs cannot entirely be attributed to cortical activity.

Morrell and Morrell[555] for example have interpreted their data as a demonstration that when (as in the adult) the rapidly-conducting thalamocortical fibres have become myelinated, evoked thalamic activity reaches the scalp after an extremely short delay, so that the short-latency cortical events occur at almost the same time as thalamic events. In the adult, they suggest, the thalamic contribution to the auditory scalp EP is masked by higher-voltage cortical components.

Studies of EPs at different levels of the auditory system show that (in cats) the auditory cortex response is more variable than responses recorded at more peripheral sites, and that prolonged stimulation leads to a reduction in the amplitudes of later components. These effects are also found to some degree at the level of the medial geniculate, but not at all at lower auditory nuclei.[536 p.219]

The maturation of visual, auditory and somatosensory EPs and problems of their quantification are discussed in Chapter 4, Section 4.2.7, and Chapter 5, Section 5.4.8.

* Auditory EPs are treated more fully in Chapter 4, Section 4.2.1.

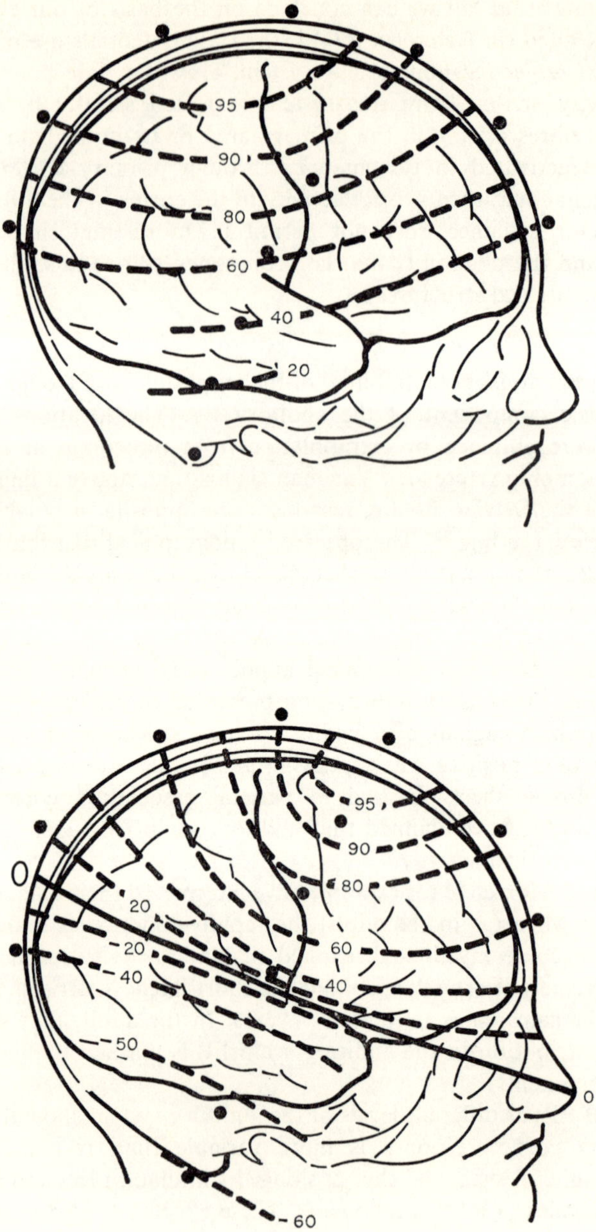

FIGURE 2.33 *Top and bottom sections show isopotential maps of AI(P200) and AII(P300), respectively. From H. G. Vaughan, Jr. and W. Ritter (1970). 'The sources of auditory-evoked responses recorded from the human scalp'.* Electroenceph. clin. Neurophysiol., ***28***, *360–367. Elsevier Publishing Co., Amsterdam.*

2.10.5 *Evoked potentials generated in the left and right hemispheres*

One problem encountered when comparing potentials evoked by stimulation of different localised retinal areas is the effect of the notorious variability of EPs (see Section 5.4.11). Since in general the EPs to successive identical trains of stimuli show considerable variability, it is difficult to decide whether an observed difference between the responses to stimulation of different retinal areas is a real difference or is merely due to variability. There is a limit to the clarification which can be obtained by extending the length of an experiment, since quite apart from increases in the amplitude of muscle artifact as the subject grows progressively more fatigued, EPs change slowly with time due to a number of factors. Among these factors is fatigue of the subject which rapidly increases if an experiment is unduly lengthy. The result of such slow changes in EPs is that if averaging is excessively prolonged the averaging process loses its effectiveness (a necessary assumption in the summation, or averaging, method of enhancing the signal-to-noise ratio is that the EP does not change appreciably with time, i.e. stationarity is assumed). One method of tackling this variability problem is to record potentials evoked by *simultaneous* stimulation of different areas of the retina.[644] This method gives a marked reduction in the effect of any part of the total EP variability which is common to the potentials evoked by stimulation of the nasal and temporal half-fields.

It is not difficult to record EPs to stimulation of an individual retinal half-field, but in normal subjects it is quite a different matter to be sure that such an EP is entirely generated within a single hemisphere. First there is the obvious possibility of contamination from scattered light. This can be minimised both by illuminating the unstimulated half-field by steady adapting light and by using stimuli of low modulation depths (low percentage change of intensity, see Section 2.3.2). A second possible complication, which is not so easily eliminated, is that signals from the stimulated half-field might be transmitted to the supposedly-unstimulated hemisphere either via inter-hemispheric neural connections or via direct neural pathways. There is one precaution which can be taken to minimise possible transmission across the corpus callosum, and this is to leave a central vertical strip of unstimulated retina. At least in monkey and baboon it is exclusively a retinal strip near the vertical meridian which is concerned with callosal connections.[135,400] Further-more, any signals which do cross the corpus callosum are likely to be in-effective in evoking scalp potentials, probably as a result of their temporal dispersion.[488]

The *bipolar* transient EPs to stimulation of either nasal or temporal half-field by pattern-reversal do not spread over the midline of the scalp for some subjects even for stimuli which extend close to the vertical meridian.[159] (Of course a bipolar EP of small amplitude may mean either that both electrodes are inactive *or* that both are active to almost the same extent.)

Monopolar steady-state EPs to monocular pattern-reversal stimulation of nasal and temporal half-fields (with a centrally located 1° vertical strip left unstimulated) show considerable spread over the midline in some subjects but not in others.[643, 645, 649] Superficially, this intersubject difference would seem more likely to be due to different spatial orientations of the EP generators than to the influence of passive conduction. On the other hand the spread might be due to signals being transmitted to the supposedly unstimulated hemisphere. Callosal transmission seems unlikely for the reasons outlined above and there is evidence against bilateral macular representation.[788]* However, the possibility of signal transmission along pathways other than the classical geniculocalcarine pathways is difficult to rule out.†

The presence or absence of pattern-reversal in one half-field does not seem to affect the response to pattern reversal in the other half-field either for transient[159] or steady-state[642] stimulation. To this extent, nasal and temporal half-field stimulation seems to evoke independent EPs.

2.11 Evoked potentials and the processing of sensory information at 'high levels'

2.11.1 *Evoked potential correlates of perceptual suppression and of 'fade out' of stabilized images*

A number of stimulus situations can result in suppression of perception of a part or of the whole of a visual field. Perhaps the most familiar of these situations is retinal rivalry. This phenomenon is commonly observed when dissimilar contours are viewed by the left and right eyes, as for example when the left eye views a pattern of horizontal lines while the right eye views a pattern of vertical lines. Under these conditions perceptual suppression occurs alternately for the pattern viewed by either the left or right eye, in other words vision takes place alternately through the left and right eyes. A less familiar example of perceptual suppression can result from stabilizing the image of the outside world on the retina so that the movements which normally result from small eye movements and tremor are prevented, thus each

* Vastola has compiled a formidable list of structures other than dorsal lateral geniculate body and striate cortex which are implicated in visuosensory functions. These structures include the ventral lateral geniculate body, superior colliculus, central grey, subcollicular tegmentum, pretectal area, reticular formation, large celled nuclei of the optic tract, pulvinar, and the posterior, lateral posterior, ventral anterior, central lateral and anterior ventral nuclei.[814 p.454.] Even this list excludes the structures involved in oculomotor functions – whose activities are just as likely to be locked to many forms of stimuli as are sensory processes. It is difficult to be sure that signals from, for example, the right retinal half-field could not evoke slow potentials in the left hemisphere by routes involving the above structures. A further point underlined by the length of Vastola's list and by the presence of oculomotor pathways is that it is unsafe to assume that all EP components necessarily reflect neural activities which are directly related to sensation.

† In addition, Halliday and Michael (personal communication) have compared the results of stimulating a strip adjacent to the vertical meridian with the results of stimulating the half-field without this strip. They have failed to find evidence of a component which could be attributed to the bilateral occipital projections of the paramedial strip.

part of the retina receives an unvarying stimulus. The result of stabilizing the retinal image in this way is that the perception of a patterned field soon 'fades out' to leave a visual impression of diffuse, uniform luminance. As the physiological basis of neither of the above two forms of perceptual suppression is understood at the present time, an electrophysiological method of studying suppression in cooperating human subjects could clearly have a part to play. In considering the suitability of EP methods for this purpose, the first question to be answered is whether changes occur in the EP which parallel the suppression of perception. This question will be discussed in the following pages.

MacKay has pointed out that the evidence so far available suggests that EP experiments on suppression might with advantage be divided into (*a*) those which studied the suppression of pure contour-sensitive EP components, and (*b*) those in which blank-field components were also recorded. However, it does seem to be the case that the results of the former class of experiments are much more clear-cut than the results of the latter class.

Cobb *et al.*[157] recorded contrast-specific responses* to pattern-reversal stimuli. The left eye was stimulated by a horizontal and the right eye by a vertical reversing bar pattern. The difference between the contours viewed by the left and right eyes established a state of perceptual retinal rivalry. Subjects were instructed to press a key so that EPs were directed to channel one of an averaging computer when the right eye was dominant, and directed to channel two when the left eye was dominant. It was arranged that a further distinction could be made between EPs to stimulation of the left and right eyes by setting the relative phases of the stimuli to the left and right eyes so that the EP to stimulation of the left eye alone was 180° out of phase with the EP to stimulation of the right eye alone. The results of this experiment suggested that stimulation of a dominant eye evoked potentials of much larger amplitudes than stimulation of a suppressed eye (Fig. 2.34).

This experiment does however leave one uncertainty. Similar findings might result if, when an eye was suppressed, its accommodation became less sharp since a slight blurring of the retainal image (equivalent to no more than 0·3 to 1·0 dioptre) can provide a marked reduction of the amplitude of the pattern-specific EP.[157, 359, 671, 748, 801, S23]

The conclusions of Cobb *et al.* were confirmed by van der Tweel *et al.*[800] in an experiment where the effects of accommodation changes was eliminated. Only a *part* of the visual field of one eye was subjectively suppressed, while the rest of the visual field in that same eye remained unsuppressed. This was made possible by using the checkerboard mirror stimulator (Chapter 5, Section 5.1.8).

In the experiment of van der Tweel *et al.*[800] the right eye saw a rhythmically-reversing checkerboard pattern. The left eye viewed an identical reversing pattern in part of the stimulus field, but in the remaining part there was a static

* These EPs were shown to be predominantly of the contrast-specific type by demonstrating (*a*) their sensitivity to visual accommodation and (*b*) the characteristic shape of their amplitude *versus* frequency curve (see Section 2.4.1).

(nonreversing) checkerboard pattern of high contrast. When the checkerboard mirror was viewed in fused binocular vision the subject saw the top half of the visual field as a static nonreversing pattern while the bottom half was seen as a rhythmically reversing pattern. In other words there was suppression of the perception of pattern reversal in the top half of the visual field of the right eye; however, some impression of diffuse flicker remained. The perceptual suppression seemed therefore to be specific to contour information. This interocular suppression effect could persist for at least several minutes, and

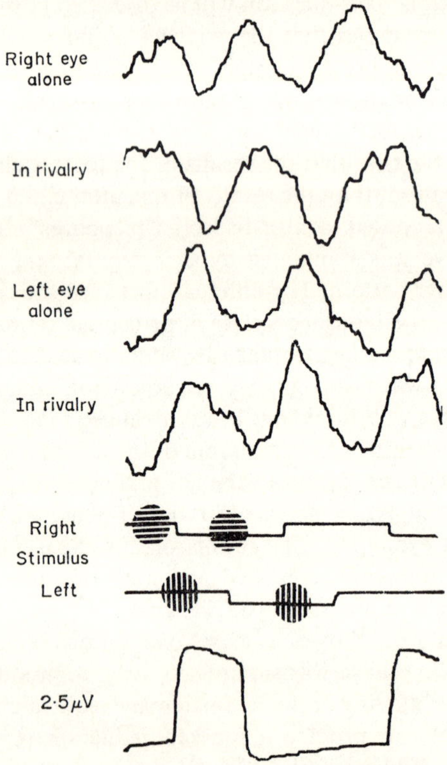

FIGURE 2.34 *Pattern reversal in visual rivalry. Each trace is the average of 128 sweeps and lasts 250 msec; response frequency, 12 c/s. The targets, 6 mm in diameter (56′), have alternating black and white bars 0·48 mm wide; for the right eye they are horizontal and move vertically by one bar width; for the left eye they are vertical and move laterally. The two traces above the calibration signal, if viewed at 37 cm, show the actual size of, and change in, the targets and the temporal sequence of their movements, which are arranged so that the responses from stimulating the eyes separately are 180° out of phase (channel 1 = right eye, channel 3 = left eye). When the eyes are stimulated together rivalry occurs and the subject sorts the responses by pressing either of two switches, according to whether the right eye (channel 2) or left eye (channel 4) is dominant. It will be seen that the responses during rivalry are as large as or larger than during single-eyed viewing, which suggests that the non-dominant eye has not contributed to the trace. From W. A. Cobb, H. B. Morton and G. Ettlinger (1967). 'Cerebral potentials evoked by pattern reversal and their suppression in visual rivalry',* Nature, ***216****. 1123–1125. Macmillan (Journals) Ltd.*

could occur for small retinal areas of only a few pattern elements (one pattern element was roughly 15′ of arc).

Van der Tweel *et al.* found that the EP virtually disappeared when perceptual suppression of the whole visual field occurred, as in the experiment of Cobb *et al.* Furthermore, when only the upper or lower half-field was suppressed the resulting EP changes were the same as those produced by physical occlusion of the corresponding halves of the stimulus field. This could be shown by utilising the fact that in some subjects it was possible to distinguish between the EPs due to stimulation of upper and lower half-fields by differences in both topographical distribution and amplitude.[355, 412, 413, 800, 825]

The amplitude of the EP to pattern reversal therefore correlated with perceptual suppression in accord with the conclusion of Cobb *et al.*,[157] but with a further point that in this case the EP changes could not be due to changes in ocular accommodation. It is worth remarking that this correlation has been demonstrated to be valid for the two possibly different suppression phenomena of spontaneous retinal rivalry and 'forced' stable interocular suppression.[534, 800] These results add to those of MacKay in suggesting that whatever switching mechanisms are associated with interocular perceptual suppression, they lie peripheral to the origin of the pattern (contrast)-specific component of the EP.[534]

Suppression experiments in which the EPs recorded have been predominantly due to changes in stimulus luminance have not so far led to such clear conclusions as the pattern-EP experiments. The experimental designs used have not avoided confusions due both to technical artifacts and the influence of uncontrolled factors such as, for example, motor activity or these psychological parameters which have been shown to influence EPs. It seems that some spatial structure must be present in both left and right stimulus fields if retinal rivalry is to take place, so that it is difficult to design a method of studying the EP correlates of retinal rivalry in which the EPs contain only 'blank field' components. In a number of investigations on retinal rivalry so-called 'unstructured (diffuse) field' EPs have been recorded which, however, were in all probability contaminated by contrast-specific components.[39, 443, 474]

The effect of perceptual suppression on EP components to unstructured (diffuse) field stimuli has been studied,[534] not in the case of retinal rivalry, but during stable interocular suppression. MacKay found that the perception of an unstructured field, flash-presented to one eye, could be suppressed by presenting a visual noise field* to the other eye providing that the two fields were presented within a few tens of milliseconds of each other. When perception of the blank field was suppressed by the flash-presentation of the noise field then the characteristic waveform of the blank-field response was found to be absent from the resulting EP. Furthermore, when the time interval between the noise and blank stimuli was increased so that perception of the flashed noise field no longer occurred, then the EP was found to show the

* Visual noise is a randomly arranged pattern of small figures or dots.[531]

characteristic blank-field response. This experiment demonstrated therefore that the amplitude of the characteristic unstructured-field EP correlates with the suppression of perception of the unstructured field when this perceptual suppression is caused by a spatially-structured field.

Perhaps the most satisfactory suppression experiments concerned entirely with the potentials evoked by unstructured (blank) fields are those of Cobb *et al.*[156] in which the luminance of two targets were square-wave modulated at a frequency of 10 Hz. In order to produce retinal rivalry, a pattern of horizontal lines was placed in front of the target viewed by one eye, and a

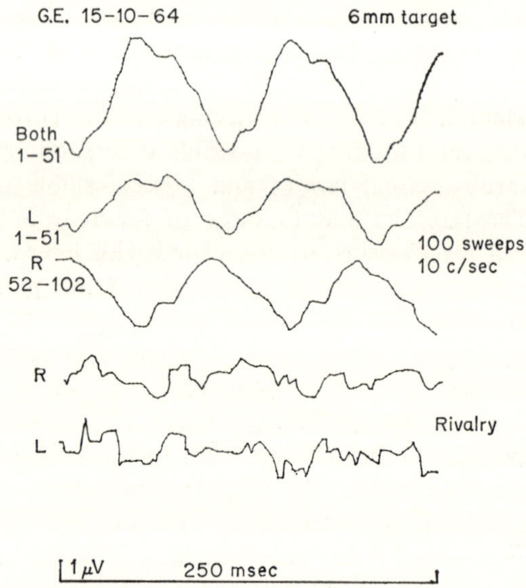

FIGURE 2.35 *The first channel shows the occipital response to square wave stimulation of both eyes simultaneously at 10 c/sec (the period is actually 102 msec in order to cause drift with respect to the 50 c/sec mains supply). The second and third channels show responses to stimulation of the left and right eyes, respectively, alone, the stimuli being 180° out of phase. The fourth and fifth channels are the responses to simultaneous out of phase stimulation of the two eyes, sorted by the subject into right and left eye dominant respectively. From W. A. Cobb, G. Ettlinger and H. B. Morton (1967) 'Visual evoked potentials in binocular rivalry'.* Electroenceph. clin. Neurophysiol., Suppl. *26, 100–107. Elsevier Publishing Co., Amsterdam.*

pattern of vertical lines was placed in front of the target viewed by the other eye. Although the patterning presumably introduced some contrast-specific components into the EP, this contamination would seem at first sight to be unimportant since Cobb *et al.* concluded that the amplitude of their EPs did not correlate with perceptual suppression during retinal rivalry (contamination of the EP by contrast-specific components would tend to result in the opposite conclusion). The above conclusion was based on the finding that EPs of similar amplitude were recorded when either a dominant or a suppressed eye was stimulated (Fig. 2.35). However, their experimental method may be insensitive if the site of suppression were peripheral to the saturation stage of the EP (see Fig. 2.13). If this were so then for the high stimulus modulation depth used by Cobb *et al.* a very considerable reduction in the signal immediately before the saturation stage might be required before producing any reduction in the amplitude of the EP (e.g. an attenuation equivalent to an eightfold reduction in stimulus modulation depth might give no change in the amplitude of the EP if saturation set in at the realistic figure of 15% modulation depth and the squarewave stimulus contained a fundamental component of 120% modulation depth). The above reservation about the conclusion of Cobb *et al.* would be met if the experiment were carried out using stimuli of low modulation depth.

The conclusion discussed above appears to conflict with that of van Balen[39] who controlled eye dominance by instructing his subjects to read with one specified eye. He compared the potentials evoked by stimulating one eye by a flash when it was reading (and therefore dominant), and when the eye was suppressed by instructing the subject to read with the other eye. The amplitude of the EP was found to be a little larger when an eye was reading than when it was not reading. However, it does seem possible that this difference might be due not to suppression but to the intrusion of contour-specific EP components which would presumably be of greater amplitude when the sharply-accommodating reading eye was stimulated than when the suppressed eye was stimulated. This suggestion is consistent with the finding of Cobb *et al.*[156] that van Balen's results could be repeated for some subjects (2 out of 6) whether the eye read or merely fixated on one letter of the text, but could not be repeated when the eye fixated on a single letter isolated on a white ground.

Other investigations which have been entirely concerned with unstructured fields are in general less satisfactory than that of Cobb *et al.* Lansing used a sharply tuned filter to extract evoked potentials to flickering light from the EEG.[474] By stimulating at the alpha frequency he was especially prone to confuse changes in alpha activity with changes in the EP. He presented a patterned target to one eye for periods of a few seconds, while continuously stimulating the other eye with a flickering field. Presenting the target to one eye markedly reduced the output of the filter, and at the same time produced changes in eye dominance. Lansing suggested an association between the EP changes and the changes in eye dominance, although he left open the possibility that the presentation of the contoured target to the unstructured eye might *in itself* have caused changes in the potential evoked by stimulating the fellow eye (such an effect was in fact reported by Lehmann and Fender[487] and by Riggs and Whittle[675]). If this effect were an important contaminant in Lansing's experiment, then it might be expected that, in a situation where the rival target was continuously presented and the subject indicated which eye was dominant, then much smaller differences would be found between the EPs to stimulation of the eye during its dominant and suppressed phases. In fact this was indeed found to be the case: the residual difference might have been due to changes, not in the EP, but in the alpha activity passing through the filter.

Martin[515] investigated spontaneous changes in interocular perceptual dominance by simultaneously presenting different stimulus patterns flashed to the left and right eyes at a rate slower than 1 Hz. The central idea of his experiment was to use the differences between waveforms evoked by different stimulus patterns as an index of which eye was dominant. Unfortunately a flash-presented pattern stimulates the eye both by a luminance change and by a pattern presentation; there is evidence that the potentials evoked by these two constituents of the stimulus have quite different properties. In particular the two types of EP seem to relate differently to eye dominance (see above). Martin's failure to find a consistent EP correlate of subjective eye dominance cannot, therefore, be clearly interpreted. Martin also found that, in fused binocular viewing, the EP was often dominated by the response of the eye which under monocular viewing gave the weaker response. A similar finding had previously been reported by Kaufman *et al.*[443] Once again, and for the same reason, the finding is difficult to interpret. However, it certainly points towards a further study in which responses to spatially unstructured fields and to changes in the contrast of patterned fields are explicitly compared.

Some experiments on interocular rivalry give a further warning that the recording of transient EPs is especially prone to artifacts due both to the motor action of key pressing[S28] and to such psychological states as 'decision making' and 'uncertainty resolution' (see Chapter 3, Section 3.3). In one experiment, simultaneously presented rival targets were continuously illuminated by steady light.[156] The subject pressed a key when either eye became dominant, and a flash immediately resulted. The flash was delivered to either eye at random. It was found that the EP to the flash was the same whether the stimulated eye was dominant or suppressed.

Cobb *et al.*[156] cited the result of this experiment in support of the conclusion they had drawn from their flicker experiment described above. However, when Donchin[243] carried out an experiment similar in all respects to that of Cobb *et al.*,[156] except that flashes were delivered at random intervals (i.e. not locked to changes in dominance), then very small EPs were recorded to stimulation of both the dominant and suppressed eye. In contrast, EPs of much larger amplitude were recorded when the experimenter attempted to make the subject 'attend to the flashes' by instructing him to press a key in response to every tenth flash.[S28] Donchin pointed out that 'large amplitude' in both Cobb *et al.*'s and his own experiments applied only to EP components of 250–300 msec latency. Earlier components were very small under all conditions. Donchin suggested that the late EP components were related, not to the perception of the flash, but to changes in the psychological state of the subject.

While it is surely correct that in experiments such as that described above there is a danger of confusing EP components which are closely related to the stimulus parameters with EP components which are loosely related to the stimulus, there is, nevertheless, an alternative possibility. This is that the EPs recorded by Cobb *et al.* may have been contaminated by components associated with the motor action of pressing the key which sorted the EPs into those recorded during suppression and those recorded during dominance. Any potentials of this type would have been averaged since the averaging computer was locked to the motor actions (see Chapter 3, Section 3.4). Although of course the subject's instructions ensured that there was a correlation between making a decision and pressing a key in both Donchin's and Cobb *et al.*'s experiments, the motor potentials recorded at the scalp need not necessarily have been immediately connected with anything other than physiological activity associated with motor action.

It should be emphasised, however, that Donchin's criticism applies to only one of the experiments reported by Cobb *et al.*[156] and does not apply to the experiment in which repetitive flashes were used (Fig. 2.35).

STABILIZED RETINAL IMAGES

Visual perception may 'fade out' when the image of the outside world is held completely still (stabilized) on the retina.[523] Image stabilization has commonly been achieved by mechanical devices (for example by mounting the target on a contact lens worn by the subject), although for the peripheral retina and even for the fovea perceptual fade out can be produced by voluntary fixation.[144,523] Perceptual fade out is not maintained indefinitely, and some parts at least of the image reappear from time to time, even in spite of heroic efforts to ensure that the stabilising contact lens does not slip. Although it has often been suggested that the cause of the perceptual fade out is retinal adaptation, there is some evidence that more central mechanisms are also involved. For example, if a geometrical pattern is 'burnt' on to the retina by a brief Xenon flash, the resulting after image must necessarily be completely stabilized, and any fluctuations in perception cannot be due to losses of image stabilization. Nevertheless fade-outs and reappearance of after images do occur, and moreover the reappearances occur in a significant manner. The geometrical image frequently reappears not as a whole, but in part, and the parts which reappear are often organised systematically.[70] This latter observation suggests that retinal adaptation cannot give a complete account of the fade-out and reappearance of the stabilized image. The further question of what physiological processes determine perceptual fade out has been approached not only by psychological methods, but also by the use of evoked potentials. As with studies of retinal rivalry it is useful to distinguish between contrast-specific EP components, and components evoked by areal changes in stimulus luminance. This distinction is especially important in the present case, since it is difficult to see how anything other than contours could be stabilized.

Riggs and Whittle[675] stimulated with an alternating bar pattern and with a flickering blank field. They found it necessary to use stimulus repetition frequencies in excess of 10 Hz, since it was difficult to achieve fade-out for lower rates. The result of this experiment was surprising. The amplitude of the EP during fade-out of the image was the same as when the image could be seen clearly. This finding held both for the alternating bar stimulus and the blank flickering field. A similar result was reported by Lehman *et al.*[486] using blank flickering fields, although their conclusion applied more to central than to retinal changes associated with perceptual fade-out.

This reported lack of correlation between EP amplitude and the perceptual fade-out of stabilized images is consistent with previous findings for retinal rivalry and interocular suppression in the case of blank-field EPs. On the other hand the lack of correlation for the alternating bar stimulus appears to conflict with the results of other experiments involving contrast-specific EP components (see this section, above). However, this may not be a real conflict, since Riggs and Whittle used a reversal rate for their bar pattern which was so high (24 Hz) that genuine contrast-specific responses were probably very small[157, 748] However, for a 24 Hz stimulus EPs to luminance flicker have been reported to be particularly large (see Section 2.8.3). The frequency of these responses would be *twice* the stimulus repetition frequency, so their waveform would mimic that of the genuine contrast-specific components. Moreover, since adjacent bars of the pattern were modulated in antiphase, the doubled-frequency (second harmonic) response to luminance changes of each individual bar would be in phase, so that they would add rather than cancel. There is strong evidence that such high-frequency responses to luminance modulation do not correlate with the perception of flicker, and may easily be recorded to stimuli whose flicker is well below perceptual threshold (Section 2.8.3). All this suggests that the potentials evoked by Riggs and Whittle's reversing bar pattern might have been contaminated by components evoked by areal changes in stimulus luminance, so that their findings would not be applicable to contrast-specific EP components and would then be consistent with the findings of other workers.

As an explanation of their finding that EP amplitude was not affected by perceptual fade-out Riggs and Whittle suggested that the neural representation of contour information may not be time-locked to a flickering stimulus, so that these 'sensory' neural signals would be inaccessible to the averaging method. Neural signals due to stimulus contours must presumably be the activity whose attenuation leads to perceptual fade-out in image stabilization, since stabilization can affect little other than contour signals. On this view, the EP components recorded by Riggs and Whittle would not be relevant to flicker perception, though just as with the high-frequency EPs (see Section 2.8.3) the question remains 'what function if any is reflected by these EP components?' Riggs and Whittle further suggested that although a dissociation between EP amplitude and the 'fade-out' of stimulus contours could be accounted for if the presence of contours were signalled by neural activity which was not time-locked to the stimulus, on the other hand this would not explain the finding that the EP remained unaltered while flicker subjectively disappeared. On the other hand it is not essential to assume that flicker must necessarily be signalled by neural activity which is time-locked to the stimulus. On the contrary, changes have been recorded in the optic nerve activity of the cat which correlate with the presence of flicker and yet are not time locked to the stimulus flicker.[299]

2.11.2 *Potentials evoked by visual stimuli during eye movements*

Visual perception is suppressed during rapid voluntary eye movements. Whether suppression is due to central or to peripheral mechanisms has been the subject of controversy. It has been suggested that this suppression is a consequence of 'retinal blurring',[232] the operation of a central inhibitory mechanism,[389] a corollary discharge,[879] mechanical shearing,[662] or that it would be predicted by the 'matching response' model of perception[532] (see Section 2.1.1). MacKay[538] has questioned whether eye movements are necessary at all since he has demonstrated a threshold elevation for flashes that occurs whenever the retinal image of a visual field is abruptly displaced, even though the eye remains stationary. MacKay[538] suggested that the displacement of the visual field generates a transient 'neural disturbance' which interferes with the detection of the subsequent flash. Conflicts in earlier reports have been explained by distinguishing between the suppression of *pattern perception* and the suppression of the *perception of a flash.*

Attempts have been made to use EPs as an objective index of the suppression of perception during eye movements. At the onset of an eye movement suppression is 'virtually complete' for the EPs to reversals of the luminance contrast of a fairly narrow (30′) bar pattern.[131, 342] This observation correlates with the strong suppression of pattern vision during an eye movement.[342] In contrast, there is little suppression of the EPs to brief flashes which are brighter than 0·5 log units above threshold,[131, 342, 546] or to stripes whose widths are 1·5° or 3°.[131] This observation in turn correlates with psychophysical findings that eye movements elevate the threshold for light flashes by no more than 0·5 log units,[470, 836] especially in view of the evidence that patterns whose elements are very large give EPs which may resemble unstructured-field EPs more closely than structured-field EPs (Section 2.4.3). Vaughan and Gross[342] interpreted their results as indicating that an inhibitory mechanism must exist which is specific for contour shift as opposed to change in luminance. Vaughan[819a] suggested that both the suppression of pattern perception and the attenuation of the EP to pattern reversal are related to the neural effects of pattern displacement at the *onset* of a shift in eye position, and that this initial strong visual excitation sharply reduces the responses to stimuli which occur during and immediately following a saccade. In contrast, Chase and Kalil[131] implicated the eye movement itself rather than merely the displacement of the retinal image, since they found marked suppression of pattern perception and pattern EPs to occur during saccades even when the subject was almost in total darkness.[S20]

2.11.3 *Evoked potentials and interhemispheric differences; meaningful stimuli*
The sensory losses which may follow unilateral brain injury have historically provided much evidence of the lateralisation of a number of sensory functions. For example, in strongly right-handed individuals it seems that the integrity of the left cerebral hemisphere, though not that of the right, is essential for speech and for the ability to draw geometrical shapes accurately.[558, 884] New insights into the physiological basis of hemispheric dominance and functional lateralisation might be possible if EPs to stimuli ranging from geometrical figures to words could be separately recorded from the left and right hemispheres.

Some endeavours have already been made in this direction. Eason *et al.*[256] tried to emphasise the activity of a single hemisphere by stimulating the appropriate retinal half-field and by recording from an electrode located 3 cm lateral to the inion. They concluded that in right-handed subjects the EP to flashes was of significantly shorter latency for the dominant than for the nondominant hemisphere. A subsequent study,[195] however, failed to confirm their finding.

John *et al.* looked for EP correlates of a higher level of information processing than the emphasis (abstraction) of simple contours.[422] They claimed that potentials of different waveforms were evoked by circles and squares. Crucially, the circles and squares evoked individually characteristic EPs *independently of the sizes of the circles and squares.* In a second report from John's laboratory[378] it was claimed that the waveshape of the EP to squares and circles corresponded 'to what the subject was thinking and not to what stimulus is actually present in the visual field'. In view of the importance of these claims, it is disappointing that independent validation and development have not yet followed these studies.

Although no attempt was made to study lateralisation, responses to meaningful stimuli were studied by Lifshitz[499] who used coloured pictures whose contents were neutral, erotic or offensive. Lifshitz reported differences between the waveforms of his EPs, but a major difficulty in such a study is the possible contaminating effects firstly of physical stimulus parameters such as differences in colour or contours, and secondly of central oculomotor activity due to pupilliary changes caused by changes in the interest value of the stimulus.[379] At the present time the available systematic knowledge of EP correlates of physical stimulus parameters is hardly sufficient to allow experiments such as that of Lifshitz to be unambiguously interpreted. Partly in order to avoid the difficulties peculiar to visual stimulation, EPs have been recorded to words of different 'affective' content.[66] Once again it is difficult to find a clear interpretation of the data since the psychological state of the subject is not easy to control under such circumstances. For example a 'taboo' word may indeed carry a shocking meaning to some subjects, but to others its familiarity might render it meaningless. Again, any differences which were found between the EPs to different words might conceivably be due to an alerting reaction which might be related to the 'affective content' of words, but probably not as directly or as importantly as implied by Begleiter[66] or Lifshitz.[499]

Buchsbaum and Fedio[102] searched for EP correlates of an even higher level of information processing than that studied by John *et al.* Transient EPs were recorded to brief presentations of random patterns of dots, geometrical figures and words. All stimuli were made up of similar dots, and for each word there was a corresponding random pattern which was made up of the same number of dots as the word. The use of identical dots to build up different figures went some way to preventing the occurrence of different responses due merely to different lengths of contour in the stimulus. No attempt though was made to stimulate the left and right retinal half-fields, and the responses of left and right hemispheres were differentiated entirely by the rather weak technique of monopolar recording from the left and right sides of the head. For right-handed subjects the EPs to words and designs was found to differ more for the left electrode than for the right electrode and, furthermore, EP variability was greater for the left electrode than for the right electrode. However, it is difficult to rule out the possibility that scalp potentials associated with lateralised activity of the motor cortex might have contributed to the findings of lateralised EPs. Such 'motor potentials' might have been associated with conscious or unconscious movements or preparations for vocalisation stimulated by the visual presentation of words.[S26, 31]

The study of interhemispheric differences by EP methods is a challenging and exciting prospect. Although the problems of experimental design are severe, this is an area in which the successful use of cooperative normal human subjects might well bring worthwhile rewards. The bulk of present-day knowledge in this area has so far been obtained by studying sensory losses caused by unilateral brain damage. Such studies clearly indicate that some sensory functions are principally associated with activity in the dominant cerebral hemisphere and other functions are principally associated with the minor hemisphere.[787, 788, 858, 884] However, the method of studying functional changes caused by injury is a valuable complement to, but surely not a replacement for, the study of the normally functioning brain. If the methodological problems can be solved, then this may prove to be an area where EP recording could assume an important role.

2.11.4 *Evoked potentials and intelligence*

The present chapter shows clearly that, although there are good grounds for optimism, our understanding of the relations between scalp EPs and the most basic 'feature filtering' in the sensory pathways of the brain is still little more than primitive. Bearing this in mind, it would be a fortunate research worker whose EP experiments yielded comprehensible information on the physiological basis of intelligence. Nevertheless, there have been a number of attempts to relate intelligence to some feature of the EP. These attempts have been criticised by Vaughan[817] on the grounds that they are based on nothing more substantial than the fact that brain processes underlie both intelligence and EPs, and he is certainly correct in that hypotheses relating psychological measures of intelligence to the underlying neurophysiology have been little more than speculations.

Starting from the idea that the speed of information processing is related to 'behavioural intelligence', and progressing to the notion that the latency of EP components might be inversely correlated with I.Q.,[125, 279, 280] Chalke and Ertl[125] measured the latencies of a number of EP components for a population with widely dispersed I.Q.s. They found that the subjects with the shortest latencies had the highest I.Q.s. Ertl's reports certainly demonstrate that waveforms for subjects of widely varying I.Q.s are quite different to visual inspection.[279]* In a different context, however, Rémond has pointed out the difficulty in deciding whether, in comparing a number of different waveforms, one is seeing the same components at different latencies, or one is seeing different components.[536]

Callaway and Stone[109] have correlated various I.Q. and performance measures with EP features. They used both two-tone auditory stimuli and sinewave-modulated light; the EP features measured included: (*a*) the difference between EP amplitudes on the left and right sides of the head, (*b*) the ratio between the amplitudes of the EPs to 20 and 5 Hz stimuli and (*c*) the latencies of auditory EP components. Little relation was found between any of these EP measures and whether or not a child was attending a clinic for specific learning disorders.

Shimizu[728] reported that severely retarded patients showed a marked inconstancy of auditory EP components, which were also of lower amplitudes and longer latencies than in normal subjects. Sleep-type components were frequently observed. However, it is not clear whether Shimizu's observations reflect specific malfunctions in the mechanisms which underlie intellectual activity, or whether they reflect more general damage to the CNS.

In an interesting note on a single aphasic patient, Shimizu[728, 729] found that during the aphasic phase the auditory EP could not be detected even though behavioural tests showed that the subject's hearing was not affected. In contrast, when the subject regained language function, auditory EPs were found to be clearly detectable. If this observation can be confirmed it raises the possibility that EPs offer access to the high-level nervous activities which correlate with the generation of words and the attachment of words to objects. More speculatively still: since words and concepts seem to be intimately related, and possibly interdependent, then if Shimizu is correct, EPs may eventually cast some light on the neural activities which underlie conceptual thinking (i.e. the neural activities which *represent* concepts and the relationships between concepts).

* A. M. Halliday has drawn my attention to the possibility that some of the gross differences evident in Ertl's published records might be due to the inclusion of people with brain damage at the lower end of the IQ scale. If this were so then it might be expected that there would be a discontinuous rather than a continuous distribution of latency for any given EP component due to the inclusion of some atypical responses at the lower end.

3

Evoked potentials and psychological variables

3.1 Introduction

There is conflict between the various interpretations and even between the reported results of experiments which deal with the *evaluation of* rather than the *responses to* sensory stimuli. This area of research presents a confusing picture. Some of the factors which lead to this confusion are as follows: (*a*) inadequate control of stimulus parameters; (*b*) vague or ambiguous definitions of psychological quantities (for example, disparities between definitions of 'attention' might account for much of the apparent conflict between the conclusions reached by different investigators); (*c*) scalp recordings may lump together responses which reflect dissimilar processes in different cortical areas (see below).

There are indications that a more coherent viewpoint is gradually emerging from the welter of experimental and interpretative claims. Central to this viewpoint is the hypothesis that the EP waveform is not a single indivisible entity. In a currently popular version of this hypothesis, the EP waveform is classified into 'early' and 'late' components. This classification is principally on latency grounds but topographical distribution is also taken into account by a number of writers. The 'early' components of the EP, it is suggested, relate most closely to the physical parameters of the stimulus (e.g. intensity or spatial patterning) while 'late' components ('association cortex potentials')[819] relate most closely to psychological parameters. There seems to be a considerable problem in defining these psychological variables with any precision; they have been variously described as 'stimulus evaluation', 'task relevance', 'information delivery', 'resolution of uncertainty', 'decision making' and 'meaningfulness'. It seems clear that this 'latency' variant of the general hypothesis that the EP is a composite response will gain in predictive sharpness when both the 'early' *versus* 'late' distinction and the psychological parameters are more clearly defined.

Doubts as to the value of such an 'early' *versus* 'late' criterion for analysing the EP waveform have, however, been raised by the reports of Grey Walter and his colleagues. They recorded from wires which had been implanted in the brains of human patients and found that EPs which habituated on repeated stimulation could be clearly distinguished from EPs which did not habituate. This distinction could be made on the grounds of *location*, but not so clearly on the basis of *latency*.

It is now well established that a complex of scalp potentials is initiated some time before motor activity of the body. The electrical events which precede movement of arms, legs and tongue have so far been most extensively studied. It has been suggested that certain components of this complex of potentials are associated with activity in the region of motor cortex which relates to the particular part of the body which is moved, and that other components are associated with the preparation for motor action and the initiating command for motor action.

Grey Walter first reported that in a stimulus situation where a warning signal is followed by a second stimulus which demands a motor response, a slow (d.c.) negative wave builds up before the occurrence of the second stimulus. This anticipatory electrical sign can be recorded both from scalp electrodes and from intracerebral electrodes; it has variously been called the CNV (contingent or conative negative variation) or the E (expectancy) wave. The suggestion has been made that CNV is in fact one component of the complex of motor potentials described above; not entirely disparately Grey Walter has interpreted the CNV as reflecting preparations for motor activity and has claimed that in the CNV experimental paradigm the amplitude of the CNV, correlates with the subject's expectancy.

Evoked potentials have been used as a tool to study learning and memory. On the basis of animal experiments, John has proposed that the waveshape of the EP can reflect both the release of information which has been stored in neural tissue and the nature of the information stored. He has further claimed such stored information can be simultaneously released from many separate and functionally disparate structures within the brain.

3.2 Habituation, attention, distraction and vigilance

3.2.1 *Habituation*

Some or all of the components of the scalp-recorded transient EP have variously been reported to decline in amplitude as stimuli are successively and monotonously repeated. Such 'habituation' has been reported for EPs to visual auditory and somatic stimulation.[847] The rate and degree of habituation seems generally to be less for auditory than for visual responses;[847, S34] this finding has been attributed to peripheral factors[71, 561] (but see below). Bogaez *et al.*[85] reported that the amplitudes of scalp potentials evoked by regularly repeated flashes (0·5 to 1 Hz) showed a cyclic waxing and waning which was superposed on a progressive decline (very roughly 50% fall in 6 minutes). Their observations that in some subjects all components habituated, but in others only the later components did so, and that the phenomenon was more pronounced in central and temporal regions than near the inion are consistent with Grey Walter's findings with intracerebral electrodes (see below and Reference 847).

Grey Walter found that EPs recorded from wires accurately implanted in human primary visual cortex did not habituate, even though they consisted of both 'late' as well as 'early' components. Pagni *et al.*[591] confirmed this finding for potential deflections of roughly 100–200 msec latencies. The implication of Walter's work is that in primary visual cortex *all* VEP components are determined exclusively by stimulus parameters. This appears to conflict with reports by Hernández Peón and his colleagues that VEPs recorded from wires implanted in human brain are reduced in amplitude during mental calculation.[369, 370, 374] However, one reason for this apparent disagreement might be that the Mexican workers' electrodes were, perhaps, not precisely located in primary visual cortex and therefore did not exclusively record signals destined for primary cortex; Walter had found that the only recordings which showed an absence of habituation were those from electrodes located precisely within the primary visual cortex. Further points are that the accuracy of the subject's visual fixation and the sharpness of his accommodation might have varied during mental calculation more than at other times. These factors might have caused some reduction in EP amplitude during mental calculation which was due merely to changes in retinal stimulation.

There is some disagreement about the role of peripheral mechanisms in EP habituation. García Ausst[301] claimed that variations in pupilliary diameter must be of little importance, since he had found habituation to be similar not only for subjects viewing through a natural pupil and through a 2 mm artificial pupil but also for subjects who either either had no iris or suffered from ocular paralysis. On the other hand an Italian group reported that the habituation of the VER could be *entirely* attributed to changes in the intensity of the light reaching the retina which were caused by changes in pupilliary diameter.[71, 73] These workers came to the opposite conclusion to García Ausst partly on the grounds of their contradictory findings with patients who had no iris; Bergamini *et al.* found that the VERs of those subjects did not habituate![72, 71 pp.33–38] It would be rather surprising in any case if changes in pupilliary diameter were *entirely* responsible for so great a reduction in EP amplitude as that reported by García Ausst, since the extreme range of pupilliary diameters (2 mm to 8 mm) would change the intensity of the light incident on the retina by no more than 16 times or so. Especially at high brightnesses, the amplitude of all EP components are little affected by changes of stimulus intensity (Chapter 2, Section 2.2). As it is the different stimulation methods used in the two studies could go some considerable way towards explaining the conflicting results. In particular, the group who reported habituation effects seem to have used less intense stimuli and/or higher repetition rates than the group who did not, and these conditions seem to be more favourable for demonstrations of habituation.[29, 30, 376, 789]

A finding was described by Grey Walter[847] which might go some way towards accounting for the conflict between reports of the habituation of scalp-recorded EPs. Grey Walter found that the amplitudes of EPs recorded from electrodes implanted within human primary visual cortex were determined *only* by the physical parameters of the stimulus ('specific' responses), in contrast to EPs recorded from cortex outside the primary visual area. These EPs were determined not only by the physical properties of the stimulus but *also* by additional psychological factors such as the subject's alertness. As already mentioned, the EPs recorded from primary visual cortex did not habituate, even though EPs recorded from wide areas of cortex outside this small region showed marked habituation. When recordings were made from implanted wires, EPs which did habituate could therefore be distinguished from EPs which did not habituate on the grounds of *localisation*. However, due to the diffusion of current caused by the structures which overly the cortex it seems likely that EPs recorded *from the scalp* are compounded of both habituating and non-habituating components.

A second finding of Grey Walter's discourages the suggestion of using *latency* as a criterion to distinguish between the components of scalp-recorded EPs which originate in primary visual cortex and those components which do not. Grey Walter reported that early and late components originate *both* in primary and non-primary cortex. This finding suggests that only limited success awaits attempts to associate late EP components exclusively with parameters other than the physical nature of the stimulus, and conversely to associate early EP components entirely with physical parameters of the stimulus,[239, 536, 741, 775] although differences in emphasis may often be demonstrable.[726] Indeed this raises the further question of what correlations can reasonably be expected to exist between *scalp* EPs and psychological variables in view of the very local nature of much cortical activity.[175]

3.2.2 *Attention and evoked potentials in animals: peripheral blocking (gating) of sensory signals*

Before the habituation of slow waves to repeated identical stimuli had been described in man the phenomenon had been extensively studied in animals. Several workers had tried to associate the objective finding of slow-wave habituation with changes in the animals state of 'attention'. An important point is that in these studies 'attention' was in practice defined by the experimenter's choice of method of manipulating 'attention'. In one study Hernández-Peón and his colleagues recorded (from the dorsal cochlear nucleus of the cat) bipolar EPs to tone bursts while distracting the animals attention with a variety of stimuli.[369, 372, 373, 593] Distracting stimuli were of several modalities: visual (the sight of mice in a bottle), olfactory (the smell of fish) and somatic (electric shocks). The amplitude of EPs recorded while the animal was distracted from the stimulus were found to be smaller, than those recorded from the undistracted animal. On the basis of these and similar findings Hernández-Peón and his colleagues suggested that while the animal was distracted from the stimulus, *the sensory input from that stimulus was blocked at a peripheral level.*[371]

Both the findings and the conclusions of Hernández-Peón and his colleagues have been criticised. One criticism was that no attempt was made to prevent the cat's turning it's head when it's attention was distracted by the sight of the mice or the smell of the fish. In themselves such changes in the position of the ears would be sufficient to result in considerable changes in the physical stimulus, and this might lead to changes in the amplitudes of EPs to tone bursts.[391] Näätänen[561] has raised further objections, one being to Hernández-Peón's claim that the amplitudes of the potentials evoked in one stimulus modality are reduced when the animal directs his attention to stimuli in a different modality. A second objection was to his suggestion that this attenuation reflects modality-selective blocking of sensory signals. This latter view amounts to the hypothesis that the brain, in effect, attenuates its own inputs from stimuli outside the focus of attention. Näätänen's central point, which had previously been raised by Jane *et al.*[409], was that Hernández-Peón had failed to exclude the possibility that his finding might be due to the effects of *nonspecific* alerting reactions, rather than being an attenuation which was selective to a particular modality. One way of eliminating this possibility would have been to demonstrate that when an EP to, for example, a visual stimulus was attenuated by an auditory distraction there was no accompanying attenuation of auditory EPs. In other words it was necessary to demonstrate that the attenuation of EPs during distraction was *modality-specific* and not an attenuation common to all modalities. Although in the majority of the reports of Hernández-Peón's group there was no mention of such a control experiment, attention was paid to this question by Palestini *et al.*[593] In their control experiment a cat was stimulated by flashes of light while its attention was distracted by a stimulus in the same visual modality (the sight of a rat). The amplitude of the visual EP was found to be attenuated by the visual distraction. Palestini *et al.* interpreted their finding as demonstrating the effects of *selective attention within a single modality*. However, as Näätänen pointed out,[561] since the attenuation found by Palestini *et al.* was mainly restricted to the later components of the EP, their observations could still be explained as due to nonspecific phenomena, for example an alerting process, and this would be in agreement with the conclusions of Jane *et al.*[409]

There is a general ambiguity in studies of attention, both in animal and in man, where the amplitude of EPs is used as an objective measure. A reduction in the amplitude of the EP even to a single stimulus cycle does not necessarily mean that a sensory input has been blocked. It could mean that the incoming burst of impulses, though unchanged in total number, were more dispersed in time, or changed in spatial patterning.[391] These criticisms would apply with even greater force to the studies in which attention has been correlated with the amplitudes of *averaged* EPs in man, since in such studies spurious changes in recorded amplitude could be introduced by changes in the variability of EPs. An additional explanation for some of the changes in EP amplitude recorded in both human and animal experiments of this type might be the alterations in pupilliary diameter which have been shown to occur in response to changes in the relevance or interest of stimuli.[379, 809, 810] In the absence of further evidence it seems possible that some part of the observed electrical changes at the scalp might be due to central activity associated with the changes in pupil size. The change in retinal stimulation caused by the change in pupil size might also produce scalp responses, although the latency of these responses would be made up of the pupilliary latency in addition to the EP latency so that they would be expected to appear as very late components of the EP.

One cause of uncertainty in both animal and human studies of attention concerns the question of how irrelevant the 'irrelevant' stimulus really is.[391] An animal whose attention is distracted from visual stimuli by, for example, a smell or sound may *look* towards the source of smell or sound and so introduce an element of visual searching into the supposedly nonvisual distraction. Indeed Horn and Blundell[393] found that attenuation of EPs to visual stimuli occurred with auditory distraction, but only when *visual searching* also took place. However, in these circumstances it also seems possible that head and eye movements, and changes of accommodation might change the physical light stimulus to the animal's eye.

Probably a fair summary of the findings of the various investigations described above of EP correlates of attention in animals is Näätänen's Finnish equivalent of the Scottish 'not proven'.[561 p.43]

3.2.3 *Attention and EPs in man: Introduction*

Just as with the animal experiments described above, one question which underlies many of the experiments on EPs and attention in man is the validity of the 'peripheral gating' hypothesis in the form that 'when attention is directed from stimuli B, C, D, etc. towards stimulus A, then the signals elicited by stimuli B, C, D, etc. are attenuated or blocked at a peripheral level whereas the signals elicited by stimulus A pass unattenuated'.

Two of the principal contributors to the confusion surrounding the question whether there are EP correlates of attention are (*a*) the difficulty of defining 'attention',[S44] and (*b*) the subsequent difficulty of manipulating 'attention' so defined. These difficulties are commonly encountered as a pair since the choice of the method for manipulating 'attention' has in practice had the further effect of defining 'attention'. A gross distinction should be made between 'attention' changes which are controlled by the experimenter's instructions to the subject, and 'attention' changes which are initiated by sudden changes in the stimulus. States of the former type of 'attention' may be more stable than states of the latter type of 'attention' which may change rapidly as the stimulus is repeated. However, as will be seen below, even the type of 'attention' which is determined by instructions seems to depend on the particular set of instructions.

One widely used experimental design for directing the subject's attention to, for example, the auditory modality has been to instruct the subject to press a key in response to auditory stimuli, and to ignore other 'irrelevant' stimuli. As will be seen below this procedure introduces numerous complications. Firstly, there is the question of scalp potentials which are wholly related to motor activity *in itself* and which may both precede and follow the motor action of button pressing. Then there are problems arising from 'arousal' or 'preparatory set'. In other words, if the stimulus delivery is so regular that the subject can anticipate whether or not the next stimulus will require him to make a discrimination he may arouse and alert himself accordingly. As this would suggest, the effect on the EP of arousal seems to depend on how difficult the *individual subject* finds the discrimination or task. Thirdly there are problems caused by the possibility of contamination of the EP by components due to oculomotor activity or changes in retinal illumination. These might accompany changes in the diameter of the eye pupil which have been reported to occur in response to shifts in the 'interest value' of the stimulus. The effects of such contaminating potentials might go some way to explaining the finding that, although task relevance has no effect on EPs to clicks, there is a marked effect on the amplitudes of later components of visually evoked potentials. However, such potentials do not account so easily for the reports that the *direction* of the amplitude change varies from subject to subject.

A number of difficulties of experimental design are at first sight simpler when human rather than animal subjects are used. It seems reasonable to suppose that human subjects could easily supply reports of their states of attention, and furthermore that their state of attention could easily be controlled by the design of the experimental procedure. For example, a subject might be instructed to attend alternately to either stimulus A or stimulus B in a randomised sequence such as ABAABABB . . . Several workers have used this paradigm. On the face of it this procedure should enable the hypothesis of modality-selective attention to be more sharply tested than is possible with supposedly less-controlled animal procedures. However, the superior credibility of such experiments with human subjects rests on the assumptions firstly of satisfactory subject cooperation in faithfully carrying out the experimenter's instructions and *no more* than these instructions, and secondly on the feasibility of determining the subject's psychological state by an appropriate experimental design. In practice, satisfactory control of the subject's psychological state has so far proved elusive, and especially so when the experimenter has tried to control a vaguely defined state such as 'attention'.

3.2.4 *Attention and EPs in man*

Haider *et al.*[346] claimed that in man the amplitude of a negative EP component's peaking at approximately 160 ms gave a fair measure of the subject's state of attention or vigilance. Their subjects were instructed to press a key in response to any flash which they judged to be dimmer than the preceding flash. It turned out that *both* the amplitude of the 160 msec component and the percentage of correctly detected dimmer flashes progressively declined throughout the $1\frac{1}{2}$ hour experiment, and also that short-term fluctuations in detection efficiency were paralleled by changes in EP amplitude. Furthermore, the potentials evoked by correctly identified flashes were larger than the EPs to those dimmer flashes in response to which the subject failed to press the key.

Haider *et al.*[346] claimed to have demonstrated an important relationship. However, Uttal[809] has detailed a number of unsatisfactory features of their study. As a general point, the reported correlation between a reduction in EP amplitude and detection efficiency does not and cannot demonstrate a *causal* connection between the two. A second criticism is that the subject's pupilliary diameter was neither monitored nor controlled. Uttal[809] has commented that changes in pupilliary diameter due, for example, to an altering reaction[379] might cause the amplitude of the EP to change in the same direction as that which Haider *et al.* attributed to the direct effect of changes in the subjects attention.

Ritter and Vaughan repeated the experiment and found, contrary to Haider *et al.*, that a late (350 msec–550 msec) positive component was prominent in the response. This component was associated with detected signals but was not observed for undetected signals. Ritter and Vaughan suggested that the reason why Haider *et al.* had failed to observe this late component was that they had used a bipolar electrode derivation only and that the late component was common to both electrodes. Ritter and Vaughan's observation of a late positive EP component both when the subject was actively attending to the stimulus and in response to unpredictable changes in stimulation led them to suggest that a common neurophysiological mechanism might underlie both phenomena.[S35] (See Section 5.4.7).

A widely used stratagem for directing a subject's attention towards modality A and away from modality B is to give the subject a task which involves stimuli in modality A. EPs both to stimuli of modality A (task-relevant stimuli), and to stimuli of modality B (task-irrelevant stimuli) are then recorded. Näätänen[561] suggested that two factors might influence the EP in this experimental situation. The first was attention, directed towards a specific modality. However, in the conditions used by a number of investigators important EP changes might be due to a second factor, namely a nonspecific arousal or alerting reaction which influenced all modalities similarly. Näätänen[561] carried out a series of experiments designed to distinguish between the effects on the EP of these two factors. By preventing arousal reactions from influencing the EPs he attempted to identify the effect on the EP of modality-specific attention. His method was to maintain his subjects in a state of *constant* high alertness by presenting 'relevant' and 'irrelevant' stimuli in a random order and at irregular intervals. Clicks and flashes were used; sometimes clicks were 'relevant' and at other times flashes were 'relevant'. A randomised presentation ensured that the subject did not know whether the next stimulus was 'task relevant' or not. Consequently his state of anticipatory arousal could not differ for 'relevant' and 'irrelevant' stimuli.

Näätänen found that *when the subject was in a constant state of alertness* the EPs to click stimuli were similar whether or not the clicks were task-relevant. This means (for click stimuli) EP amplitude did not correlate with 'attention' *as defined by task-relevance*. However, results were quite different when the experiment was repeated with the modification that stimuli were now presented regularly in a fixed predictable sequence rather than irregularly and in random order. In this experiment all stimuli were auditory and consisted of loud or soft clicks. The result of presenting stimuli in a fixed predictable sequence was that EPs to clicks which were task-relevant were now quite different from EPs to similar clicks which were task-irrelevant. Näätänen attributed the difference between these EPs not to the influence of attention, since this explanation was discounted by his earlier experiment, but the effect of an *arousal or alerting reaction* which preceded the task-relevant stimuli.[561, 563]

In contrast with his findings for auditory stimulation Näätänen found that the amplitudes of long-latency components (250–400 msec) EPs to flash did depend on whether the flashes were task-relevant. Some subjects showed an increase in amplitude to task-relevant stimuli and some subjects showed a *decrease*, in accord with earlier findings.[409, 700, 701] This occurred even when stimuli were presented at irregular intervals in a random order. At first sight these findings with visual stimuli suggest the selective effect of 'attention' (as defined by task-relevance) operating within a single modality. Näätänen, however, discounted this interpretation on the grounds that if 'attention' influenced visually evoked potentials it should therefore influence click evoked potentials in a similar manner, but it demonstrably did not. He attributed the differences between his visual and auditory results to 'peripheral factors' and suggested that his subject's fixation might have been steadier for relevant than for irrelevant stimuli. This does not seem likely however as his subjects had no prior warning of the relevance of any stimulus. Moreover in this case, changes in pupil size which have been reported to accompany changes in the 'interest value' of the stimulus[379] do not seem to be a likely explanation of the difference between Näätänen's auditory and visual results, since such pupilliary change might be expected to occur in both situations.[S37] Näätänen's conclusion contradicts the claim made by a number of workers that increased 'attention' to a stimulus enhances the amplitude of the EP to that stimulus. Näätänen suggested that the disagreement was due to differences in experimental design which in previous reports allowed the effects on the EP of an arousal or alerting reaction to be confused with the effects of task-relevance. Indeed, as already mentioned, when he eliminated EP effects due to changes in the state of arousal, he found that task relevance (which was assumed to control the subjects 'attention') had no effect on EPs to *clicks*. Sutton has pointed out that Näätänen's use of a 1 Hz lower cutoff frequency in his amplifiers would have the effect of distorting late components of the EP. In any case, as mentioned above, Näätänen's evidence was much less compelling for visual stimuli than for auditory stimuli. His experiments therefore leave open the possibility that 'attention' (*as determined by task-relevance*) has an influence on the amplitudes of *visually* evoked potentials and especially on the later components of visual EPs. In assessing Näätänen's conclusions Lindsley has raised the further question whether it is in fact possible to maintain an 'attentive' set towards given stimuli in such circumstances that it is impossible to *organise* and regularise one's internal responses to stimuli because of their irregular presentation.[248 p.33]

Two methods which have been used to direct a subject's attention into a particular modality are instructing him either to press a key or to count in response to stimuli in the designated modality. This experimental design has the advantage that attention can be directed first to one, then to another modality. In several studies of this type successive stimuli have been presented *regularly* in a fixed sequence so that the subject knew when the next stimulus would occur and also whether or not he would press the key.[223, 345, 756] As a consequence his alertness and preparatory state would most likely be different before the delivery of relevant stimuli than before the delivery of irrelevant stimuli. This could have accounted for some part of the differences that were reported between the resulting EPs. This same criticism that relevant and irrelevant stimuli were delivered alternately applies to the experiments of Satterfield and Cheatum[701] (shocks) and Satterfield[700] (clicks and shocks). These workers also attributed their observed changes in EP amplitude to modality-selective effects of attention, e.g. that attention to 'relevant' visual stimuli would diminish the amplitudes of EPs to 'irrelevant' click stimuli. It is therefore curious that they found the *direction* of this change to vary from subject to subject.

As in the experiments described above, Davis[197] delivered stimuli to his subjects at a regular rate, and in a predictable sequence. EPs were recorded from the vertex with a mastoid reference. There was a constant interval of 2·5 secs between stimulus tones. The first and fourth tones served as warning and control respectively. The subjects' task was to judge whether or not the third tone was louder than the second and press a key accordingly. The intensity difference between the second and third stimuli was never large (0 or 3 db) so that responses to these stimuli could be compared without the difficulties which arise when comparison stimuli are physically very dissimilar. Davis found that for five out of his six subjects the response to the third (test) tone in this fairly difficult discrimination task was significantly larger than the response to the second tone. On the other hand, when the subject performed the much easier task of merely responding to the third tone there was no difference between the EPs to the third (test) tone (to which they presumably attended) and to the standard second tone (to which they presumably did not attend). The EP changes which Davis observed during the discrimination task were much clearer for later components (roughly

200 msec latency) than for earlier components and clearer for recording sites near the vertex than for sites near the inion. One of the subjects differed from the other five in showing no EP differences related to the task for either the simple or the more difficult task. An explanation of this curious disparity is suggested by Davis' report that this subject gave an unusually good performance in the discrimination task, thus *both* tasks may have been indifferently easy to her so that she may have attended indifferently to all stimuli. This leads on to a criticism which applies to all experiments in which the subject is left in a supposedly 'neutral' state for part of an experiment. It is a real possibility that a subject with no task may invent his own so that his state of attention for 'irrelevant' stimuli is in fact uncontrolled and unknown rather than neutral. The criticism that, as a result of a predictable and regular stimulus presentation, the observed EP changes might be largely due to some form of preparatory arousal reaction rather than to attention applies also to Davis' experiment. Näätänen[561] investigated this crucial question whether, when stimuli were presented in a regular and predictable manner, the differences between the EPs to task-relevant and task-irrelevant were greater for more difficult tasks. He found that changes in the EP were indeed greater when the subject was given a task which *to him* was difficult rather than a task which *to him* was simple.[561 pp.163–166] In addition, both slow negative shifts (i.e. CNV which, Näätänen argued, reflected activation of the nonspecific arousal systems of the brain[563]) and flattening of the spontaneous EEG (which, Näätänen argued, reflected increased nonspecific cortical activation)[563] were observed immediately *before* the delivery of the relevant stimuli in the more difficult situation (but not in the simple task situation). Neither of these anticipatory differences were found for relevant and irrelevant stimuli when the stimulus delivery was arranged to ensure that stimuli could not be anticipated. Näätänen interpreted his finding as a confirmation that although there was no EP correlate of *intermodality selective* attention, on the other hand a clear EP correlate of an anticipating alerting reaction could be observed when stimulus delivery was predictable. The way in which 'task difficulty' and individual skill *jointly* determine the EP correlates of an anticipatory alerting reaction might also go some way towards explaining why, when attention was supposedly elevated by such simple task as counting stimuli, some workers found that in many subjects there was no EP change,[385, 386, 756] while others found EP amplitude increased during counting.[301, 302, 303, 341, 431]

EPS AND THE SPEED OF REACTION TIME

Some studies have ascribed fluctuations in the speed of reaction time to fluctuations in the level of arousal or attention, and have pointed to concomitant variations in the waveform of the EP.[247, 556, 872] Contrary to the conclusions of other workers,[872, 873] Bostock and Jarvis reported a strong correlation between the speed of reaction time and the amplitude of a negative wave with a latency of peak of roughly 250 msec.

Barlow[44, 45] put forward evidence that oculomotor reaction time may be less than 40 msec although there may be little EP evidence of components whose latencies are as short as 40 msec.

3.3 'Task relevance', 'meaningfulness', 'information delivery', the 'resolution of uncertainty', 'decision making', etc.

3.3.1 *Introduction*

Components of the transient evoked potential (especially late components) have been reported to show systematic changes in amplitude in a large number of experimental situations in which the internal state of the subject is manipulated. Almost as many psychological terms have been used to explain these observations as experiments have been carried out. Sutton gives a list which, although incomplete, includes no less than twenty-nine different terms.[775] However, many concepts in Sutton's list overlap to a large extent, and others are so unsharp as to be of little scientific value.

There is growing evidence that in many situations the slow (200–550 msec) positive vertex waves first described by Davis are less closely coupled to stimulus parameters than are earlier EP components. A full and clear definition of the pscyhological quantities which determine these late components has however proved to be elusive. It has been suggested that a positive wave of roughly 300 msec latency (P300 wave)*[S35] is evoked by stimuli which *resolve the subject's mental uncertainty*.[245, 779] If the subject makes a judgement in response to a certain stimulus, then so long as he is certain of his judgement, a P300 wave will be evoked by that stimulus whether the judgement is correct or incorrect. The *absence* of a stimulus can also evoke a P300 wave which again has been attributed to the resolution of uncertainty (Fig. 3.1).[779, S33] 'Task relevant' stimuli have been found to evoke larger responses than 'task irrelevant' stimuli.[128, 129, 726] However, the closely related notions of 'information delivery', 'task relevance' and 'resolution of uncertainty' now seem to have less value in EP research than was at first thought.[775, S35] Furthermore the later parts of the transient EPs do not always have such simple structures as the EPs analysed by Sutton and Donchin.[239, 778, 779]

3.3.2 *Information delivery and uncertainty resolution*

The notion of 'information delivery' has been used to explain a number of EP findings.[778, 779] In one study the subject was instructed to guess whether the next stimulus would be a high-pitched click or a softer lower-pitched click.[775] The lower-pitched clicks were introduced between high-pitched clicks without warning. The amplitude of the positive 300 msec evoked by the low-pitched clicks was found to *increase* when the mean frequency of the low-pitched clicks was *decreased* (while keeping the frequency of the higher-

* It is difficult to find a clear statement of the range of variability of the latency of the 'P300' wave. A range of roughly 230–360 msec seems to be a roughly appropriate estimate for a number of stimulus situations.

pitched standard clicks approximately constant). This effect was interpreted as showing a correlation between the amplitude of the positive 300 msec wave and the 'information delivered' by the stimulus. The justification for this view was that a decrease of the mean frequency of the lower-pitched clicks was equivalent to a decrease in the probability of the lower-pitched clicks, and could therefore be described as an increase in the information delivered to the

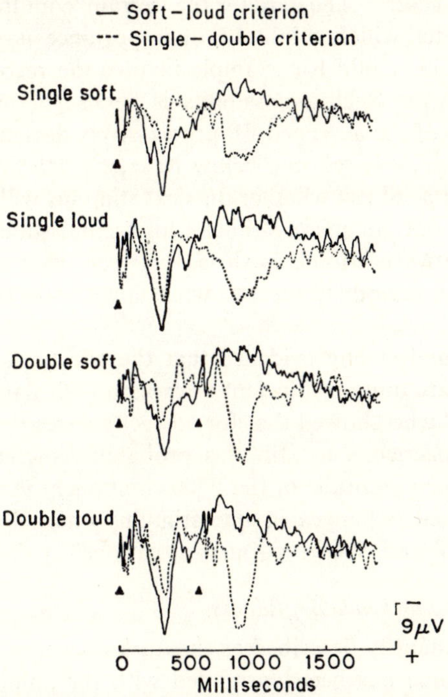

FIGURE 3.1 *Average response waveforms obtained to four types of clicks (as labelled) for one subject. Waveforms —— obtained when the subject is guessing soft* v. *loud; waveforms --- obtained when the subject is guessing single* v. *double.* ▲ *Points at which clicks were delivered. Labels at the left specify the physical characteristics of the stimuli. When a single* v. *double criterion was used a late positive component was recorded whether or not the second stimulus occurred. From S. Sutton, P. Tueting, J. Zubin and E. R. John (1967). 'Information delivery and the sensory-evoked potential', in* Science, ***155****, 1436–1439.*

subject by each low pitched click. The P300 wave was found to be of very small amplitude when the subject knew in advance whether the next stimulus would be a low-pitched or high-pitched click. This is consistent with the 'information delivery' explanation since the information supplied by the soft clicks was then presumably zero. However, under these conditions of zero uncertainty the amplitude of the 300 msec wave although small, was not zero. More importantly, when the experiment was repeated of varying the probability of occurrence of the low-pitched clicks by altering the relative frequencies of the low-pitched and high-pitched clicks, but this time *warning the subject in advance whether the next click would be low pitched or high pitched* then the amplitude of the 300 msec wave again increased as the probability of the low-pitched clicks (F soft) was decreased. The fractional change in amplitude of the 300 msec wave turned out to be roughly the same whether the subject had prior knowledge of the stimulus or whether he had not (Fig. 6.6 in Reference 775). This suggests that explanations utilising the notions of 'information delivery' or 'uncertainty resolution' may not provide a complete explanation in this case.[775] The data for the 'certain' condition suggest that an additional parameter which might be of importance is the mean interval between stimuli. This could for example involve the recovery rate of some peripheral mechanism. Such a possibility is also suggested by reports that late positive waves of the averaged EP progressively decrease in amplitude as the interstimuli interval is reduced below 10 secs.[205, 547, 678] A further possibility is that telling a subject whether the next stimulus will be low-pitched or high-pitched does not adequately control his mental state in an experiment where the time between stimuli is varied between what might seem to the subject rather short periods (2 secs) to what might seem rather long periods (7 secs).

On the other hand strong evidence that the effects of changes of interstimulus intervals are quite insufficient to explain their data was put forward by Tueting *et al.*[793] who showed that for correct guesses the amplitude of the P300 component *decreased* as stimulus probability increased, whereas for incorrect guesses the amplitude of the P300 component *increased* as stimulus probability increased. Changes in interstimulus interval were common to both 'correct-guess' and 'incorrect-guess situations' in this experiment.

3.3.3 *Task-relevance and meaningfulness*

A psychological quantity described as the 'task-relevance' or the 'meaningfulness' of a stimulus has been correlated with the amplitude of transient EP.[128] Chapman and Chapman and Bragden[129] presented letters and numbers in a regular alternate sequence through a window. When numbers were task-relevant the subject was instructed to say which of two numbers was larger; when letters were relevant the subject stated which of two letters was earlier in the alphabet. Task-relevant and task-irrelevant stimuli were presented alternately. The main result of this experiment was that responses to either numbers or letters were found to be larger when the stimuli were task-relevant than when they were task-irrelevant. This distinction held over a wide range of brightness. However, the differences in amplitude which were observed were not great, and no attempt was made to analyse the responses into components of different latencies. In these early experiments some reservation must also be made about the *regularity* of stimulus presentation which might have enabled the subject to alternate attention and inattention. An additional reservation concerns the possible effect of *contour-related* potentials which may have been important components of the EPs recorded and which are known to be very sensitive to changes in accommodation of the eye.[359, 748, S8] (See Section 2.4).

A sharpening of accommodation for each task-relevant stimulus could have resulted in an increased amplitude of contour-specific EP components. Chapman[128] later confirmed his findings for stimuli presented in randomised order. This experiment was, therefore, not open to the objections raised above about possible anticipatory effects. A final general point is that although a subject has been assigned a task involving numbers for example, it is not entirely safe to assume that the alternate stimuli (in this case letters) are in fact task-irrelevant, since the subject might have devised himself a task involving letters and might even be unaware of this.

Only the last criticism is relevant to a later study by Donchin and Cohen[245] in which auditory stimuli were used and in which the greatest amplitude enhancement to 'task-relevant' stimuli occurred for a positive component of roughly 300 msec latency. Donchin and Cohen avoided problems arising from the effects of accommodation on contour-sensitive EP components. They presented their relevant and irrelevant visual stimuli at irregular intervals which varied between 2 and 3 seconds in order to maintain their subjects in a state of constant alertness. Donchin and Cohen reported that the same conditions which gave an enhanced late positive component (250–300 ms) to the task-relevant stimuli gave an attenuated component to the task-irrelevant stimuli. Although the differences seem clear to eyeball inspection in only 3 out of 8 subjects (see Fig. 3, Reference 245), recordings from the occipital region only were presented, whereas the late positive waves seem generally to be most pronounced near the vertex. Näätänen, Donchin and Cohen subsequently exchanged a number of 'letters to the Editor'.[562] Näätänen claimed that Donchin and Cohen did not present their stimulus in a sufficiently irregular manner to prevent their subjects' anticipating the next stimulus. Therefore the reported changes in EP amplitude could not be unequivocally interpreted as being due to task-relevance, since they might also be due in some measure to various kinds of anticipatory reaction. In reply Donchin and Cohen challenged Näätänen's arguments that periodic changes of 'cortical activation' had occurred during their experiments and pointed out that 'task-relevance', *as defined by their experimental paradigm* was in fact the psychological quantity discussed in their paper.

This exchange of letters serves to confirm that any ambiguity or imprecision in defining the psychological terms used in EP research is a most potent source of misunderstanding and confusion.

'Task-relevance' is a notion which overlaps to some extent with 'information delivery'. Both terms have been used to define a psychological correlate of the (idealised) 300 msec EP wave. In practice the operational meaning of both terms has been largely determined by the choice of experimental procedures, rather than the reverse. It is not only the psychological terms, however, that are vague here. The 300 msec positive EP component also seems not to be such a general phenomenon as had been suggested,[775] at least within the narrow definition of P300 described above.

Evidence that the late positive wave is in fact related to 'decision-making', on the part of the subject and not as was suggested by Sutton *et al.*[779] to 'information delivery' was given by Smith *et al.*[741] using auditory stimuli. They found that when a subject was instructed to press a key in response to clicks delivered to only *one* ear, then all clicks delivered to *either* ear gave rise to similar late positive vertex waves which were larger than when the subject transferred his attention to a simultaneously-occurring verbal message. Smith *et al.*, however, did not indicate whether the degree of irregularity of their stimulus presentation was sufficient to allow the anticipatory alerting reaction described by Näätänen[561] to constitute an explanation of their results alternative to 'decision making'.

Donchin and Smith have suggested that the amplitude of the P300 wave and the amplitude of the CNV (Section 3.4) might be *physiologically* related.[249] In marked contrast Donald and Goff[236] pointed out that the amplitudes of the CNV and the amplitude of the P300 component might, in some circumstances, be related for *instrumental* reasons. The experimental paradigms used in some experiments designed to investigate the relation between some psychological variable and the amplitude of the P300 component are quite similar to the basic CNV paradigm (Section 3.4). In some P300 experiments, therefore, a steady negative d.c. potential might be expected to develop in the intervals before a certain stimulus (e.g. before a task-relevant stimulus); this negative d.c. potential would then abruptly fall to zero shortly (roughly 300 msec) after the occurrence of the stimulus. Donald and Goff[236] pointed out that when a.c.-coupled preamplifiers are used (as they are in many EP experiments) an abrupt reduction of a steady negative d.c. potential is seen as a transient positive wave. They showed that such contamination of the P300 wave may be serious in classical P300 paradigms, but that the occurrence and the dependence on stimulus relevance of the P300 wave cannot by any means be explained as an instrumental artifact of the CNV.[S41]

The necessity for careful experimental controls is seldom clearer than in the experiments described in this section, and yet here such controls are peculiarly difficult. In a number of reports which attribute EP changes to changes in the subject's psychological state, alternative explanations such as potentials associated with the act of button pressing, changes in visual accommodation, or changes in stimulus periodicity have not been convincingly eliminated. When a subject's instructions leave him without a task he is unlikely to be in a neutral state.[536, 775] On the contrary a subject may alleviate boredom by devising himself some task or game, and in so doing make a nonsense of the experimental design. This danger is perhaps at its most acute in the type of experiment described in this section. It is undeniably difficult to design clear-cut experiments which test questions relating to subjects' internal states.[S15] Progress towards sharper experiments may perhaps follow more careful attempts to frame subject instructions in such a way that the number of options open to a subject is reduced much more drastically than has commonly been the case.[775] More speculatively, a hint of the possibilities of a completely different approach to this area of EP research is given by reports of the way in which the amplitude of EPs at a specific latency can be reversibly changed by operant conditioning (for example, References 293, 293a).

3.4 Electrical activity which precedes the stimulus

At first sight electrical activity which *precedes* a stimulus might imply extra-sensory perception by the subject. Although such a daring interpretation of the results of an EEG experiment is not unknown,[252] the slow negative-going wave which has been found to anticipate the stimulus in certain experimental situations has so far been associated with such comparatively mundane parameters as the 'contingencies between stimuli' and 'readiness for motor action'.

Scalp potentials which occur before and immediately following the onset of motor activity have been investigated by recording the EEG on one track of a multi-track tape recorder, while recording on another track a signal synchronous with the onset of muscle activity (e.g. a pulse triggered by an EMG burst). By using this technique a series of waves can be identified and associated with movement (Fig. 3.2). Recordings from electrodes within the brain have confirmed the intracerebral origin of these potentials. The relative amplitudes of the different waves show substantial variations from person to person, vary between different movements executed by the same person and vary with the speed and vigour of a particular movement. The whole complex of potentials was labelled the 'motor potential' by Vaughan[319, 816] since he found that *all* components in the complex were bilaterally asymmetrical and were largest over those contralateral areas of motor cortex which represented the moving muscle groups (Fig. 3.4). Vaughan based this claim on his findings that: (*a*) the distributions over the scalp of the potentials associated with voluntary movements of the hands, feet and tongue were in fair agreement with the locations of the various cortical areas whose electrical stimulation results in movements of hands, feet or tongue (Fig. 3.4), and (*b*) the field distribution of the motor potentials over the scalp are similar to the field distribution due to a body of roughly the same size as the motor cortex – the eye in this case.[820]

In contrast, Kornhuber and Deecke reported that only *one* of the components of the complex was largest over the area contralateral to the moving muscle groups. The potentials which have been reported to be associated with movement are:

(*a*) the *readiness potential* (Bereitschaftspotential),[467, 468] a negative wave that builds up slowly in the period (1 to 2 seconds) preceding the onset of movement. This potential is maximal at the vertex and, according to Kornhuber and Deecke, bilaterally symmetrical.[224, 467, 468, S31, 32]

(*b*) the *pre-motion positivity*, a potential which (for finger movements)[818] begins some 80 msec before the onset of movement. According to Kornhuber and Deecke this potential is, like the readiness potential, bilaterally symmetrical but, in contrast, its amplitude is larger over parietal than over precentral regions.[224] This potential is not always observed.[818]

(*c*) the *motor potential.* (Vaughan[319, 842]) This is a sharp, negative-going wave which is bilaterally asymmetrical, and is the only component whose topographical distribution is closely related 'to that part of motor cortex which is active in a specific movement'.[224] This 'motor potential' precedes movement by an interval which depends on the particular muscle group being contracted. For face and tongue movements the interval is 30–50 msec, for hand movements 80–100 msec and for foot dorsiflexion 150–200 msec (see also Chapter 2, Section 2.6.3).

(*d*) A final large positive wave which usually begins shortly after the onset of contraction, but may sometimes precede it is included under the term 'motor potentials' by Vaughan.[224, 319, 698, 818]

Vaughan has suggested that intersubject variability could be one reason for the conflict between the finding of his laboratory that all components of the motor complex have bilateral asymmetries which suggest origins in motor cortex, and the reports of Kornhuber and Deecke that only one component of the complex is bilaterally asymmetric. Gerbrandt *et al.*[313] suggested that other possible explanations for the conflict might be differences in electrode sites, differences between the indifferent electrodes used, differences between the intervals separating successive movements and differences between the method of defining the 'amplitudes' of the components of the complex of potentials. Furthermore they claimed that an abrupt negative component which is maximally asymmetric in front of the Rolandic line biasses the measurements of all other components making them appear bilaterally asymmetric. This negative wave was the only component they suggested to be motoric, although even for this component some doubt was raised by their finding that its largest amplitude was some distance in front of motor cortex.

The interpretation of their findings given by Kornhuber *et al.* is as follows. The readiness potential reflects bilateral activity in the parietal and precentral areas. This activity is connected with planning and preparing for action. The command for movement corresponds to the start of the pre-motion positivity. This message travels to the motor cortex where the motor potential appears some 25 msec after onset of the pre-motion positivity.[224, 468, 466b, S36] On the other hand Vaughan has cited evidence that steady negative shifts may appear both in motor cortex and in sensory cortex, depending on whether the subject's task permits the establishment of a preparatory motor set or whether the task requires a purely sensory discrimination. Furthermore, he has argued for a close relationship between the sharp negative component of the motor complex and synchronous single unit firing in the pyramidal tract.[818]

Grey Walter has attached a quite different significance to a slow negative wave which he found to *precede* stimuli in a variety of experimental situations at about the same time (1964) that Kornhuber and Vaughan first recorded the complex of potentials associated with motor action. There is some conflict about the relation between Walter's data and the complex of potentials just described.

The first few presentations of a novel stimulus produce an alerting response in addition to the EP. The alpha rhythm is blocked, electrical changes may be recorded at the skin, and an 'orienting potential' may appear at the vertex.*[163, 347, S33, 39] The amplitude of the orienting potential rapidly falls as stimuli are successively repeated.[298] Walter found that in man as in animals when the response to a monotonously repeated stimulus has habituated, its initial amplitude may be temporarily restored if an association is established between the stimulus (A) and a second stimulus (B). This restoration is particularly effective and long-lasting if the subject is *motivated* to produce a motor action in response to the second stimulus (B).[163] Under these conditions the negative-going components of the response to the second stimulus (B) appear to be diminished when a.c. coupled preamplifiers are used ('contingent negative habituation'). However, when d.c. coupled preamplifiers are used, the real reason for the apparent attenuation of the second response can be seen to its being 'submerged' under a slow, negative-going wave which precedes the second stimulus and abruptly terminates immediately on the occurrence of the second stimulus.[849, 851] This finding would be in line with the speculation that the cortex may have a fixed capacity for negative shifts so that the slow negative wave may run into this 'ceiling'.[459] According to Cohen, while the association is being established between stimuli A and B, the orienting potential can be seen to fuse into the early part of the slow negative wave.†[163] The onset of this slow negative wave has variously been claimed to be some 200–400 msec[163] or 'greater than 400 msec'[631] after the occurrence of the first stimulus; it is often difficult to distinguish the early part of the slow wave from the late components of the vertex EP to the stimulus.[631] The shape of the slow wave shows marked intersubject variability, and in any given subject depends on the interstimulus interval.[S41] Even though a clear wave will not be sustained unless the subject is *motivated* to produce the motor response, nevertheless the amplitude of the wave is increased when the subject responds with a greater mechanical force.[404, 405] The most widespread controversy has been over the factors which determine the form and amplitude of the slow

* Ritter *et al.*[678] reported that a *positive* wave of peak latency roughly 350 msec correlated with a shift of attention or orienting response, whereas Haider *et al.*[347] associated a *negative* wave with the orienting response. Vaughan (personal communication) was unable to account for this discrepancy. Ritter *et al.*[678] further reported that an N1 (*c.* 100 msec) to P2 (*c.* 180 msec) measure did not correlate with the orienting response and that its observed short-term decrement as the stimulus was repeated was unlikely to be a genuine habituation effect. Ritter *et al.*[678] suggested that the N1–P2 decrement for stimuli following the initial stimulus of a sequence was more probably the well-known effect that longer interstimulus intervals can give larger responses.

† Cohen's statement presumably refers to the *negative* orienting potential described by Cohen[163] and Haider *et al.*[347] and is difficult to relate to the *positive* orienting potential described by Ritter *et al.*

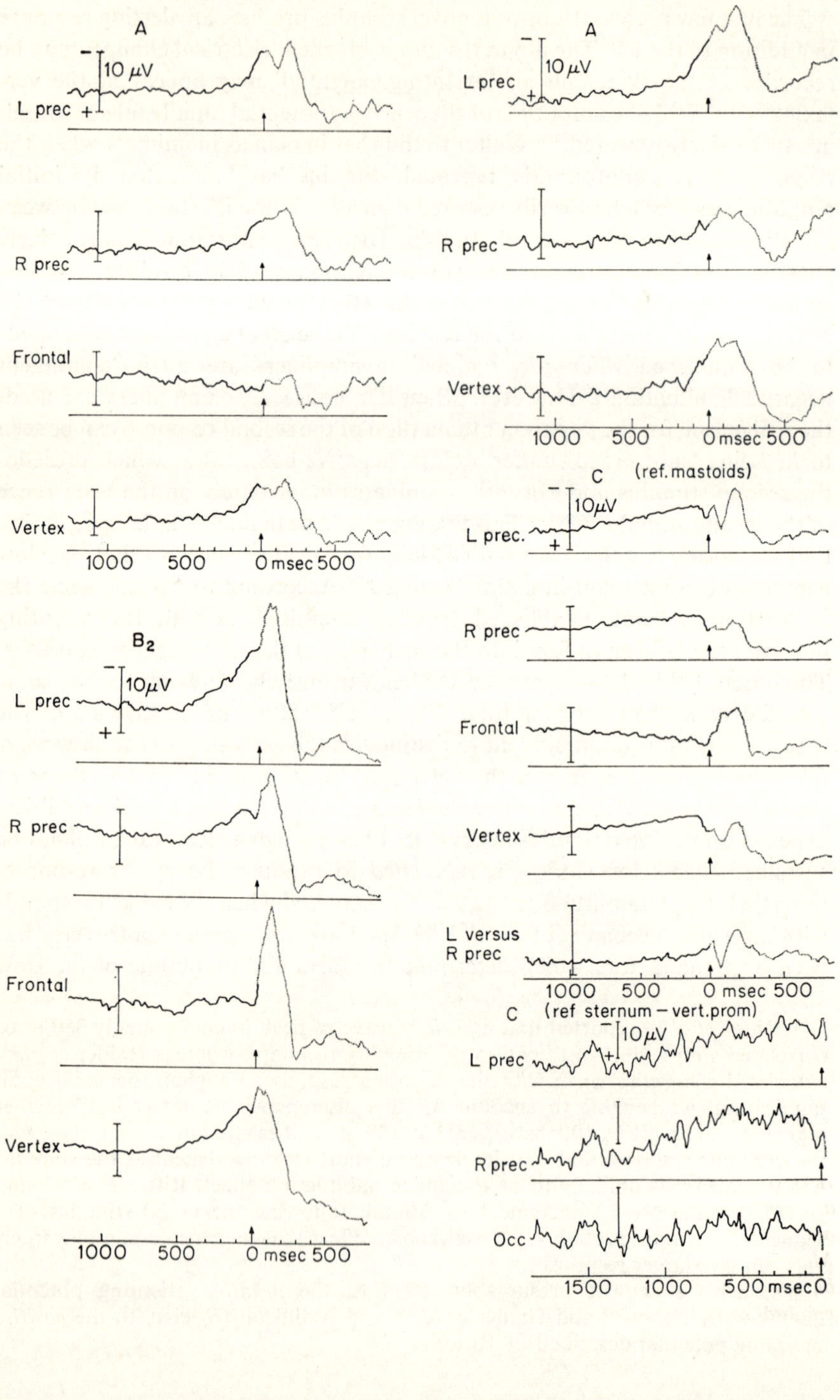

A
10 μV
L prec
R prec
Frontal
Vertex
1000
500
0 msec 500
A
10 μV
L prec
R prec
Vertex
1000
500
0 msec 500
B2
10μV
L prec
R prec
Frontal
Vertex
1000
500
0 msec 500
C (ref. mastoids)
10μV
L prec.
R prec
Frontal
Vertex
L versus R prec
1000
500
0 msec 500
C (ref sternum – vert.prom)
10μV
L prec
R prec
Occ
1500
1000
500 msec 0

negative wave[606] (see below), and even over whether it has a neural basis,[504] but there has in addition been disagreement on how it should be measured.

Walter and his colleagues have described a number of experiments in which they have studied this slow, negative-going wave by using the following paradigm. A click (conditional stimulus) is followed 1 second later by a train of repetitive flashes (imperative stimulus). This pairing is repeated twelve times. The subject's prior instructions are that 'when the flashes start you should press a button as quickly as you can'. Some modest encouragement is provided by arranging that the flash train should be ended by pressing the button. The averaging computer is triggered by the first (conditional) stimulus and *not* by the onset of the motor response. Walter considered that the slow, negative-going potential was governed by the statistical relationship between the first and second stimuli of the stimulus pairs, and for this reason proposed that the name *contingent negative variation* (CNV) or *expectancy wave* (Fig. 3.3). Later evidence that the CNV is related more closely to 'arousal' than to conditional expectancy[509, 510] is difficult to evaluate because of the vagueness and ambiguities of operational definitions of 'arousal'.

Recordings from implanted wires (on the dura) showed the CNV to be synchronous over wide areas of frontal cortex,[S41] so that the amplitude and waveform of the CNV recorded at the scalp is little influenced by the diffusing effect of skull and other overlying material.[848] For the CNV, therefore, in contrast with some EP components,[175, 312, 366] scalp recordings will give a good indication of local cortical potentials.

The CNV is subject to contamination by potentials arising from vertical eye movements, even when the eyes are shut, and even when stimuli are entirely nonvisual.[404, 405, 510] However, such contamination does not entirely account for the CNV, since a clear CNV has been recorded in a subject with no eyes, similar in form to the CNVs which can be recorded in normally sighted subjects when care is taken to control ocular fixation,[510] or when eye artifacts are electrically 'balanced out'.[522] Furthermore, similar CNVs may be recorded from scalp and intracerebral electrodes.[847, 851, S41]

Vaughan has contested Grey Walter's interpretation of the CNV as

FIGURE 3.2. *Original recordings representing 3 of the 4 types of subject. Arrow: onset of the mechanogram. A, left: Type A with additional negativity at all points, but most left precentral and least right precentral. Subject H.J. (left-handed) 181 samples, linked mastoid reference. A, right: Another type A, subject F.K. (right-handed) 227 samples, linked ears reference. B_2: Type B_2 with PMP right precentral and vertex, and negativity left precentral. Subject W.S. (right-handed) 202 samples, linked mastoid reference. C (mastoids): Type C with positivity at all leads, less left precentral. Subject H.B. (right-handed) 180 samples, linked mastoid reference. C (sternum): Type C with a sternum-vertebra prominens reference, showing positivity in all leads including occipital, less at the left precentral electrode. Subject U.F. (right-handed) 287 samples. More noise due to ECG. From L. Deecke, P. Schneid, H. Kornhuber (1969). 'Distribution of readiness potential, premotion, positivity and motor potential of the human cerebral cortex preceding voluntary finger movement', in* Exp. Brain Res., *7, 158–168. Springer-Verlag, New York.*

'reflecting the probability of association between the two stimuli comprising a pair', and has suggested that on the contrary, the CNV might be *no more than* a reflection of 'physiological preparation for motor activity' (in this case, button pressing), though these two interpretations do not appear to be logically inconsistent, and indeed Vaughan's suggestion is not dissimilar to an early interpretation due to Walter that the CNV is 'an electrical sign of cortical priming' whereby 'responses to associated stimuli are economically accelerated'.[851] Conversely, Cohen has suggested that the motor potential of Gilden *et al.*[319] might be *no more than* a CNV where both the stimuli of the CNV paradigm have been internalised.[163]

Evidence which at first sight weighs against suggestions that the CNV is no more than a potential which depends on motor activity is the finding that a CNV can be sustained in the absence of any overt motor action, and even in the absence of external stimuli.[165, 510, 519, 849] On the other hand it might be claimed that physiological preparations for motor action might occur, with their associated electrical signs, even though an overt motor response did not result. Indeed it has been suggested that the common factor in all conditions where a slow negative shift of potentials is observed is a 'mental preparation to make a response', and that CNV should in fact denote 'conative negative variation'.[510, 519] This interpretation is not dissimilar to Walter's earlier view that the 'expectancy wave (E – wave) —— reflects very accurately the attitude of the subject to the stimulus association *and his intention to act on it*' (author's italics). Donald[235] has suggested that the CNV occurs during any period of intense short-term concentration and does not occur only during anticipatory states. He further suggested that the CNV may reflect the activity of a functional system distinct from the general arousal system. Rebert and Knott[631] pointed out that their value for the latency of the CNV (roughly 470 msec) was close to the 500 msec interval (between the conditioned stimulus and the unconditioned stimulus) which gives the most rapid rate of learning in classical Pavlovian conditioning. They suggested that simultaneity of CNV onset and the occurrence of the unconditioned stimulus might be 'an important conjunction in classical conditioning'.[S45]

The conclusion of Irwin *et al.*[404, 405] that, in human subjects, motivation is a more important determinant of the CNV than conditional expectancy may not be far removed from Kornhuber and Deecke's view[468] that the amplitude of their readiness potential is increased by the 'intentional engagement' of the subject, and decreased by his 'mental indifference' and accords with McAdam and Seales'[521] evidence than the amplitude of the readiness potential increases when the subject's motivation grows. Evidence linking Kornhuber's readiness potential with the CNV was reported by Walter.[850] When it was arranged that the motor act of button pressing is followed by an 'interesting' consequence after a delay of 1 second or so, then the negative-going readiness potential persists until the result of the motor action has been observed. Under these circumstances, therefore, the CNV and the readiness potential are very similar (at a single electrode at any rate).

There is some discrepancy between the descriptions offered by different laboratories of the relation between CNV and the potentials associated with motor action. Vaughan claims that the distribution of the slow negative shift observed in the classical CNV paradigm (see above) is consistent with a generator site in motor cortex contralateral to the responding muscles.[818, 820]

Vaughan's account stresses the similarity of the (asymmetrical) distribution of his slow negative motor potentials and the distribution of his CNV-like response. This conflicts with the account of Walter and his colleagues who found the CNV to be bilaterally symmetric;[847] and (as described above) also conflicts with Kornhuber and Deecke's findings. Unless eye movements were a serious contaminant in Walter's and also in Kornhuber and Deecke's experiments, and unless the effects of intersubject variability had been underestimated by these workers, then it would seem that Vaughan on the one hand, and Walter, Kornhuber and Deecke on the other hand are discussing different 'CNV's'.

In disagreement with the published views both of Walter's group and Kornhuber's group, Vaughan has suggested that slow (approximate to d.c.) potential shifts, of which Walter's CNV is one example, may comprise at least three components. These are (1) vertical eye movements,[510] (2) the *readiness potential* of Kornhuber and Deecke and (3) d.c. shifts generated in or near primary sensory cortex.[461b] Slow potentials shifts of the type originally described by Kohler[461b] have received little attention since their discovery twenty years ago – partly due to the technical difficulties of d.c. recording. There is, however, recent intriguing evidence that slow negative shifts of potential can be observed, not over the vertex, as when the classical motor-orientated CNV paradigm is employed, but displaced towards the occipital region when the subject's task is one of purely visual discrimination.[163, 818]

3.5 Evoked potentials and learning

Roy John and his colleagues have been particularly active in the search for slow-wave neuroelectric correlates of learning. Over many years they have recorded evoked potentials from wires implanted in the brains of animals while the animals learnt a sensory discrimination task. John reported that the processes of learning and recall were paralleled by changes in evoked potential waveshapes.[418–421, 423, 424, 426, 693]

John's central claim is that two processes influence the waveshapes of the potentials evoked by sensory stimuli. These processes are (*a*) 'exogenous', in other words determined entirely by the physical parameters of the stimulus, and (b) 'endogenous', that is *released* in the brain by the triggering action of the stimulus and determined by the present state and prior experience of the organism. These latter components are of greater latency than the former components.

The triggering action of a single type of stimulus causes the same released waveshape to appear in many functionally different brain structures including cortex, thalamus and mesencephalon. To within a millisecond or so the released waveshape appears *simultaneously* in these different structures. The most obvious explanation of such a widespread distribution – that is, 'salt solution' conduction – is not tenable, since although released waveshapes may indeed be of large amplitude in adjacent structures, they may nevertheless be separated by a region in which the response is comparatively small.

An early example of an experiment in which exogenous and endogenous EP components were distinguished is as follows. An animal was trained to perform a conditioned response on presentation of a conditioned stimulus (flicker at frequency F_1 (7·7 Hz)). John found that when the animal gave correct responses, then the EPs recorded from various brain structures were of periodicity F_1 Hz. When the animal was subsequently stimulated by flicker of frequency F_2 (10 Hz), which differed from frequency F_1, the animal sometimes performed the previously learned response. (This phenomenon of an animal performing a conditioned response on presentation of a novel stimulus which has some similarity to the conditioned stimulus is called 'generalisation'.) When generalisation occurred, the EPs recorded from various brain structures appeared (to visual inspection) to be composed of a component whose periodicity was the same as that of the physical stimulus (F_2) and a second component of periodicity F_1.[418] The EPs evoked by flicker of frequency F_2 were however of quite different waveshape when the animal had subsequently learnt to differentiate behaviourally between flicker stimuli of frequencies F_1 and F_2. Under these conditions, flicker of frequency F_2 evoked potentials whose periodicity was the same as that of the stimulus.[418]

John's view is that when generalisation occurs, a stored representation of prior experience (i.e. conditioning to perform a response on presentation of the conditioned stimulus F_1) is recalled by the novel stimulus F_2.[249] The neural activity underlying the recall of this prior experience was, John suggested, reflected by the released EP components.[418, 693] This conclusion was at first based on visual inspections of EP waveshapes,[418] but in order to establish a more quantitative basis John later used statistical analysis, and factor analysis (Chapter 5, Section 5.4.11[418 pp. 336–343]) to describe waveshape differences.

The essence of John and his colleagues' thesis is that slow waves can reflect the storage and retrieval of information. The neural representation of information stored in the brain is not on their view the activity of certain hypothetical coded cells which 'stand for' specific items of information, but is rather certain spatiotemporal patterns of organised activity (specifically coherent activity) in enormous aggregates of neurons.[418 p. 419] John has assembled evidence to support his view that 'released' (endogenous) slow waves, by influencing the probability of spike firing within a local region of the brain, thereby indicate the time course of the average spike activity of a population of neurons.[418 p. 414]

4
Clinical applications of evoked potentials

4.1 Introduction

This chapter is divided into two sections. The first is a sober account of what has so far been achieved in the clinical application of EP methods. The second section includes a more roseate discussion of what might be achieved in the future and an outline of the fundamental research whose clinical possibilities have not yet been much explored.

It seemed worthwhile to present the text of the first section of this chapter under two headings. The first covers EP methods of testing sensory pathways which might be used to advantage in conjunction with, or in place of, conventional subjective testing procedures. At the present time the need for objective tests most commonly arises when examining uncooperative patients such as young infants. The second heading covers the use of EPs in fundamental clinical studies of disease processes.

Both in diagnostic and research applications, EP methods are likely to be of most value as one of a battery of tests rather than in isolation.

At the present time EP techniques can claim no more than minor clinical importance, except perhaps in testing the hearing of infants and children. The following pages discuss why this is so and argue that EPs may soon come to play a number of valuable roles in diagnosis and clinical research.

Given the indications of Chapter 2 that EPs show considerably greater promise than is indicated by their achievements to date it might still be asked *why* there has so far been little clinical return from EP research to match the expenditure of effort and money invested in the field. The following factors may have contributed to this situation (1) since a large number of variables exert complex influences on the EP, and since some variables are not clearly defined, the field demands exceptional rigour in experimental design. This has not always been evident. Furthermore, the 'suck it and see' experimental approach seems to be almost as fruitless in EP work as an experimental programme designed along too inflexible preconceived lines; (2) since EP recording is still a developing research technique it has seldom been practicable to market the simplified, stereotyped devices which could easily be operated by technical staff after a short training course. Research workers may enthusiastically develop a new clinical technique but are likely to have moved on to some fresh problem when the time-consuming routine application of their technique is called for (reference 454a gives an illuminating insight into this point); (3) again, partly because of their flexibility, commercial averaging devices are still too expensive for other than the largest and richest hospitals. Even in these the use of experimental stimulation and recording procedures may be severely restricted by limited workshop and technical resources.

A supporting argument is sometimes advanced that EP recording is the only practical means of access to the electrical activity within the sensory pathways of the intact human brain. This chapter argues that EP methods may both reflect perceptual events (see Section 33)[S35] and offer access to the 'feature filters'[23, 50, 51, 283, 399, 489, 527] which shape the content of perception. On the other hand it is by no means established that scalp EPs are not 'blind' to the particular aspects of central brain activity which underlie thought processes and intelligence.

The clinical future of evoked potentials can be said, almost without exaggeration, to depend on only one factor. This factor is the degree of reliance which the clinician places on the technique. The scientific, technical and financial obstacles to the clinical application of EP methods would assume the significance of 'problems to be overcome' rather than 'reasons for not trying' if it became clear that EPs could give information to the clinician which was decisive in his choice of clinical management of patients. Morrell and Morrell[555] have suggested that evoked potentials may come to play a role in bridging the gap between neurology and psychiatry by providing methods of assessing the functional integrity of brain systems which process information, and thereby offering to the neurologist objective access to the hypothetical minimal brain damage 'which results in reading disorders, speech difficulty, distractibility and some forms of mental retardation'.

It may well be true that the major scientific obstacle encountered in applying EP methods to clinical problems is the shallowness of our basic understanding of scalp potentials. At the present time there is an urgent need to strengthen the internal consistency of EP data and to relate it more fully to the general store of neurophysiological knowledge. Perhaps the first priority in clinical research is to study the effects of a much wider range of stimulus parameters than has hitherto been customary, and furthermore to select those parameters more on the basis of clinical or 'physiological appropriateness' than on the basis of how easy they are to measure. Among the gaps in our basic knowledge of EPs are: (1) a firm understanding of the sites of EP *generators* (e.g. cortical sites) (see Chapter 1, 1.2 – 1.2.4 and Chapter 2); (2) a knowledge of the neuroanatomical sites at which different EP features are *determined*, as distinct from generated (e.g. retinal sites); (3) specifications of the norms and the normal intersubject variability of different EP features in each of a wide variety of stimulus situations; (4) specifications of the norms and normal intersubject variability of a variety of EP features at different stages of maturation of the CNS, again using a wide variety of stimuli; (5) specification of the EP changes which, in a wide variety of stimulus situations, together define pathological changes in a particular neuroanatomical region, and (6) an established basis for distinguishing between on the one hand the effects on the EP of changes in the internal psychological state of the subject (e.g. attention, anxiety) and on the other hand the effects of lower level activity (e.g. information processing at retinal level). Such a method of discrimination between different EP components might be based on, for example, latency differences, differences in topographical distributions, or different rates of habituation (see Chapter 3).

4.2(a) Sensory testing

4.2.1 *Sensitivity to stimulus intensity; audiometry*

INTRODUCTION

At the present time the major clinical application of evoked potentials is, by a long way, the assessment of hearing in uncooperative or uncommunicative patients. These patients may be adults who may be suspected of malingering, as for example in tests for industrial hearing injury,[377] but for the most part are infants and children. It is difficult to decide whether an infant who shows no behavioural response to sound really is deaf, and more difficult still to determine whether its apparent deafness is due (*a*) to peripheral damage, or (*b*) to brain damage, mental retardation or psychosis. It is important to detect peripheral hearing loss at an early stage so that a hearing aid can be prescribed or appropriate education arranged. Davis considers that EP audiometry, particularly when used in conjunction with behavioural audiometry, justifies its expense by allowing vital early decisions to be made about the handling of young children and infants.

Rapin has cited cases of infants who, were it not for EP audiometry, might have been thought completely deaf or autistic. She describes how residual hearing was detected in these multiply-handicapped patients. As a result, effective hearing aids were prescribed and tested, again by EP audiometry (Fig. 4.1).[452,627,628]

THE AUDITORY VERTEX POTENTIAL

In 1938 Loomis *et al.*[505] reported that a response to auditory stimulation could be observed in the raw EEG during sleep. The first negative component was followed by a large positive wave at a latency of some 750 msec; they called this response the 'K complex'. One year later Pauline Davis described a diphasic negative-positive 'on response' which started 50–100 msec after tonal stimulation.[206] Its amplitude grew larger as subjects became drowsy. In the same year H. Davis reported that in light sleep the 'on response' was followed by a much larger wave, maximal at the vertex. This series of waves (V potential)[40, 306] was similar to the K complex[201] and could be detected to tones only 20 db above subjective threshold. Davis reported that similar vertex potentials were evoked by visual and tactile stimulation so that the reponses appeared to be nonspecific; Hrbek *et al.*,[398] however, has reported that in neonates at any rate, and probably in adults too (referencing Grey Walter),

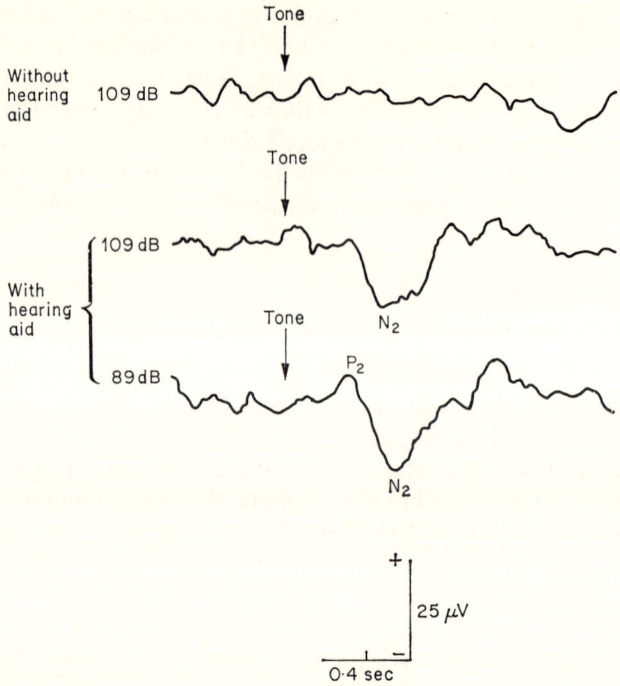

FIGURE 4.1 *Improvement in threshold for the auditory-evoked response by the wearing of a hearing aid. All traces obtained on the same day in a 21-month-old girl with rubella sedated with chlorpromazine. Stimuli: 500 Hz. Derivation: left temporoparietal to mastoids. Analysis time, 2 seconds; prestimulus delay, 0·5 second. From I. Rapin and L. J. Graziani (1967). 'Auditory-evoked responses in normal, brain-damaged and deaf infants', in* Neurology, *17, 881–894.*

that the visual vertex potential is quite different in form from the somatosensory or auditory vertex potentials. The auditory vertex potential generally takes the form of four major waves: P1 (vertex-positive, 50–60 msec), N1 (vertex-negative, 95–105 msec), P2 (vertex-positive, 170–200 msec) and N2 (vertex-negative, *c.* 200 msec)[203] (Fig. 4.2). The latencies and relative amplitudes of the peaks depend strongly on age and behavioural state, on the rise and fall-time of the stimulus tone burst,[547] and probably also on the stimulus duration.[200, 203]

S38

THE RECORDING OF AUDITORY EPS

The recording of auditory EPs to low sound levels became a routine clinical procedure with the advent of the averaging computer.[198] In adults and children the most pronounced feature of the V potential is the N1–P2 deflection and this is the measure which is most generally used. Some investigators, however, use quite different measures of amplitude. Keidel's group measure the amplitude of a 150 msec peak (more recently the area under this peak) from a baseline. The use of a baseline avoids the problem of confounding the behaviour of two quite different peaks (e.g. N1 and P2). Such confusion is a

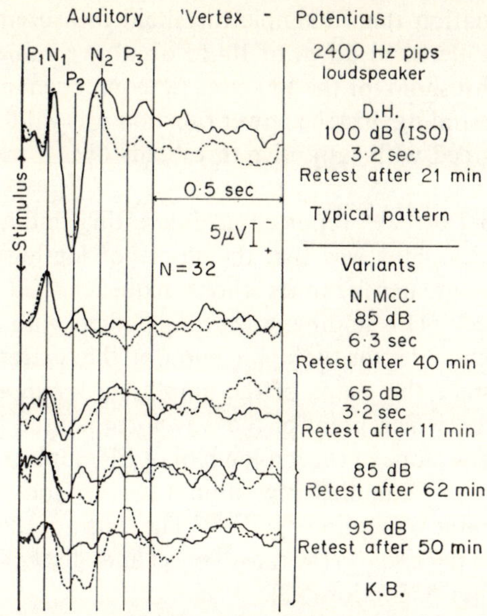

FIGURE 4.2 *Typical pattern and variants of slow-evoked response (V potential) to auditory stimuli. Upward deflection means vertex more negative. 2400 c/sec pips were presented by loudspeaker at regular intervals. K.B. is a subject with variable patterns. D.H.'s and N.McC.'s patterns are very different from one another but both are very consistent. From H. Davis, T. Mast, N. Yoshie and S. Zerlin (1966). 'The slow response of the human cortex to auditory stimuli:recovery processes', in* Electro-enceph. clin. Neurophysiol., ***21**, 105–113. Elsevier Publishing Co., Amsterdam.*

danger of the peak-to-trough amplitude measure. On the other hand with the baseline-to-peak measure there are serious problems in defining the baseline. In the neonate the two most constant waves are P2 and N2, and the P2–N2 measure has been used in Rapin's group.

Averaged auditory EPs have been described both by Rapin and by Davis *et al.*[203] as consisting of two parts, neither of which originates in primary cortex. The early part is mainly myogenic in origin, as described by Bickford (Chapter 5), (although Davis *et al.*[203] suggested that a small, early [30 msec peak latency] wave may be neurogenic in origin). The second part of the auditory EP is a 'nonspecific'* K complex. Drowsiness enhances the K complex and attenuates the myogenic component (probably due to muscular relaxation).

Keidel, Spreng and colleagues reported that one particular component of the auditory EP in the waking adult, defined by its negativity at the glabella (relative to a temporal electrode) and latency of 150 msec, could be shown to be modality-specific, and not of myogenic origin. Their evidence was that a plot of log (EP amplitude) *versus* stimulus intensity in db was a straight line whose slope was the same as that of the Stevens sensory magnitude plot (see Chapter 2, Section 2.2).[446–448, 450] They claimed that the form of these curves

* See Sections 5.4.8 and 4.3.3 for discussions of 'nonspecific'.

gives more information than a simple threshold measurement.[763] Although EPs could only be detected down to 10–15 db above subjective threshold,* the extrapolated threshold for the 150 msec EP component could be estimated from the graph (assuming that the power function was valid to threshold) and these estimates agreed with subjective thresholds over a wide range of tonal frequencies.[107, 450]

Tyberghein and Forrez[804] reported an interesting finding which calls for confirmatory studies. This was that the slopes of log-log amplitude *versus* intensity plots were greater for tones whose frequencies fell in the range most important for speech. This finding, however, conflicts with other reports.[447]

Some care is demanded in the application of the 'extrapolation to threshold' procedure since the shape of the amplitude *versus* intensity function depends strongly on which point of the waveform is used for the amplitude measurement.[764] The slope of the log-log plot of EP amplitude *versus* intensity depends markedly on stimulus repetition rate, as does the slope of the psychophysical loudness function.[450, 547, 630] The shape of the amplitude *versus* intensity curve also depends on the rate of onset and offset of the stimulus tone burst[547] (see Chapter 5, Section 5.3).

If a reliable assessment of an infant's or child's hearing is to be obtained, it is essential to pay close attention to details of the recording procedure. This point is extensively discussed in the literature, which gives the impression that in audiology there is no substitute for experience. Commercial recording equipment which is specifically designed for EP audiology is available (see Appendix) and recording techniques have been thoroughly discussed.[627, 762] However, adequate recording equipment is not enough. With children older than $1\frac{1}{2}$ years or so sedation is not necessary, but it is essential to have a skilful nurse who can apply the electrodes and ensure that the child is in the correct psychological state for audiometry.[628; 248 pp. 322–324] Roughly 40 minutes working time is the maximum with awake children. The criteria for the EP detection threshold are not easy to quantify, especially if the individual peculiarities of the patient's waveform are not known; it can be helpful to record a visual or (better) a tactile EP so as to define the characteristic waveform for the individual patient.[248 p. 323] Confidence in recognising the EP waveform in the presence of noise can be increased by the use of the $\pm$ reference.[627]

* The 'detection threshold' for the V potential is the least stimulus intensity which gives a visually-recognisable potential waveform. In general the value of the detection threshold for an EP has most probably little physiological significance since it depends strongly on instrumental factors such as, e.g., number of sweeps. An alternative method of estimating EP threshold is to plot EP amplitude *versus* stimulus intensity with axes chosen so that a straight line is obtained. An estimate of threshold (the 'extrapolated threshold') can then be obtained by extrapolating the graph to zero stimulus intensity. The use of extrapolated thresholds does, however, involve an assumption which often is untested by experiment. This assumption is that the functional relationship between EP amplitude and stimulus intensity which can be experimentally demonstrated for high EP amplitudes also holds for the lower EP amplitudes where experimental verification is less straightforward.

In infants and children the amplitude of the V potential is larger in certain stages of sleep than in the awake subject.[55, 627, 679] In some mentally retarded subjects the EP threshold may be considerably (25 db or more) above behavioural threshold.[682]

The N1–P2 amplitude of the response to auditory stimulation depends on temporal features of stimulation. A large increase in amplitude can be obtained by increasing the length of the interstimulus interval from 0·5 to 2·5 secs. Rothman and Davis found[686] the amplitude of the EP to increase more slowly as the interstimulus interval was increased beyond 2·5 sec, but Rau[630] reported appreciable gains up to a frequency of one stimulus per 30 secs. Milner[547] reported that EPs saturated at medium stimulus intensities for repetition rates faster than 0·3 Hz, but not for rates appreciably slower than 0·3 Hz. A small increase in amplitude results when stimuli are presented irregularly rather than regularly. There is, however, conflict about the size of this effect.[446, 447, 686, 804] This conflict might partly be due to the effect of varying mean interstimulus intervals, since mean interstimulus interval depends on the method of randomisation. Overlapping and/or interactions between the neurophysiological responses to the onset and to the offset of an auditory stimulus can lead to confusion when comparing the results of studies where stimuli of different durations have been used since the waveform of the EP can depend on stimulus duration.[452, 759, 763] As a further complication, the relation between the onset and offset EPs are different for tonal and noise stimulation.[452] It has been suggested that certain differences between EP measurements for binaural and monaural stimulation might offer possibilities for distinguishing between peripheral and central defect.[452]

There is not one but several reasons why the amplitude of an averaged EP may be small. These include (*a*) small individual responses and (*b*) variable latency of individual responses. Point (*b*) has been discussed by Spreng.[760]

EP AUDIOMETRY

A number of workers have carried out EP audiometry by determining EP detection thresholds defined as the least stimulus intensities which give recognisable nonspecific V potentials. Good correlations have been reported between the results of EP audiometry and conventional pure tone audiometry in adult patients with peripheral hearing loss.[161, 162, 780]* Evoked potential audiometry is capable therefore of supplying the useful clinical information that hearing loss is greatest in some particular frequency range.

Davis validated the detection threshold method of EP audiometry for children between 4 and 10 years old by comparing EP and behavioural thresholds in 162 children. No drugs were used, and the children were fully conscious. The average difference, case by case, between the EP and behavioural thresholds was 5 db.[198, 199, 202] Evoked response audiometry was validated for infants under one year of age by Rapin.[627, 628] Recordings were made during sleep in order to obtain a favourable signal-to-noise ratio for

* See supplementary footnote No. 35 for a quite different approach to EP audiometry.

the EP. Threshold was defined as the stimulus intensity which gave a recognisable EP in 50% of the records. In most cases sleep was spontaneous; when sedation was necessary chlorpromazine was found suitable since it had little effect on threshold.[627, 628]

Thresholds to pure tones of frequencies between 250 Hz and 800 Hz are similar in neonates and adults.[274] In sleep, EP detection thresholds are roughly 15 db higher than behavioural thresholds.[628] In most cases brain damage does not interfere with EP audiometry, although severe brain damage can be a hindrance. Rapin considers that EP audiometry rarely underestimates the severity of an infant's peripheral hearing loss. If, therefore, a behaviourally deaf child shows only moderate impairment when tested with the EP, then the clinician can feel confident that the child's deafness cannot be explained by severe peripheral damage.[628] Rapin has further emphasised the point that the presence of clear auditory EPs does not necessarily mean that the child can 'hear' in the sense of utilising the auditory signals to modify its behaviour.[627]

4.2.2 *Tests for the integrity and special functions of a sensory pathway*

VISUAL ACUITY

Evoked potential studies of patients with poor vision have been made using both spots of light and patterned fields for stimulation. The results of these studies indicate that *both* these types of stimuli should be used routinely in EP assessments of visual function, since some of the most valuable clinical information is obtained only by comparing the two types of EP.

In a group of patients with normal vision in only one eye Copenhaver and Perry compared the results of stimulating the affected and the 'good' eye with flashes of 2·5° subtense.[178] All patients had lesions peripheral to the chiasma. These included retinal detachments, macular scars, and optic neuritis. In most cases the EPs elicited by stimulation of the affected eye were much smaller than the EPs due to stimulation of the 'good' eye (by factors of 2 to 10 times). In contrast, stimulation of an eye whose poor vision was entirely due to refractive errors gave EPs little different from the control EPs in which the 'good' eye only was stimulated. If, therefore, when an eye with poor vision has its fovea stimulated by a light spot the resulting EPs are markedly depressed, then a neural lesion is suggested and the impaired vision is unlikely to be due merely to defects in the imaging structures of the eye. Conversely, a defect of the imaging structure alone is suggested when a foveal stimulation by a small spot of light is found to give EPs of normal amplitudes.[178, 731] Perry and Childers[604] confirmed EP depression in amblyopia for small foveal targets, but found no effect for large (20°) stimulus fields.[S55] Shipley's[731] method for ensuring good fixation in EP studies has obvious clinical value (see Chapter 5, Section 5.1.2). His observation that in amblyopic patients, but not in normal subjects, the EP for the 'good' eye is markedly depressed by stimulating the fellow eye with diffuse light suggests that there is an abnormal interaction between the eyes or an abnormal sensitivity to diffuse light in amblyopic patients.

The sharpness of the retinal image has a marked effect on EP amplitude when spatially patterned stimuli are used, in contrast with findings when small light spots are employed. In normal subjects the amplitude of the EP to pattern-reversal is very sensitive to ocular accommodation; it has been claimed that a 50% change in amplitude can result from only a 0·3 dioptre disaccommodation.[157, 748, 801, S8, 17, 23] The amplitude of EPs to transient flash presentations of checkerboard patterns are also sensitive to defocusings which do no more than blur the edges of the pattern elements without destroying the structure.

Harter[359] reported that defocusing a checkerboard pattern produced different effects on the two prominent components of the transient EP which have latencies of roughly 100 msec and 200 msec.[S49] Nevertheless, either of these components could be used to carry out an objective refraction procedure for the correction of defective vision.[359, 363] Fig. 4.3 shows the results of this EP procedure. The EP test predicted correcting lenses whose powers were the same as those prescribed by conventional subjective testing. The point can be made here that if the EP were to be routinely used in refraction, steady-state EPs might have some advantage over transient EPs since by using Fourier Analysis (Chapter 5) a considerable improvement in speed and precision ought to be possible; in addition, cheap, special-purpose equipment could be used. These might be worthwhile advantages in the clinical situation.[S52]

There are two points which demand attention when recording pattern-EPs. Firstly, the potentials evoked by stimulation of upper and lower halves

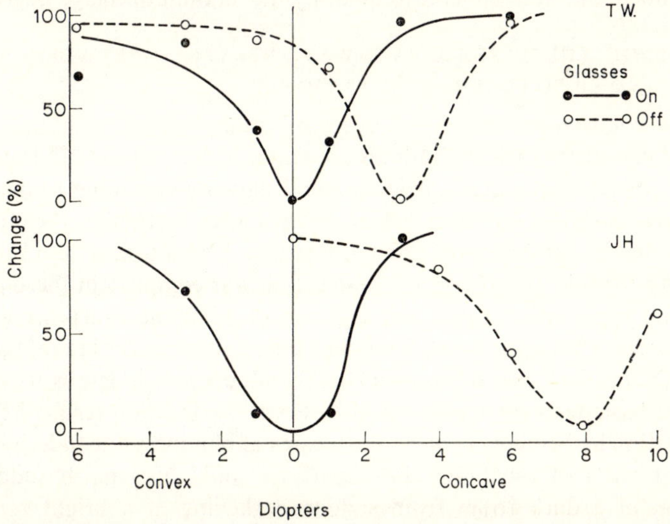

FIGURE 4.3 *Variations in component 'A' (90–100 msec latency) as a function of viewing lenses and whether corrective glasses were worn for 2* Ss *who required relatively large refractive corrections. When these* Ss *wore their glasses, their response functions resembled those of* Ss *requiring little or no correction. From M. R. Harter (1968). 'Effects of contour sharpness and check-size on visually evoked cortical potentials', in* Vision Res., ***8****, 701–711. Pergamon Press, Oxford.*

of the retina are largely independent and in many subjects have opposite polarities, especially when transient stimuli are used (Chapter 2, Section 2.10.2). As a result the use of full-field stimulation can result in waveform changes because of cancellation between EPs from upper and lower half-fields,[413, 414] and although this does not seem to have hindered Harter's refraction procedure, it might introduce unnecessary difficulties with some subjects which could be avoided by stimulating either the upper or lower half-field alone.*[S16]

The second point applies to control data obtained from studies of subjects with normal vision. A commonly-used method of investigating the effect of degrading the retinal image is to place lenses in front of the eye. This method has the disadvantage that the eye has some range of accommodation and so may take up some of the error. Also the eye will then be 'hard against' one end of its accommodation range, and this might lead to undesirable complications in some experiments. The method of briefly presenting the stimulus in a dark environment seems to overcome this problem,[363] but it is restricted in its application to transient EPs. For steady-state recording, the eye can be accommodated on a mark outside the plane of the stimulus, and the effective disaccommodation calculated (in dioptres).[801] However, this method is limited to small disaccommodations, and is difficult to use with binocular stimulation. All these difficulties can be avoided by defocusing the target itself, either optically (when the target is a projected transparency) or by constructing degraded targets. On the other hand, this method carries the disadvantage that it is difficult to quantify the amount of image degradation.

LESIONS OF THE VISUAL PATHWAY. RELATION BETWEEN SITE OF LESION AND EP TO FLASH STIMULATION

There is controversy about the effect of brain lesions on human vision. Cases of complete cortical blindness are scarce in the literature.[98] In the great majority of reported cases cortically blind patients were able to distinguish light from darkness by some hours or days after sustaining their occipital wounds during combat, even though many had been totally blind for some time after the injury.[97] If cortical destruction was complete in these patients, the above observation raises the question of what the functions might be of the 20–30%[76] of optic nerve fibres which do not run to the lateral geniculate nucleus,[S50] but few case reports of cortical blindness include details of other than the most basic tests for visual function. Some clarification resulted from the investigation by Brindley *et al.*[98] of two cases of blindness due to lesions of the posterior parts of the brain. Both patients could distinguish sudden illumination of a dark room from sudden darkening of a bright room, but completely failed a number of other tests of visual function, including the discrimination of steady light from steady darkness. There is sharp conflict between these findings for brain-injured man, and reports on the behavioural

* Furthermore, for EPs, the central 1° and parafovea are weighted differently in upper and lower half-field.

effects of brain lesions in monkeys. The removal of striate cortex leaves a monkey able to reach accurately for objects using visual cues only, and able to make a number of discriminations between visual stimuli. The monkey's rapid response to moving visual stimuli contrasts dramatically with its apparent blindness to static objects.[182, 183, 320, 402, 598, 707, 859, 876] Such findings form part of the body of evidence which supports the hypothesis that there are two neural mechanisms for visuomotor control, one concerned with locating and the other with identifying objects.[403]

It is hardly surprising that behavioural tests of brain-damaged laboratory primates have produced much more information about subtle sensory losses than has subjective testing of brain-damaged human patients, the latter often carried out in difficult circumstances (e.g. see Reference 387). This disparity may be at least partially remedied by psychophysical studies on sensory losses in brain-damaged war veterans which are currently in progress.[664] In any case the conflict between the human and monkey data might be due to incomplete or diffuse brain damage in the human patients, rather than reflecting a genuine inter-species difference. This uncertainty about the subjective effects of occipital lesions does not necessarily detract from the importance of efforts to correlate changes in scalp potentials with the sites of focal lesions in brain-damaged monkeys.

Vaughan and Gross[821] recorded potentials evoked by flash stimuli from epidural electrodes over striate, prestriate, inferotemporal and frontal cortex before and after brain injuries. These included unilateral striate lesions, unilateral optic tract section and unilateral inferotemporal lesions. The results are summarised in Fig. 4.4. They concluded that the wavelets in the striate cortical EP reflected the geniculo-calcarine input, but that the slower components were derived in addition from a contralateral input (possibly cortico-cortical via the left and right prestriate cortices and the corpus callosum). Parietal EPs were similar to striate EPs except that they had smaller amplitudes and longer latencies. The early negative component of the inferotemporal EP was attributed largely to subcortical input; the later components were attributed only partly to subcortical input. The EPs from frontal cortex were 'something of a puzzle' since they were not affected by any of the lesions listed above.

In man, lesions which are sufficiently severe to result in hemianopic field defects give in most cases decreased alpha activity over the damaged hemisphere.[64, 166, S47] Such a lesion also produces changes in visually evoked scalp potentials which, in contrast to the EEG changes, offer considerable possibilities for the location of the lesion to some site along the visual pathway (see below).*

There certainly seems to be a real clinical need for such a supplement to the established EEG and ERG procedures in the diagnosis of visual lesions.

* There seems to be insufficient direct evidence to support any worthwhile discussion on whether EP methods can distinguish between similarly-sited but different types of brain lesion, e.g. tumours and infarcts.

FIGURE 4.4 *Summary of effects of lesions**

Lesion	on Striate Response		on Prestriate Response		on Inferotemporal Response	
	ipsilaterally	contralaterally	ipsilaterally	contralaterally	ipsilaterally	contralaterally
unilateral optic tract section	elimination of early wavelets and marked reduction in amplitude of other components	reduction in amplitude of all components except early wavelets	elimination of early wavelets, reduction in amplitude of remaining response, and earlier onset of positive wave	reduction in amplitude of entire response and earlier onset of positive wave	radical reduction of entire response	variable
unilateral striate ablation		as above	as above	as above	marked reduction in variance of late components and some decrease in their amplitude	marked reduction in variance of late components
unilateral inferotemporal lesion	no effect	no effect	effects seemed dependent on presence or absence of contralateral striate cortex			effects seemed dependent on presence or absence of contralateral striate cortex

The evoked responses recorded from frontal cortex were unaffected by the experimental lesions

* H. G. Vaughan and C. G. Gross (1969). 'Cortical responses to light in unanaethetised monkeys and their alteration by visual system lesions', in *Exp. Brain Res.*, ***8***, *19–36*. Springer-Verlag, New York.

Jacobson and Hirose[407, 408] have discussed the point that such a conventional diagnostic procedure as an examination of the fundus does not reveal the cause of many children's visual problems. In such cases the ERG has proved to be a valuable clinical tool and has been used to differentially detect functional disease involving the retinal receptor and bipolar layers. Photopic and scotopic components of the ERG can be discriminated either by high-frequency flicker (flicker ERG), or by distinguishing between the photopic b-wave (x-wave) and the scotopic b-wave.[333a, 407, 408] At the present time some cases fall outside the scope of the ERG. Examples of these are firstly cases where the seat of the lesion is either in the retinal ganglion cells or more centrally in the brain, and secondly the group of conditions in which there is no recordable ERG. Because of the requirement of good fixation, ERG methods are difficult to use in children with small macular lesions.*[S48] This can be a serious limitation of the ERG since there are a number of clinical situations where it is important to establish whether the retina is the site of the disease and where no retinal abnormality is apparent to visual inspection.[407, 408]

According to Vaughan and Katzman,[824] by recording both ERG and scalp EPs, visual disorders can be classified as follows into lesions of (1) retina, (2) optic nerve, (3) optic chiasm, (4) retrochiasmal projection and (5) visual cortex by using the following criteria:[167, 289, 407, 408, 464, 465, 823, 824, 825, 835] (1) Unilateral retinal involvement – unilateral ERG changes and EP changes; (2) optic nerve involvement – EP absent when affected eye stimulated, but ERG unaffected; (3) chiasmal involvement – EP asymmetries indicating bitemporal hemianopia; (4) geniculocalcarine involvement – EP asymmetries indicating hemianopic defects in either both left or both right half-fields.[824]

Vaughan and Katzman[824] reported that complete blindness associated with pregeniculate lesions produces complete loss of all cortical responses to flash stimulation, whereas in bilateral geniculocalcarine lesions the 'later' (roughly response 40–80 msec peak) may persist, although the 'early' response (roughly 35 msec peak) is lost. A similar observation was reported by Crighel and Botez.[191]

Vaughan and Katzman further reported that a criterion of 50% asymmetry in the amplitude of visual EPs from the left and right sides of the head can distinguish between normal controls and patients with hemianopic field defects involving the central 10°. Some patients with diffuse cerebral disease and hemianopic defects show large (6 msec) latency and amplitude asymmetries.[824] Jonkman,[430 p.113] however, in his extensive study reported cases of hemianopia accompanied by an asymmetry of less than 50%, and conversely, cases in which no clinically demonstrable visual defect was accompanied by highly asymmetric EPs. Cohn also reports that asymmetric changes of EP amplitude do not always occur despite undisputed visual field defects, and that he observed amplitude asymmetries in normal controls when a sufficient number (100) were examined.[170, S47]

* EP methods can detect a quadrantic defect of 2° radius.

Oosterhuis *et al.*[582] found that the abnormality of the EP was generally more marked as the cerebral lesions was more extensive, even without there being an impairment of the visual fields. The correlation between EP abnormality and the severity of a cerebral lesion is better for a parieto-occipital derivation than for an occipital-to-ear derivation; the combined use of both placements has been recommended.[582]

Interestingly, Jonkman sometimes found markedly asymmetric EPs in the presence of tumours which, because of their nature and localisation, had produced few clinical or EEG changes.[430 p.67] Again, subthalamic and thalamic lesions have been reported to give asymmetric flash EPs even when they have not produced hemianopia.[192] Jonkman found no correlation between the nature of a lesion and the asymmetry of different transient EP components,[430 p.118] and in normal subjects no correlation between asymmetry and hemispheric dominance[71] (see also Chapter 2, Section 2.11.3).[S26]

Bergamini and his colleagues[73, 74, 71 p.64] found that asymmetric visual EPs could be the result of space occupying lesions restricted to nonspecific cortical areas (for example frontal tumours). They reported that flash EPs can be affected by tumours in a number of different ways; in some cases all components of the EP were attenuated, and in other cases only some components changed. These findings were attributed to the varying sites of lesions in different patients. [71, p.64]

The stimulus used by Kamphuisen[439, 440] in his clinical study was a spatially-unstructured (blank) stimulus field whose brightness was modulated, not in short pulses (flashes), but with a sinusoidal waveform (the complementary nature of the responses to these two types of stimuli is discussed in Chapters 2 and 5). Patients fell into two rather broad categories. In cases of 'hypofunction'* of the posterior cortex the saturation curves for the EP (Chapter 2) were of similar shapes; in other words any asymmetry of the EP did not depend on stimulus modulation depth. On the other hand, in cases of unilateral 'irritative disturbances'* Kamphuisen often found that on one side of the head the amplitude of the EP levelled-off (saturated) at high modulation depths, whereas on the other side of the head the amplitude of the EP was maximal at some intermediate modulation depth and fell off both at high and low modulation depths. In other words the asymmetry of the EP depended on modulation depth in these patients. Kamphuisen's study indicates that the effects of varying modulation depth as well as the effects of varying stimulus intensity should be routinely explored in symmetry studies in patients.[S15]

For children at any rate, absent or severely depressed flash EPs during a period of cortical blindness are compatible with the ultimate return of normal or nearly normal vision. Normal or nearly normal EPs during the period of severe visual impairment may herald the onset of rapid clinical recovery.[56] There seems to have been no extensive longitudinal-in-time EP study which

* Kamphuisen regarded hemiparalysis, hemiparesis, pathological reflexes or asymmetry of reflexes as indicative of 'hypofunction', and symptoms of epilepsy as indicative of 'irritation'.

might have revealed whether there is an EP counterpart in man of the temporary elimination of the EP after brain damage reported for monkey.[169]

It should be remembered, of course, that all the studies mentioned so far were carried out exclusively with unstructured-field stimulation.

As mentioned earlier, blindness due to geniculocalcarine lesions is associated with loss of early EP components, but with *retention* of late components.[824] Crighel and Botez reported that bipolar EPs to flash, recorded from leads in front of an occipital lobe carrying a well-demarcated surgical lesion, were similar or even larger in amplitude than the EPs recorded from the undamaged side. In contrast, the EPs recorded from the damaged region were either absent or much smaller than on the unimpaired side.[191]

These findings lead to the question whether the site of a lesion can be identified by the latencies of the affected EP components. This point is not discussed by Crighel and Botez;[191] Vaughan and Gross have presented evidence against the possibility.[821 p.32] Cohn's[169] evidence is not encouraging. He reported that the immediate effect of focal injury to monkey visual cortex is a marked decrease in the amplitude of the EP to flash, leaving the waveform and the latencies of components little affected. Nevertheless, visual field defects could be detected by behavioural methods. After some time the EP returned to its control amplitude, *but the visual field defect remained.* Moreover, in the presence of clear visual field defects produced by destruction of the optic tract (accompanied by minimal cortical damage), no immediate nor late changes in the EP could be detected. Cohn concluded that the immediate reduction of EP amplitude following brain injury is an expression of gross injury to neural tissue, rather than a reflection of a specific visual lesion. Cohn suggested that since almost normal responses could be recorded after ablation of striate cortex, the visual EP to flash in the intact animal does not reflect conduction along the classical anatomical visual pathway to the striate cortex.[169] Cohn claimed that his findings could most probably be extrapolated to man, thus predicting a dismal future for EP methods of mapping visual field defects. Against this, Corletto *et al.*[180] reported that total ablation of the occipital pole in man, although leaving earlier and later waves unaffected, greatly reduced the amplitudes of the prominent EP components with peak latencies from 50 to 110 msec (i.e. Corletto *et al.*, in conflict with Cohn, found waveform changes in the EP).

At first sight, then, it seems that the presence of non-specific EP components, possibly varying in prominence from subject-to-subject, might indeed create a serious obstacle to the clinical application of EP methods of visual field investigation. However, it should be noted that all the studies so far reported have mainly restricted their attention to the analysis of EP waveform with perhaps some consideration of the distribution of EP amplitude over the scalp. In all these studies only one form of stimulation has been used – flash presentation of spatially-unstructured visual fields. The clinical possibilities of utilising a variety of stimuli in attempts to investigate different functions of the visual pathways and to emphasise neural activities at different anatomical sites have hardly been explored (Chapter 2) in spite of the fact that microelectrode recording in primates provides abundant evidence that spatially-unstructured flash stimulation is not an appropriate stimulus for the majority of primary cortical neurons.

Scalp potentials evoked by changes in the brightness contrast of sharply-accommodated spatially-structured visual stimuli are quite different both in topographical distribution and in characteristics from the potentials evoked by changes in the brightness of a spatially-unstructured (blank) field (Chapter 2). This suggests that these two types of EP reflect the activities of neuronal populations whose functions and anatomical sites are different. Attempts have been made to identify the neuroanatomical sites at which pattern-EPs are generated (Chapter 2, Section 2.10.2), but there have so far been few attempts to use pattern-EPs in clinical work. Apart from a few studies in which red and blue stimuli have been used to distinguish between optic nerve damage to the macular and peripheral bundles[609, 688] there has also been little exploitation of stimulus colour in clinical investigations. Perhaps the effects of changing stimulus colour might appropriately be studied in patients during the evolution and recovery of optic neuritis. Motion-EPs do not seem to have been used at all in clinical work.

The EP measures which show the most clinical promise are, perhaps, those of left *versus* right symmetry. Such measures have the important advantage that they reduce the problem of intersubject variability by comparing two different EPs from the same subject; intersubject variability is such that it is only in rare cases that a single EP can be said to be abnormal.[582]

In all the studies described so far the symmetry of EP amplitude or latency has been assessed by recording simultaneously from the left and right sides of the head while stimulating the eye with a centrally-viewed patch of light. Central-retinal stimulation has the disadvantages that the EPs due to ipsilateral and contralateral signals are confounded by volume conduction, and can be separated to some extent only by placing electrodes on either side of the head. If, on the other hand, the responses to *focal stimulation* of the left and right retinal half-fields were recorded, then an enhanced sensitivity to differences between the ipsilateral and contralateral responses might be expected. The result would be that the sensitivity of the EP to the presence of asymmetric lesions would be considerably improved. This method brings with it two difficulties. The first is the problem of ensuring that stimulation really is restricted to a single retinal half-field. The second is that if the EPs to stimulation of left and right half-fields are recorded on separate occasions, the reliability of their measured asymmetry is sharply limited by the effect of EP variability. The first problem can be alleviated by stimulating one half-field with changes of mean brightness of no more than 20% or so, while at the same time brightly illuminating the other half-field so as to further reduce the effects of scattered light.[644] The second problem, the effects of variability, can be minimised by recording EPs to left and right half-field stimulation *simultaneously* as follows. If left and right half-fields are stimulated simultaneously at almost identical frequencies, so that the stimulation frequencies for the left and right half-fields differ by 0·3 Hz or so, then two Fourier Analysers or a single off-line averager can record the two separate EPs simultaneously from a single electrode. A frequency change of 0·3 Hz generally has little effect on the EP, so that any difference between the EPs to simultaneous stimulation of left and right half-fields is due to differences between the ipsilateral and contralateral pathways, and is not due to the 0·3 Hz difference in stimulation frequencies. This method provides a 'baseline' in that the responses to stimulation of an abnormal part of the visual field can be compared with the responses evoked by the simultaneous stimulation of a 'reference' area of the same eye. In practice the effect of variability is reduced typically by a factor of six; this corresponds to reducing the recording time by at least thirty-six times.[121a, 644]

This procedure of simultaneous stimulation and recording has been used to investigate a hemianopic visual field defect due to occlusion of the left posterior cerebral artery.[643] EP contributions due to transcallosally-transmitted signals were minimised by leaving a central 1° strip unstimulated, and steadily illuminated (in monkey, baboon and cat callosal connections relate directly only to areas close to the vertical meridian).[135, 400] Two quite different forms of stimulation were used (*a*) the left and right retinal half-fields were stimulated by unstructured fields whose brightnesses were sinusoidally modulated, and (*b*) the left and right retinal half-fields were stimulated by contrast-reversal of a checkerboard pattern.[S48] The EPs to stimulation of the left and right half-fields by flicker were found to be very different in amplitude; in contrast, the pairs of EPs to pattern-reversal were similar. Since pattern-reversal EPs are due almost entirely to stimulation of the central 3°–4°,[S8, 16, 17, 47] whereas flicker EPs have appreciable extrafoveal contributions, the EP data were interpreted as indicating a hemianopic field defect with macular sparing. This prediction was verified by subjective perimetry. However, this interpretation is open to the criticism that the accuracy of the subject's fixation was not monitored by an objective method. An alternative explanation for the EP findings may be that the pattern and the flicker EPs were generated in different cortical regions by signals which had traversed different pathways.

A number of workers have attempted to chart visual fields by successive focal stimulation of different retinal regions.[176, 408, 564, 708] Potts and Nagaya[613] used a 0·06° red target in order to emphasise the responses due to foveal cones. In agreement with other reports[564, 604, 731] they found that the foveal EP is diminished or absent in strabismic amblyopia and went on to show that there is no such loss in hysterical amblyopia (see Section 4.2.2).

SOMATOSENSORY EPS. LESIONS OF THE PERIPHERAL NERVES AND OF THE SPINAL CORD

Three features of transient EPs which are both quantifiable and recognisable to visual inspection are the waveform, the amplitude and the latency of the response as a whole. Halliday claimed that these three features are affected independently of each other by lesions of somatosensory afferent pathways and suggested that this might reflect different mechanisms.[348–350] A lengthening of latency of individual peaks may be due to a decreased conduction velocity of damaged afferent fibres, whereas an increased duration (width) of individual waves may reflect an increased temporal dispersion of the afferent volley.[71 p.68] Peripheral nerve lesions can result in any of these EP changes. Only with severe sensory losses is the EP quite undetectable.[317, 348–350] Lesions to the spinal cord can also change the amplitude, latency and waveform of somatosensory EPs.[12, 71, 317, 352] For both spinal cord and peripheral nerve lesions, however, normal sensation may be experienced in the presence of grossly abnormal somatosensory EPs. In spinal cord disease where pain and temperature sense alone have been impaired, the somatosensory EPs are normal.[317, 325, 565, 566]

Bergamini and Bergamasco reported that somatosensory EPs were affected not only by (*a*) peripheral nerve lesions but also by (*b*) damage of root and posterior medullary column.[71 p.69] Lesions in these regions (*a*) and (*b*) above may be differentiated by the following criteria: a lesion of an afferent peripheral fibre increases the latencies of the EP components, and exaggerates the durations of the individual waves, but the waveform is little affected. In posterior column and root lesions, on the other hand, there are marked changes in the waveform of the somatosensory EP.[71 p.70] With the aid of these criteria and recordings of peripheral nerve action potentials, somatosensory EPs have been used to determine the sites of lesions in a number of diseases of the peripheral nervous system.[71 p.71]

Halliday and Wakefield[352] concluded that both early and late components of the somatosensory EP were due to signals travelling up the dorsal column pathways (see also Chapter 2, Section 2.10.3).

The application of EPs in neurological diagnosis may be limited by Cohn's finding that (in monkey at any rate) EP changes following cortical injuries are *temporary*, not only for visual EPs but also for somatosensory EPs.[170] Cohn was unable to confirm (in monkey) Golding's finding that in man the result of ablating the cortical projection area for one hand was to abolish somatosensory EPs to stimulation of the affected hand. In monkey, after ablation of the hand area (actually the area firing to contralateral median nerve stimulation) there is full recovery of the EP[170] in the course of 6 to 8 weeks.

Perhaps the most celebrated and certainly the most dramatic clinical application of somatosensory EPs to date is a happy case in which scalp recordings demonstrated that a pair of Siamese twins had no spinal nerves in common. Subsequent surgery, decided by the EP findings, was completely successful.[71, 75]

SOMATOSENSORY EPS. CENTRAL LESIONS AND FUNCTIONAL LOSSES
(See also Chapter 2, Section 2. 10.3)

Unless a central lesion involves primary somatosensory cortex, the somatosensory EP is little changed.[317] Giblin reported that in some cases there may be a dissociation between sensation and the EP, so that clear EPs may be recorded to stimuli which the subject does not perceive. Williamson *et al.*,[874] however, found this not to be the case; there was a good correlation between EP change and clinical sensory loss. Again, Liberson[494] found the somatosensory EP to be abnormal in 10 of his 15 aphasic hemiplegic patients; the severity of the aphasia correlated with the degree of EP change. In cases of hysterical anaesthesia and hypnotically induced anaesthesia, the somatosensory EPs have variously been reported to be unaffected[12, 71, 353] or, in contrast abolished.[375] Levy and Behrman[490] put forward evidence that this conflict may be due to the use of different stimulation procedures and in particular that (*a*) when stimulation is restricted to peripheral receptors, the anaesthetic side produces a consistently smaller EP regardless of stimulus intensity, and (*b*) when stimuli are applied to peripheral nerves the amplitudes of the contralateral EPs are equal at high intensities, but at low intensities stimulation of the anaesthetic side produces a smaller response than stimulation of the normal side. Levy and Behrman explained their findings by suggesting that hysterical anaesthesia was accompanied by both a depression in peripheral receptor sensitivity, and central alterations of sensitivity.[490]

EVOKED RESPONSES IN VIIITH NERVE LESIONS

Shimizu[727] has emphasised that early diagnosis of an VIIIth nerve lesion such as a neurinoma is of the first importance because of the danger to life when it enlarges from the internal auditory meatus to invade structures in the posterior fossa. Auditory dysfunction is the earliest symptom, but the results of auditory tests are inconsistent in a large percentage of cases. In such a situation the use of a battery of clinical tests helps towards early diagnosis. In four patients with VIIIth nerve lesions every auditory EP to stimulation of the impaired ear showed longer latency and smaller amplitude than the EP to stimulation of the 'good' ear.[727] In contrast Menière's disease produced either shorter latency or little difference in latency, coupled with an increase of EP amplitude to stimulation of the affected ear. It therefore seems that auditory EPs show promise as a tool for differentiating VIIIth nerve lesions from cochlear lesions, although Shimizu did not quote the range of variability of normal control subjects so that it is not clear how far his patients fell beyond the normal range.

4.2.3 *Evoked potential methods for identifying structures within the brain; stereotactic surgery*

Neurosurgical methods for the treatment of tremor and abnormal movement involve the placement of lesions in the brain by stereotactic techniques. Hypotheses of the basic mechanism of abnormal movement stress the role of central structures, although inputs from peripheral receptors may also play a part (Reference 476 lists source material). The globus pallidus (GP) and ventrolateral (VL) nuclei have been the most popular targets. In practice, stereotactic location of these nuclei has been found to be hampered by neuroanatomical variability from one patient to another, even when electrode placement has been assisted by X-ray photography of the brain with the stereotactic apparatus in place.

Evoked potential methods have proved useful in providing additional positional information.[13, 14] Low-frequency stimulation of the VL nucleus elicits repetitive waves in the ipsilateral cortical area. This procedure has been used to delineate the VL prior to its surgical destruction.[883] More recently it has been reported that it is muscle tone that is primarily determined by VL, and that tremor is influenced only secondarily; destruction of a small circumscribed area immediately beneath VL is sufficient to relieve tremor, and this procedure also can be assisted by EP recording.[332, 581, 807] Criteria have been established for identifying the responses of a number of thalamic nuclei evoked by peripheral shock stimulation to the median nerve, the sciatic nerve and the infraorbital nerve.[698] These nuclei can then be used as landmarks to assist the subsequent placement of surgical lesions.

On the grounds of the known close connection between the amygdaloid nucleus and the olfactory system, olfactory stimulation has been used as a means of checking the location of the electrode tip during surgical destruction of the amygdaloid nucleus undertaken for the relief of behavioural disorders.[570, 571]

EP methods have been successfully used to assist the placement of stereotaxic lesions for the relief of trigeminal pain.[15]

Sances and Larsen[698] refer to previous recording of single unit potentials during stereotactic surgery and comment that although EP recording is of greater practical value during surgery, single unit records are more likely to aid the basic understanding of dyskinesia. In this connection. Sances and Larsen's undeniably complex block diagram of some of the known interconnections between a few of the many identifiable brain structures gives the impression that such a basic understanding will not be gained easily; as Sances and Larsen blandly put it 'analysis of the many circuits of the brain ---- presents a tremendous challenge to the systems engineer'.

4.2(b) The use of evoked potentials as a supplement to other techniques in research into specific clinical conditions

4.2.4 *Evoked potentials in psychiatry*

INTRODUCTION

Vaughan has cautioned that to reason from the fact that brain processes underlie both EPs and psychiatric illness to the suppositions that EPs might provide an objective index of psychoses is hardly to reason at all. However, this stricture does not by any means apply to all attempts to apply EP recording to the solution of problems in psychiatric medicine.

It has been suggested that a basic difficulty encountered by many schizophrenic and autistic children is that their perceived world lacks certain elements of constancy which we normally take for granted.[586] If this is the case, the physiological basis of the inconstancy might be that the pattern of neural activity in the CNS which *represents* (i.e. stands for) some feature in the external world is not constant, but varies from moment-to-moment.[496, 497] On the basis of this notion, a number of workers have attempted to use EPs as a means of access to the internal neural representation of features of the external world, reasoning that if EPs can be used for this purpose, then the moment-to-moment variability of scalp potentials evoked by identical stimuli might give a measure of the lability which is supposedly basic to schizophrenia. However, it might be wise to bear in mind when reviewing variability studies that variability measurements can present special problems in eliminating instrumental artifacts.

A second systematic approach has stemmed from the suggestion, based on psychological studies, that the capacity for establishing major 'sets' is impaired in schizophrenic individuals.[723] 'Set' here means the strategy which an individual develops for categorising sensory inputs and for directing action. Schizophrenics are marked by their tendency to develop multiple, unarticulated sets; this is called 'segmental set'. Its manifestations include a poor capacity for sustained attention and a preoccupation with minor details. On these theoretical grounds a group of workers introduced an EP method (two-tone EPs) which was designed to detect this preoccupation with minor details which is supposedly basic to schizophrenic malfunction.

A third approach to psychiatric research is also not without rationale. Work with normal subjects had led to the suggestion that the CNV is a measure of the capacity to distinguish relationships between stimuli, that is the capacity to predict future events (Chapter 3). Clearly, such a measure might have value in psychiatric conditions accompanied by an impaired capacity to detect and act on relationships between events.

Vaughan's call for rationality in the application of EP recording to psychiatric problems has some force, and certainly a 'suck it and see' experimenter would need great luck to stumble upon a worthwhile finding. On the other hand neither does it seem that success in research is guaranteed by sticking rigidly to a preconceived theoretical plan; there are many historical examples of major advances brought about as much by opportunism as by planning.

A caution addressed by Vaughan to those who use EPs in psychopathology[817] applies with almost equal force to EP research in general. Vaughan points out the real danger of using correlation measures as a search procedure rather than a method of testing hypotheses. If the $p = 0{\cdot}05$ confidence level is one's chosen criterion, then a significant correlation can be found by chance on (more or less) one occasion out of twenty. Now the different components of evoked potential waveforms generally offer a number of possible measures of amplitude and latency. It is easy to see how an ingenious search through an array of twenty measures of the EP for significant correlations on the basis of a $p = 0{\cdot}05$ confidence limit could easily lead to embarrassing consequences!

A special difficulty in assessing EPs recorded from psychiatric patients must surely be the influence of attention, which is so notoriously difficult to control even in normal subjects (Chapter 3).

EPS TO UNPAIRED STIMULI

A number of workers have endeavoured to find whether EPs to unpaired stimuli show any differences between schizophrenic patients and control groups. The differences reported seem to be minor and are sometimes difficult to replicate. The latency of a 46 msec peak of the EP to flash stimulation has been reported to be shorter in schizophrenic subjects.[720] Rodin *et al.* found visual EPs have different amplitudes in schizophrenic patients than in non-patients *but only when the patients were subclassified on the basis of metabolism.* The after-discharge (ringing) of the flash EP has been reported to be reduced in schizophrenic groups;[722] the interpretation of this finding is not straightforward on the basis of present knowledge. Somatosensory EPs have been reported to be larger in schizophrenic patients than in normal controls,[718, 719] but later work failed to confirm this finding, which was attributed to effects of age and sex.[714, 722]

VARIABILITY OF EPS IN SCHIZOPHRENIC PATIENTS

A method for objectively discriminating between certain schizophrenic patients and a control group was described in 1965 by Callaway and his colleagues.[112, 428] Monopolar EPs were recorded to 600 msec tone stimuli whose frequency was either 1000 Hz or 600 Hz. The two tones were presented in 'haphazard' order and were matched for loudness. In control subjects the two tones were found to elicit EPs which looked alike to visual inspection and which gave a high Pearson product moment correlation coefficient (a measure of overall waveform similarity, see below and Chapter 5, Section 5.4.12). On the other hand, the schizophrenic patients gave EP waveforms to the two tones which, to visual inspection, looked different and which gave a low Pearson product moment correlation coefficient. In other words Callaway and his colleagues claimed that *the result of comparing EPs either by visual inspection or by Pearson's statistical procedure* 'rather than by some technique which did not ignore variability' was that schizophrenic patients appeared to give dissimilar EPs to two quite similar tones, whereas control subjects gave similar EPs to the tones.

A possible complication arose from the fact that most of the schizophrenic patients either had been or were at the time receiving drug therapy. However, this seemed unlikely to have affected the results, since the two-tone EPs of control subjects were not affected by drug doses comparable to those received by the schizophrenic patients;[428, 429] it was not considered ethical to investigate the effect of drugs on two-tone EPs in schizophrenics.

In a later study Jones and Callaway[427] reported the unexpected finding that the Pearson coefficient distinguished between schizophrenic patients and controls not only when the two tones had different frequencies, but also when they had identical frequencies. This fact pointed towards a more careful consideration of the use of the Pearson coefficient in EP research.

The Pearson product-moment correlation coefficient gives a measure of the difference between two averaged waveforms, but no information as to the contributions of different components to this difference. For example, one pair of waveforms might differ mainly in their early components, and another pair might differ mainly in their later components, but the Pearson measure could describe the pairs as equally different. This 'blind-spot' could well be a serious limitation of the Pearson procedure[244] since there is a body of evidence that components of different latencies relate differently to stimulus parameters, and are possibly generated in different neuranatomical regions (Chapters 1 and 3). A second limitation of the Pearson coefficient arises from the use of averaged EP waveforms as raw data.[244] To start from averaged waveforms is to throw away information on the variability of the many segments of raw EEG which together constitute the summated EP. When two-tone EP data was analysed by a statistical procedure which does not ignore variability (Stepwise discriminant analysis in this case) it turned out that the reported differences between the two-tone EPs of normal and schizophrenic subjects was due to an increased variability of the EPs of schizophrenics rather than to a consistent tendency of schizophrenics to persist in concentrating on differences between tones.[113, 244, 427]

The reason why the above account of the work of Callaway and his colleagues is framed entirely in terms of empirical findings, is that the validity of these findings is quite distinct from the validity of any hypothesis of the basic mechanism of schizophrenia. As a matter of fact the two-tone procedure was introduced rationally in order to test a prediction of the psychologically-inspired hypothesis of 'segmental set'.[112] This prediction was that schizophrenics would show greater persistence in paying attention to small differences between stimuli than normal subjects. However, as described above, a more recent analysis carried out by the same group of workers on similar two-tone findings leads to a different interpretation of the data.[113, 244, 427] These published reports give valuable indications of the practical dangers associated with the use of statistical procedures (including averaging) in EP work.

Quite apart from the two-tone studies, there have been a number of attempts to directly assess EP variability in schizophrenic patients.* Visual EPs have been reported to be more variable in schizophrenic patients than in normal controls.[497, 498, 746, 248 p.183] Schizophrenic children showed larger changes of auditory EP wave N_2 during sleep than did normal controls; this difference was attributed to central vestibular dysfunction.[584]

Reasoning from the observation that many schizophrenic patients find

* Bergen, Czigman and Koella[75a] have reported that the variability of visually evoked EPs in the rabbit are increased, without any associated change in mean response amplitude after injection of a plasma protein fraction from schizophrenic patients.

greater difficulties in an environment rich in sensory stimuli than when sensory input is reduced, Lifshitz has attempted to develop an EP measure of the way in which schizophrenics handle several simultaneous stimuli.[248 p.357] Lifshitz recorded EPs to a number of 'simple' stimuli presented in isolation, and then recorded EPs to simultaneous presentation of more than one of the 'simple' stimuli. He attempted to predict the waveforms of the EPs to these latter 'compound' stimuli by linearly summing the EPs to simple stimuli. The accuracy of the linear prediction was assessed by the nonparametric Mann-Whitney U test.

Liftshitz reported that failures in the linearity of summation were particularly marked for stimuli within the same modality and suggested that departures from linearity might have clinical significance. On the other hand his finding was therefore in accord with previous observations on normal subjects (Chapter 2). Furthermore, Lifshitz' exclusive use of 100% stimulus modulation depths would seem to invite the intrusion of certain important nonlinearities (saturation) which could have been avoided by the use of lower stimulus modulation depths without any serious reduction of response amplitude. There is ample evidence for the presence of these nonlinearities in the EPs of normal subjects (Chapter 2, Section 2.3.3). Their presence might therefore undermine the basis of Lifshitz's present version of his 'linear prediction' method. Furthermore in view of the earlier discussion about the sources of EP components of different latencies (see Chapter 1, Section 1.2–1.2.4 and Chapter 3), the power of Lifshitz' procedure might be increased by treating EP components of different latencies separately.

CORTICAL EXCITABILITY AND THE RECOVERY FUNCTION

The notion that deviant reactivity or excitability of the CNS underlies psychopathology was the rationale behind Shagass' introduction of a well-established neurophysiological procedure into psychiatric studies. Shagass and his colleagues evoked somatosensory EPs by electric shock stimulation. They applied stimuli in pairs and explored the effect of changing the interval between the two stimuli of a pair.[16, 209, 210, 717] The size of the second response relative to the first response was taken to indicate the extent to which responsiveness had recovered after the elapse of a particular interval. The variation of responsiveness with the time which had elapsed after the first stimulus was variously called the 'recovery function', 'recovery curve' or 'excitability cycle' and was regarded as a measure of the time course of recovery of excitability of cortical neurons after stimulation. The recovery curve up to 200 msec is biphasic with an initial return to full responsiveness by 20 msec followed by a phase of reduced responsiveness and then by a second phase of full recovery, peaking at 120 msec.[717, 718]

Shagass suggested that a diminished recovery function implies that stimuli which follow the first in a sequence will not elicit the normal neural response until an abnormally long time has elapsed, and that the pathology underlying this finding might form a basis for distortions of perception and hence account for the deviant conduct characteristic of schizophrenia. More conservatively, Shagass has emphasised the need to establish a physiological basis for the recovery function by animal experimentation.

Three groups of psychiatric patients have depressed recovery curves, particularly in the early phase up to 20 msec. These groups can be classified as personality disorders, schizophrenia and psychotic depression. In contrast, the recovery curves for psychiatric patients with anxiety, depression or psychophysiological reactions do not differ from the recovery curves for nonpatients.

Shagass claimed that ten peaks and troughs can be reliably identified in the somatosensory evoked potential. In schizophrenic patients the recovery curves of four peaks are significantly depressed, and the recovery curves for three latencies significantly enhanced.[714]

However, there are some complications. Earlier studies used high-intensity stimuli of equal strengths. When weak stimuli were used in later studies it was found that a patient who showed reduced recovery with intense stimuli might show supernormal recovery with weak stimuli.[716, 722] At first sight this might seem to cast doubt on the generality of the recovery function, value as a measure of excitability of the CNS, although it has been suggested that the difference between the recovery functions for strong and weak stimuli reflects the activities of different mechanisms.[716, 722]

Further complications are that the amplitudes and latencies of some EP components vary with age,[771] and sex.[720] Recovery functions show some sex-dependent differences and these differences are more marked in patients than in nonpatients.[715]

Following Gastaut[305] and along the lines of Ciganek,[137] Shagass then tried visual stimuli to determine recovery functions. He was, however, unable to detect any difference between the recovery functions of schizophrenic patients and nonpatients.[721] On the other hand Rodin and his colleagues were able to distinguish between the visual recovery curves of schizophrenics and non-patients especially at low stimulus intensities[248 p.324] but *only after the schizophrenic patients had been subclassified on the basis of metabolism.*[681] Rodin's finding suggests that not only the absolute number of EP correlates but also their specificity to particular psychiatric conditions might be increased by subtyping psychiatric patients on some such basis as energy metabolism.

Although it seems clear that a number of the EP measures introduced into psychiatric research by Shagass and his colleagues can discriminate between nonpatients and certain general classes of psychiatric patients, at the present time none of the measures have any greater diagnostic specificity, and their application is technically difficult. Whether the measurement of recovery curves is likely to prove to be of clinical value is a question which may be resolved when the techniques can be made more specific, and when the physiological basis of the recovery cycle is clarified by animal experiments.

APPLICATIONS OF THE CNV IN PSYCHIATRY

Walter has reported that the amplitude of the CNV (see Chapter 3) is much reduced in psychopaths,[848] somewhat reduced in schizophrenia[S41] and anxiety, and enhanced in obsessive neuroses.[110, 522] The CNV would, then, seem to have promise as a clinical tool. Unfortunately, there seem to be a number of obstacles to its general clinical application. Straumanis *et al.*[772] found that CNVs measured in the same subject changed when the experimental conditions were changed, which suggested (with reservations)[772] that the CNV measured in one experimental condition does not characterise the individual. Apart from this fundamental question, Straumanis *et al.*[772] pointed out certain technical difficulties. The commonly-used vertex-mastoid electrode derivation is subject to serious contamination of the CNV by potentials due to eye movements elicited by the stimulus. These potentials are very similar to the CNV and must either be balanced out[522] or minimised by steady visual fixation if the eye artifact is to be negligible.

Vaughan claimed that Walter's CNV is largely generated in motor cortex, and primarily reflects preparation for movement (see Chapter 3). Vaughan went on to suggest that Walter's CNV data on psychiatric patients gave little more information that would have been obtained from a study of reaction times. A reaction time with a large variance would of itself result in an apparently small CNV since, in the CNV paradigm, the averaging computer is triggered by the stimulus rather than by the onset of motor activity. However, Vaughan's argument does seem to depend on the validity of his suggestion that the CNV is wholly related to motor potentials, and this suggestion has been challenged[163, 235] (see Chapter 3).

At the present time there is a deal of conflict about the factors which determine the CNV; expectancy, 'cortical priming', motivation, conation, volition, concentration and arousal have each been suggested (Chapter 3). It is not clear whether the CNV is a unitary phenomenon or whether it has multiple sources (Chapter 3). There is some problem in eliminating eye artifacts, especially with uncooperative subjects. The presence of so many uncertainties must surely obstruct immediate systematic application of CNV recording in psychiatry.

S15

4.2.5 *Epilepsy and migraine*

EPILEPSY

The problem of extracting the somatosensory EP from noise in patients suffering from myoclonic epilepsy led Dawson to devise first the superposition technique (Chapter 5, Section 5.4.10), and then the averaging computer (Chapter 5, Section 5.4.10), and thereby to initiate the study of average evoked potentials. Dawson[208, 209] found the somatosensory EP to be five to ten times larger in myoclonic patients than in normal controls. Latency was unaffected by myoclonic epilepsy. Halliday[349, 350] later found that the enhancement of EP amplitude was specifically linked with the presence of myoclonic jerks rather than with a history of the disease. In familial essential myoclonus, the jerking is not associated with EPs of increased amplitude.[349, 350] Using paired stimuli Dawson[209] found that for interstimulus intervals between 60 msec and 100 msec the response to the second stimulus was sometimes enhanced in myoclonic patients. This finding was later confirmed by Giblin.[350]

In grand mal epilepsy, visual EPs show no consistently abnormal features.[24, 430, 511] Bergamini and Bergamasco[71] reported that the visual EP may be larger during spike and wave discharge and that the after discharge may be very prominent in centrencephalic epileptics. Enhancement of the amplitude of the visual EP has been reported in photosensitive epilepsy.[95, 184, 187, 304, 383, 553, 554] Aoki distinguished two classes of photosensitive epilepsy on EP grounds, and claimed that serial recordings of visual EPs showed changes which paralleled clinical and EEG changes.[24]

Lücking *et al.*[511] have flatly stated that in epilepsy EP recording adds little to the routine EEG.

MIGRAINE

EEG abnormalities have been observed both during migraine attacks[271] and between attacks.[116, 251] However, the sources of the abnormal brain rhythms cannot be defined with any precision and, furthermore, it is difficult to quantify the EEG.

Visual stimuli flickering at most frequencies throughout the range 11–22 Hz evoke much larger potentials in migraine patients than in control subjects,[329, 744, 790] but this EP distinction persists between attacks. It may therefore have a place in studies of the predisposing factors in migraine, but since it persists between attacks it is unlikely to provide an objective index of the migraine attack, or to be of value in assessing therapy.

Richey *et al.*[665] stimulated migraine patients with centrally-viewed flashes during the intervals between migraine attacks. They found no difference between patients and control EPs for males, and only slight differences for females.

Regan suggested that EPs might be asymmetric in migraine attacks which were accompanied by asymmetrical symptoms, and that such an asymmetry could possibly provide an objective measure of the attack. In a preliminary study, patterned-reversal and flicker EPs elicited by simultaneous stimulation of the left and right retinal half-fields were recorded.[645] Between attacks some, but not all migraine subjects (3 out of 5), showed greater differences between the EPs to left and right half-field stimulation than did control subjects. In all three patients studied during migraine attacks the ratio between the EPs to left and right half-field stimulation showed significant changes which could be as large as 500%. In each case the direction of the change was the same for the flicker EP and the pattern-reversal EP, but the absolute asymmetries were generally quite different for the two types of stimuli.

4.2.6 *Demyelinating diseases*

Halliday and Wakefield[352] reported a study on two cases of disseminated sclerosis in which scalp potentials were evoked by 1 Hz shocks to the fingers. In one case the later components of the somatosensory EP were much less attenuated than the early components; in the other case, a marked increase in latency was accompanied by waveform distortion. Rather than touch sensitivity or two-point discrimination, joint position sense was used as a criterion for judging discrimination sensory loss. The reason for this choice was that joint position sense, in contrast with touch sensation, is an unequivocal index of posterior column function. The study by Baker *et al.*[38] of somatosensory EPs in fifteen cases of multiple sclerosis showed delayed onset latencies, and a monophasic response in those patients with defects of proprioception.

In a later study, Baker *et al.*[37] reported on 91 patients with multiple sclerosis. In 10 patients with no sensory loss, 5 had abnormal EPs, suggesting that EP methods might prove to be of value in supporting problematic clinical diagnoses of multiple sclerosis. Proprioreceptive sensory loss was found in 81 patients, 68 of whom had abnormal somatosensory EPs. Of the 68 patients with abnormal EPs, 59 had severe to moderate debilitating multiple sclerosis.

Baker *et al.* considered that the changed waveform and marked increase in EP latency observed in cases of multiple sclerosis were probably due to (*a*) a nonuniform increase in conduction time and (*b*) a temporal dispersion of signals in the CNS. They suggested that both of these changes were caused by the process of demyelination. The EP changes observed in cases of multiple sclerosis were also seen in patients with polyneuritis, combined system disease, tabes dorsalis and Friedreich's ataxia.

Namerow compared somatosensory EPs from 50 multiple sclerosis patients with EPs recorded from 28 control subjects. Stimulation was by shocks to the median nerve at a frequency of 1 Hz; bipolar EPs were obtained from the scalp on the side contralateral to the stimulated side. Stimulation of all 27 hands with vibration and/or position sense impairment at the time of testing gave abnormal EPs. These EP abnormalities were an absent or delayed early wave (negative 18–22 msec in normals) and a major positive peak (31–48 msec in normals) broadened and delayed beyond the 97·5% confidence limit for normals. Furthermore, stimulation of twenty-five of these 27 hands gave a simple monophasic waveform instead of the normal polyphasic waveform. There was evidence that the EP method was more sensitive than routine sensory testing in detecting demyelinating lesions.

The EP changes described above are not specific to multiple sclerosis but apparently relate in general to diseases which alter conductivity through the relevant afferent pathways.[565, 566] Namerow[565] further suggested that significant numbers of the more heavily myelinated and fastest conducting fibres had conduction blocked at the point of demyelination, so that the recorded EP was due to signals conducted along smaller and slower fibres. Further evidence for this notion was obtained in a later study of somatosensory 'recovery functions' (see Section 4.2.4), which were strikingly different in multiple sclerosis patients and normal controls.[568]

4.2.7 *Maturation of the brain*

INTRODUCTION

Abnormal EEGs are frequently recorded from mentally retarded patients, but there are few features of the EEG which correlate specifically with mental retardation. On the other hand, evidence is accumulating that EPs can provide an index of brain maturation. If EPs are to become a useful diagnostic tool in cases of retardation, a body of normative data must be established both of the EP characteristics at different stages of development and of the variability of these measures. This groundwork is presently being carried out in a number of laboratories; the results are summarised below.

AUDITORY EPS

Between 23 and 45 weeks after conception the auditory EP shows a stereotyped sequence of changes. Latencies fall progressively and there are accompanying changes in waveform and topographical distribution (Fig. 4.5).

In premature infants of post-conceptual age 23 to 29 weeks the major component (relative to linked ears) is a negative wave N1 with a peak latency of 180–270 msec. Wave N1 is usually followed by a positive slow wave P2 whose latency falls between 600 and 900 msec. Wave N1 is larger postero-laterally than either on the midline or antero-laterally. By the 30–34th week the latency of negative wave N1 is less at the posterior than at the anterior electrodes, and amplitude differences between different sites are reduced (Fig. 4.5). The latency of P2 has fallen. Major changes take place between weeks 35–37. In the medial-vertex region P2 becomes larger than N1 (Fig. 4.5). Between 37 and 38 weeks, an additional short-latency (90 msec) component and a long-latency (500–700 msec) negative wave appear in the medial-vertex region. The anterior medial electrodes show the early positive wave, but with a 110–140 msec latency. At this time the premature infant's EP in the vertex region begins to bear some resemblance to the EP of a full-term infant. By 39–45 weeks, EPs recorded near the vertex are closely similar to those for a full-term neonate[860] (Fig. 4.5). By 45 weeks, the N1 component is frequently absent, and P2–N2 have become the major waves.

At all ages a small, early (*c.* 15 msec) component can be recorded from the ear electrode. This component is much attenuated during quiet sleep and is probably myogenic in origin.

Both auditory EP and neurological reflex tests give results which correlate well with *postconception* age, but less well with birth weight, postnatal age or somatic growth.[337] Akiyama *et al.*[20] claimed that the 'patterns of the peaks' in the acoustic EP give a better indication of conceptual age than is given by the latencies.

Weitzman and Graziani[863] reported that there was a consistent difference in the latencies of the N1 and P2 components during the two EEG patterns which characterise sleep in the human infant.[860] They suggested that these EP findings may indicate short-term cyclic changes in the functional activity of the premature infant which might also take place in the foetus *in utero*.

A major complex of the auditory EP (N2–P2–N3) has been reported to be significantly different for normal infants and certain developmentally-retarded (mongoloid) infants.[55] The amplitudes of the P2–N3 component were found to be significantly greater for the mongoloid infants, and the difference could not be explained by differences in skull or scalp impedances.

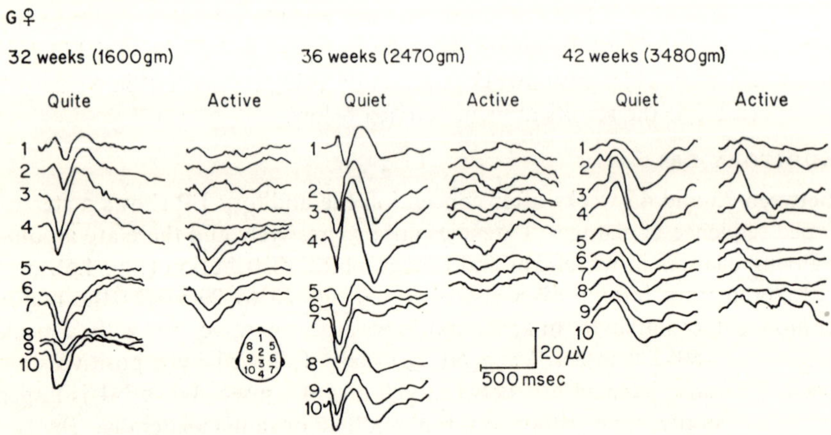

FIGURE 4.5 *Comparison of auditory-evoked response patterns in the same infant as a function of maturation and sleep state. From E. D. Weitzman and L. J. Graziani (1968). 'Maturation and topography of the auditory-evoked response of the prematurely born infant', in* Develop. Psychobio., *1, 79–89. John Wiley and Sons, Inc.*

Barnet and Lodge suggested that the EP differences between the normal and retarded infants reflected underlying differences in the brain mechanisms which govern sensory input, and furthermore that late components of the EP relate more to the regulation than to the reception of sensory input.

VISUAL EPS

The ERG of the newborn infant already has a waveform which is similar to that of the fully-developed adult ERG, though of smaller amplitude and slightly longer latency.[56, 290, 503] This similarity for the ERG contrasts with the situation for the visual EP, which shows marked progressive changes between birth and late childhood.

The ERG of neonates has maximum sensitivity towards the blue end of the spectrum, whereas the scalp EP is most sensitive in the green. This suggests that for neonates, as for adults,[29, 30] the ERG is largely scotopic while the scalp EP is predominantly photopic.

Even in premature infants, recognisable visual EPs can easily be recorded.

This indicates that the presence of a visual EP does not necessarily imply useful visual function.[290, 805] Peak latencies fall progressively with increasing age,[273, 290, 805, 857] but because of intersubject variability latency cannot be used to give a reliable estimate of post-conceptual age.[805] Only part of this intersubject variability is due to sex and race.[273]

In premature infants the visual EP is restricted to the occipital region[805] and spreads with increasing age during the first months.[264, 265, 805, 857] There

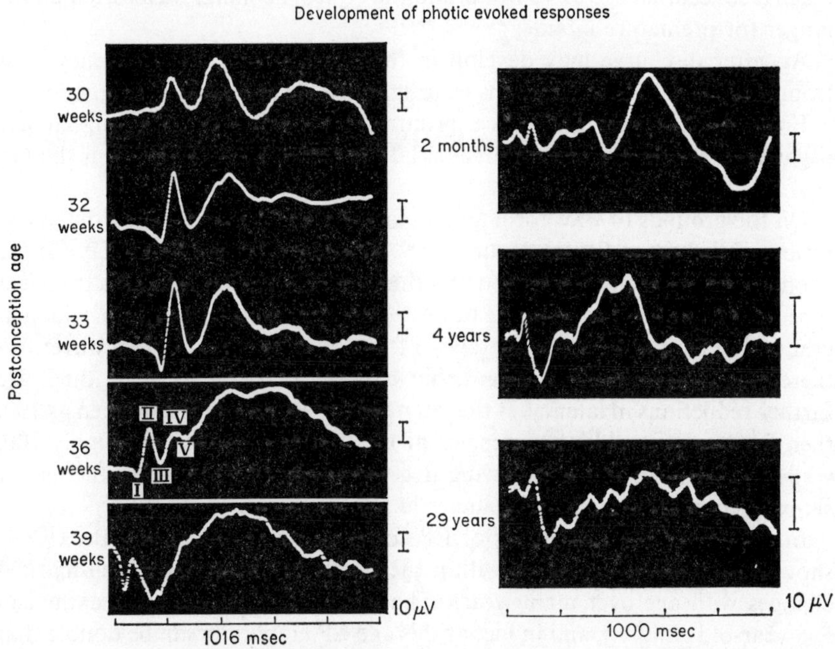

FIGURE 4.6 *Developmental changes of PERs recorded from parieto-occipital lead. Each trace is the average of 20 (left 5 traces) and 100 (right 3 traces) stimulations. All PERs recorded during non-rapid eye movement sleep except 36 week trace. Left upper 3 traces are from same subject in longitudinal study. Note the development of peaks I and III, decrease of peak latencies, and in right 3 traces, the development of the rhythmic after-discharge. From H. Umezaki and F. Morrell (1970). 'Developmental study of photic-evoked responses in premature infants', in* Electroenceph. clin. Neurophysiol., ***28***, *55–63. Elsevier Publishing Co., Amsterdam.*

seems to be fair agreement about the course of maturation of the visual EP except for some discrepancies on the polarity of the response.[290] In most cases an initial negative peak (II) is followed by a positive peak (III) and then by a large negativity containing two or three subpeaks[394, 396, 805] (Fig. 4.6). At approximately 32 weeks postconceptual age a positive peak (I) can sometimes be seen just earlier than peak II, and becomes a common feature by 35 weeks[265, 394, 396, 805, 857] (Fig. 4.6). Small wavelets preceding wave I can be seen in many neonates. Peak II is consistently the most prominent peak, and can fall in latency from 258 ± 53 msec (29–31 weeks postconceptual) via

172 $\pm$ 60 msec (38–43 weeks) to roughly 80 msec at 2–4 years.[290, 805] Waves I and III show similar latency changes.[290, 805] Scores for mental performances at 8 months have been reported to correlate with neonatal photic latency, independently of differences in birth weight and gestation age.[106] The visual EP of the premature infant of less than 35 weeks postconceptual age can be distinguished from that of the full-term infant on waveform grounds.[284, 805] Many prematurely born infants fail to show a normal latency when they reach a conceptual age of 40 weeks and the typical neonatal waveform persists longer for premature infants.[394, 396, 398]

An after discharge may develop in the third month; the frequency rises from roughly 5·5 Hz at 3 months to roughly 10 Hz at 6 years[396] (Fig. 4.6).

From the 2nd year onwards a prominent wave is seen as a long-latency negativity, and in the central areas a late negative wave develops in the 6th year.[857]

On the grounds of waveform and latency Hrbek[396] has classified the maturation of the visual EP into four stages. These are (1) the foetal EP, (2) the neonatal EP which, in the second and third months change into (3) a transient type of EP which has some features of (4) the mature EP, into which it gradually changes between the ages of one and two years. The waveform thereafter remains fairly constant, but between two and six years there are further reductions in latency. If the latencies for six year olds are taken as 100, then for two year olds the latencies of the first two waves are roughly 100, while the latencies of the following five waves are 130–145. After the age of six only comparatively small changes in latency occur.

In a study of the amplitudes of EP components Dustman and Beck[254, 255] showed that waves occurring within the initial 250 msec show well-marked changes with age over many years. The occipital responses are maximal in 5–6-year-old children, and in fact at this age EP amplitude can be double that at other ages. Amplitude declines after the age of seven until it appears to rise again at 13–14 years. There is, however, some problem in assessing the statistical significance of this 'hump'. At the age of 16 the amplitude stabilizes. Older subjects (mean age 67) show increased latencies and amplitudes for those early waves which peak within 100 msec.[254, 255]

Whether the stereotyped sequences of changes in the maturing EP reflect the development of the information-handling and organising mechanisms of the brain is an important question from the clinical standpoint but is still answered by little more than speculation. However, the groundwork is not being ignored; determined efforts have been made to relate the developmental changes of the EP to changes in the activities of individual neurons.[188, 805, 857] Morrell and Morrell[555] have reported evidence that the developmental sequence of the visual EP to flash parallels the gradual myelination of thalamo-cortical radiation fibres. Creutzfeld and Kuhnt[188] and Umzeki and Morrell[805] have further suggested that the maturation of the visual EP to flash reflects the slower myelination of nonspecific projection and association fibres compared with specific sensory afferents.[549]

SOMATOSENSORY EPS

The growing understanding of the pathways which are involved in the somatosensory EP (Chapter 2, Section 2.10.3) is an encouraging indication of a useful future for somatosensory EPs in the study of clinical problems of maturation.

In the vertex area, somatosensory and auditory EPs are remarkably similar for neonates.[398] On the other hand, visual EPs are quite different in waveform from either auditory or somatosensory EPs.

The somatosensory EP changes in form with the behavioural state of the infant.[227, 397, 398] The late ('nonspecific') waves 4 (220 msec) and 5 (380 msec) are considerably larger in regular (high voltage) sleep than in irregular (low voltage) sleep or awake states.[397, 398] The neonate somatosensory EP shows an initial negative component, followed by a positive and then a further negative component. This latter component has a slower time course than in the adult and, furthermore, there are marked waveform differences between neonate and adult.[226] The difference between adult and neonate EPs are much less marked for foot stimulation than for hand stimulation, an observation which might suggest that cortical maturation of the hand projection lags behind that of the foot.[225]

4.3 Clinical Application of evolved potentials: possibilities

The clinical possibilities of certain areas of EP research have not yet been experimentally demonstrated although they are strongly suggested by the material discussed in Chapter 2. Some of these possibilities are discussed below.

4.3.1 *Tests for the integrity of a sensory pathway*

There are prospects that not only the presence of a lesion in a sensory pathway, but also its location might in future be more accessible to EP methods. For example, it has already been shown that some information on the site of a lesion in the visual pathway can be obtained by the simple stratagem of stimulating discrete regions of the retina[824, 825] (Section 4.2.2). Perhaps this trick of stimulation may become more effective both with visual and somatosensory EPs by the use of methods developed for recording EPs to simultaneous focal stimulation of two or four retinal or somatic areas,[121a, 643, 644, 645] and by further clarifications of the neuroanatomical sites of the generators of different EP components.[355, 413, 414]

A potentially more general approach to the location of lesions is discussed below in Sections 4.3.2 and 4.3.3.

4.3.2 *Tests of special functions of a sensory pathway*

There is a growing body of evidence that EPs 'carry the signature' of the particular stimulus which evokes them. Parallel, but generally quite separate psychophysical and microelectrode studies have supported the notion that neural tissue can perform the function of 'filtering' or 'emphasising' those features of the external world which are important to the organism. Neural organisations in the visual pathway located up to and including primary and extrastriate cortical levels process incoming information in such a way that features such as the movement of the edge of an object is an adequate stimulus for some particular central neuron; this neuron can easily be activated by its own adequate stimulus, but can hardly be activated at all by any other stimulus.[399, 489] The auditory pathway seems to be organised in an analogous way.[283, 327]

By putting the EP evidence (from human subjects) together with the micro-electrode findings (from animals) the suggestion emerges that it might be possible to develop EP methods which would allow the objective investigation of the specific neural 'feature filters' which are (presumably) present in the human brain at levels up to and including primary cortex. One may surmise that the effective operation of these filtering mechanisms is necessary for normal sensory discrimination, i.e. for normal perception of the external world. It follows that future EP methods for objectively assessing functioning of 'feature emphasising' mechanisms in sensory pathways might prove to be clinically useful. There is encouraging evidence that such exciting developments are possible;[787] the clinical potentialities of these future techniques promise ample rewards for overcoming the difficulties which no doubt lie ahead.*[S56]

At a more peripheral level some progress has already been made in using the amplitude of pattern-specific EP components (Chapter 2, Section 2.4) as a measure of the sharpness of the retinal image, and of visual acuity. Subjective suppression of pattern perception has been found to be accompanied by a marked reduction in the amplitude of pattern-specific EP components (Chapter 2, Section 2.11.1); perhaps such observations may lead to the use of EPs as a measure of visual suppression in squint.[S25]

When recent reports of stereoscopic EPs are coupled with suggestions that specific defects of stereoscopic vision may be a cause of squint[663] it seems possible that the development of techniques for stereoscopically eliciting scalp potentials might provide data on squint which is often difficult to obtain by subjective clinical tests.

Evoked potential methods of recording the spectral sensitivity curve of the eye are already available, and may provide measurements which are as precise as those obtainable by psychophysical means. The wavelength discrimination curve, which describes how the eye's sensitivity to different hues varies through the spectrum, can be assessed by EP recording, and technical developments should soon shorten the procedure.

It may soon prove possible to distinguish between EPs to changes in the intensity of a tonal stimulus, and EPs to changes in the pitch of a tone of constant intensity. Such a development would enable more detailed assessment of hearing than is at present routinely available by EP recording.

Evidence has recently been put forward that EPs are specifically elicited by

* Evidence has accumulated for an EP indicator of a subject's detection of a sensory signal.[S35]

the transition from constancy to change of any one of a variety of stimulus parameters. For example, an EP of this special type would be generated if a tone, initially of constant frequency, suddenly started to rise in frequency; the stimulus for the EP would occur at the instant of transition from constancy to change (Chapter 2, Section 2.7). There is a body of evidence that our perceptual mechanisms are specifically sensitive to *changes* in the external world and comparatively insensitive to static features. Evoked potentials which were specifically sensitive to the transition from rest to change of some feature of the external world might offer a novel means of investigating what is possibly a particularly fundamental function of our sensory systems; such EPs might prove to be sharp clinical tools.

4.3.3 *The location of brain lesions by EP methods*

There are a number of procedures in everyday use for detecting and localising brain lesions. These procedures include both the subjective sensory tests used by neurologists such as visual field investigations, and various objective procedures such as ventriculography, pneumoencephalography, angiography, scanning and recording of the spontaneous EEG. Subjective test procedures are of little value with aphasic or uncooperative patients, and may have limited application with children. In some cases subjective testing may achieve little more than to indicate the presence of a lesion and may fail to provide a clear localisation. Some objective methods of localising brain lesions may involve risk to the patient, and may require the use of a surgical theatre and theatre staff. Scanning has limited value in detecting certain small lesions. Spontaneous EEG recording, on the other hand, carries no risk but gives only a diffuse picture of brain activity, and may fail to detect other than superficial lesions. If it proves possible to develop EP techniques which can provide a fresh means of locating brain lesions, then these techniques would have the advantage over such procedures as angiography and pneumoencephalography that they involved no risk or discomfort to the patient. Evoked potential methods, in contrast to conventional EEG recording, offer straightforward opportunity to selectively emphasise the activities of chosen regions of the brain.[S48] This possibly is inherent in the nature of EPs since by appropriately choosing a visual, auditory or somatosensory stimulus the resulting EP can be made to reflect activity generated in the visual, auditory or somatosensory cortex. More significantly, it seems that even though potentials recorded at the scalp may be generated almost entirely by cortical cells, the characteristics of these scalp potentials may reflect events occurring not in the cerebral cortex, but at lower levels in the sensory pathways. Furthermore, it seems possible that for any particular sensory pathway the sites of activity (e.g. retinal *versus* cortical) whose functions are reflected in the scalp EP can be selected by appropriate choices of stimulus parameters (see Sections 2.4.5, 2.4.6, 2.5, 2.8.8, 4.2.2; Figs. 2.13, 4.1). This suggests that it might be possible to use the scalp EPs recorded from a single electrode to explore different brain structures, and to test the normality of their respective functioning merely by using a battery of different stimuli. This suggestion does not ignore the power of multi-channel recording, nor of sophisticated methods of analysing the EP – quite the reverse. The purpose of these remarks is to point out that, given the groundwork of adequate fundamental research, there is good evidence that the scalp EP to stimulus A may largely reflect the functioning of the peripheral sensory organ, while for stimulus B the scalp EP may largely reflect the functioning of more central structures; by appropriately processing the respective EPs, the emphasis of peripheral or central activities may be even further enhanced.[547a]

A parallel line of argument stems from Rose and Lindsley's[684] study of visually evoked potentials in the developing cat. Even with simple flash stimulation they were able to distinguish between an EP component which reflected signals transmitted via the superior colliculus ('nonspecific' signals), and an EP component due to signals transmitted via the lateral geniculate body ('specific' signals). The latency differences which allowed these 'nonspecific' and 'specific' components to be discriminated were no longer evident in adult cats so that EPs to flash stimulation could no longer discriminate between the collicular and geniculate pathways.[551] If Rose and Lindsley's findings in cat could be extrapolated to man, then a good deal of human EP findings would be better understood. These findings include both (*a*) the common observation that short-latency and long-latency components of the transient EP have quite different characteristics, and (*b*) the differences between the characteristics of steady-state EP components in different frequency regions (Chapter 2, Sections 2.8.2, 2.8.3, 2.8.4). If it does prove possible, by manipulating the stimulus, to distinguish between EPs due to signals transmitted along the geniculocalcarine pathway and signals transmitted along other routes, then a clinical tool would be available which would have no current equivalent in routine clinical subjective testing although its feasibility is suggested by animal studies.[402, 859]

There is some advantage in putting this more formally. A theoretical analogue model of a sensory pathway (as seen via the scalp EP) could be a formal way of describing how different neural organisations (and possibly neuroanatomical structures) contribute to the EP. One proviso which should be made is that there should be an experimentally established correspondence between, on the one hand, each sequential and parallel stage of the theoretical analogue model, and on the other hand specific neuroanatomical regions in the real physical brain. At least one formal model of this type has been proposed (Chapter 2, Sections 2.8.2 and 2.8.3). Its application is restricted to steady-state EPs; there is need of a parallel effort to model the processes involved in the generation of EPs by transient stimulation. The early stages of the steady-state model have been found to correspond with definite sites in the retina of vertebrates (fish);[749] similar studies on primates might assist the development of EPs as a tool which would be effective at all levels of a sensory pathway for the location of lesions.[548]

A final point arises from the body of evidence that in some circumstances the correlations between subjective perception and certain EP features may be very poor. One explanation of this could be that EPs might allow access to populations of neurons whose functioning is not easily checked by sensory tests. Here there is a possibility that EP methods might not only *supplement* existing diagnostic procedures (and thus have a place when the indications provided by existing procedures are insufficiently clear), but might also be capable of providing information which is *not otherwise available.*

4.3.4 *Evoked potentials and pharmacology*

Appreciable efforts are being made in a number of laboratories to describe the effect of a wide variety of drugs on the EP. One aim of these studies is to find whether EP recordings could be capable of indicating the presence of a particular drug in the body. If this proves possible, then EPs might clearly be of value with certain comatose patients.

So far, most work on EPs and drugs has been restricted to the use of a narrow range of stimulation procedures. If the arguments of the preceding section ('location of brain lesions') are valid, then the use of a wide variety of stimulation procedures, coupled with parallel developments of automatic EP analysers, might enable neural function at different neuroanatomical sites to be systematically investigated. In this way scalp recordings might be capable of monitoring the effect of drugs and anaesthetics at specific local sites throughout the nervous system.

4.3.5 *Evoked potentials and psychiatry*

The recent introduction of techniques for recording the activities of single nerve cells in the brains of anaesthetised and even of normally functioning animals has led to a great advance in our understanding of the organisations of the visual and auditory pathways. So far, however, investigations have been restricted to neuroanatomical levels between sensory receptors and primary cortex. As already mentioned it seems clear that one function of neural tissue at these relatively peripheral levels is to 'emphasise' or 'abstract' those features of the outside world which are of importance to the organism. On the other hand, we still have no more than the most tenuous understanding of the central neural patterns of activity which underlie both normal and deviant mental life. It is still quite out of the question to define the aberrations of higher nervous activity which underlie specific psychiatric conditions.

In this situation it is true to say that apart from a very few cases in which intracerebral electrodes were implanted the recording of scalp evoked potentials is our only objective means of access to the activities of large neural populations in the intact human brain. At the present time, therefore, EP recording offers unique possibilities for advancing our understanding of the neurophysiological basis of mental life, and its malfunctions in psychiatric illnesses. Unfortunately there seems little doubt that this area of EP research is by far the most demanding, both scientifically and conceptually.

5

Techniques in evoked potential research

5.1 Visual stimulators and stimulation techniques

5.1.1 *The measurement of light and colour*

The first part of this chapter is devoted to advice on the basic design of stimulators, and is aimed at research workers who have little background in physics or engineering. The second part briefly surveys methods of data analysis which have been found useful in EP research.

It is essential to make a clear distinction between on the one hand physical measurements of power or energy, and on the other hand quantities which involve sensory physiology, such as for example the 'luminance' or the 'colouring' power of a stimulus light.

In addition, visual impressions which are governed by the peculiarities of the subject's own visual system should be distinguished from quantities whose definitions are based on the unique, internationally-agreed characteristics of the 'CIE standard observer'. For example, if two lights of different spectral energy distributions have the same luminances (see below), an observer who had a 'CIE standard eye' would see them as equally bright. To many people the two lights would appear to be in some degree unequally bright. Furthermore, even the individual subject who judges the two lights as equally bright at high levels of light adaptation would judge them quite different in brightness (e.g. by a factor of 100) under conditions of dimmer illumination. For such reasons it is customary in photometry to distinguish between terms which refer to the physical stimulus (e.g. luminance), and terms which refer to a sensation (e.g. 'subjective brightness' or luminosity). The term 'brightness' is an exception. It is used in an ambiguous and sometimes confusing manner to mean both the 'photometric luminance of the stimulus' and 'the subjective magnitude of the sensation of brightness'. This customary usage has, most probably, slipped into the following pages.

PHOTOMETRY

The primary source of light is a *black body* radiator at the temperature of solidification of platinum (2042°K).[839, 806]

Within a restricted range, viewing conditions have an influence on the relative spectral sensitivity curve of the eye but this influence is negligible when compared with normal inter-subject variability.[839 p.72] The limits of this range are (*a*) the retinal illumination should not fall below 100 trolands or so, and (*b*) the field should be centrally-viewed and of 2° to 3° subtense. This stability of the spectral sensitivity curve at high brightness levels is the basis of an internationally agreed system of light measurement (which, correspondingly, is valid only within a restricted range of stimulus conditions). In photometric texts the relative spectral sensitivity curve of the eye at high brightnesses (also called the 'relative luminosity' or 'relative visibility' curve) is called the Photopic V_λ curve. In order to circumvent the problems arising from inter-individual variability, a unique, internationally-agreed CIE (sometimes called ICE) V_λ curve has been defined for the 'standard observer'.

At very low levels of brightness (below roughly 1 troland) colours become less striking or even indistinguishable, and the eye approaches a condition where, just as in the photopic range, there is a well-defined relative spectral sensitivity curve. In photometric texts, this low-level curve is called the Scotopic V'_λ curve and its stability (within a certain range of stimulus conditions) is the basis of a system of low-level (scotopic) photometry which, correspondingly, is valid only within a certain range of stimulus conditions. Again, in order to avoid confusions due to interindividual variability, a unique, internationally-agreed CIE (i.e. ICE) scotopic V'_λ curve has been defined for the 'standard observer'. The scotopic relative spectral sensitivity curve has been found experimentally to be displaced to somewhat lower wavelengths than the photopic curve (the sensitivity peaks are at roughly 510 nm and 555 nm respectively).

The systems of photopic and scotopic photometry are both based on the same primary light source (see above). On the other hand the photopic system uses the photopic V_λ curve, whereas the scotopic system uses the scotopic V'_λ curve in order to define the respective photopic and scotopic units of luminous flux, luminance and illumination.

Within the intermediate range of stimulus levels (below roughly 3 cd/m^2,[334 p.11] i.e. roughly 40 trolands), the relative spectral sensitivity curve of the eye depends on stimulus brightness and assumes a form which shares scotopic and photopic characteristics. The measurement of light levels in this *mesopic* range presents special problems.[594, 595, 596]

PHOTOPIC PHOTOMETRY

The fundamental unit in photometry is one of *Luminous Intensity* (in other words 'strength of light source') and is the *candela* (cd.). The candela is defined as one-sixtieth of the luminous intensity per square cm of the primary source.[806, 839] The luminous intensities (in candelas) of lamps used as secondary standard sources are calibrated by comparison with the primary source. The *lumen* is the unit of *luminous flux*, and is defined as the flux emitted within unit solid angle (one steradian) by a uniformly-radiating point source of 1 candela. The *illumination* of a surface is defined as the luminous flux reaching it per unit area in lumens per square foot (*foot candles*), or lumens per square metre (*lux*). The *luminance* ('brightness') of a surface is its luminous intensity (i.e. 'source strength') per unit projected area, the plane of projection being perpendicular to the direction of view. The units of luminance are *candelas per square inch* (cd/in^2), *candelas per square foot* (cd/ft^2), *candelas per square cm* (cd/cm^2) and (commonly) *candelas per square metre* (cd/m^2). The *retinal illumination* is one *troland* when a surface of luminance one candela/m^2 is viewed through an exit pupil of area 1 mm^2. When calculating retinal illuminations the *Stiles-Crawford effect*[768, 839] should be borne in mind.*

Certain units used in illumination engineering are based on the notion of an ideal diffuser, that is a surface which has the same luminance from whatever direction it is viewed.[806] Many practical surfaces roughly approximate to this ideal. The luminance of an ideal diffuser emitting (or reflecting) one lumen per square foot is defined as one *foot-lambert* (*ft-L*). The luminance of an ideal diffuser emitting (or reflecting) one lumen per square metre is defined as one *apostilb* (*asb*).

SCOTOPIC PHOTOMETRY

All the photometric quantities defined for the photopic system have their scotopic analogues, and are distinguished by the prefix 'scotopic'. For example the scotopic luminance of the primary source is 60 scotopic candelas per square cm.

PHOTOMETRIC MEASUREMENTS

Under the most favourable conditions a difference of luminance of about 1% to 1½% can be detected by the eye; this ultimate sensitivity determines the limiting accuracy of visual photometry.

National standards laboratories are willing to calibrate suitable tungsten sources. Note that the calibrated value of the luminous intensity of a lamp applies to only one direction of light radiation. This direction will be marked on the lamp during the calibration procedure. The calibrated lamp should be used only occasionally for the purpose of calibrating other devices, and should be returned to the Standards Laboratory at regular intervals for re-calibration.

When comparing the luminous intensity of a test source with that of a calibrated source it is convenient to use the inverse squares method.[839] In practice, however, it is difficult to match the luminances of two lights when their colours are very different. The method of heterochromatic flicker photometry is a convenient way of minimising the effect of this problem. It is easy to demonstrate that when two differently coloured, unequally bright lights are alternately presented to the eye at a sufficiently high frequency, the colour and luminance differences between the two lights seem to disappear at different flicker frequencies. The colour difference disappears at a somewhat lower flicker frequency than the luminance difference, leaving a light of apparently constant colour which flickers in luminance. There is, therefore, a range of flicker frequencies over which brightness differences can be detected

* See page 40.

without complications due to colour differences. This fact is the basis of flicker photometry. When using the flicker technique the flicker frequency should be set (by trial and error) so as to give the most sensitive judgement. A surround field of roughly the same luminance as the test field is helpful.[839 p.304] The two lights should be presented for equal durations during each stimulus cycle. When measuring relative spectral sensitivity it is usual not to alter the comparison white standard light but instead to adjust the field luminance due to the test light. One practical technique of flicker photometry is to rotate a 90° sectored disc placed at 45° to the path of the beam. The front of the disc should be matt white. The flicker frequency should be variable over a range of roughly 10 to 20 Hz; this can easily be achieved by the type of variable-speed d.c. motor sold in toyshops.

Photometry is much more straightforward when the spectral energy distribution (i.e. colour) of the test field is similar to the spectral energy distribution of a calibrated comparison field than when colour differences exist. In commercial instruments, such as the SEI photometer and MacBeth Illuminometer this type of measurement is easily made by adjusting the luminance of a spot of light until it looks equally bright as an image of the test object.

When stimuli of identical colours are physically added, their total luminance is equal to the sum of their individual luminances. Abney's law states that this rule also applies when stimuli of different colours are physically added. There is evidence, however, that deviations from Abney's law may be marked.[839 p.390] These deviations are minimal when all luminance measurements are made by flicker photometry.[839 p. 391]

MEASUREMENT OF RADIANT POWER

The equivalent power (in watts) of a beam of light can be measured directly. On the other hand the conversion of this measure to lumens can only be accomplished by careful reference to the CIE relative spectral sensitivity (V_λ) curve for the 'standard eye'. For example, at a wavelength of 555 nm, approximately 685 lumens are equivalent to a power of 1 watt. In the ultra-violet and infra-red regions of the spectrum, the equivalent power of one lumen is effectively infinite.

Before embarking on attempts to measure radiant power, the experimenter is well advised to ask himself whether he really needs to carry out the difficult measurements of *absolute* light energy, or whether relative energy measurements or even photometric measurements would suffice.

Except within Standard Laboratories the ultimate instrument for measuring radiant power is a calibrated bolometer or thermopile. Both thermopiles and bolometers are equally sensitive to the invisible infra-red and ultra-violet radiations as they are to visible light. When calibrating a visual stimulus it is as well therefore to ensure that no ultra-violet or infra-red radiation is reaching the measuring instrument, particularly when the equivalent power of white light is being measured. This point is worthy of attention even when there are interference filters in the stimulus beam.

Thermopiles and bolometers are rather insensitive. It is often necessary to employ the absolute instrument to calibrate a photomultiplier tube which is sufficiently sensitive to detect the radiation falling on the position occupied by the subject's eye. It is sometimes possible to calibrate the photomultiplier by using the same light source and filter combinations which will be used in the physiological experiments. This method eliminates the need to allow both for the bandwidths of interference filters and the spectral distribution characteristics of sources.

THE MEASUREMENT OF COLOUR

In EP work it is usually sufficient to specify a stimulus colour by no more than its *dominant wavelength* and *colorimetric purity*. In any case, this method of specifying a colour has the practical advantage that it gives an immediate idea of what the colour will look like. The two quantities can be measured by the following procedure: one half of a bipartite 2° field is illuminated by the test stimulus. The other half of the field is illuminated by a mixture of white (illuminant B)[806] and a narrow-band monochromatic light whose wavelength is variable. The test stimulus is then subjectively matched by a suitable mixture of monochromatic light (of wavelength λ and luminance L_λ) plus white light (luminance L_w). In order to match extraspectral purple colours to white it may be necessary to add the monochromatic light (in this case the complementary wavelength) to the test stimulus, rather than to the white stimulus. The dominant wavelengths of the test stimulus is defined as λ and its colorimetric purity as:

$$p = \frac{L_\lambda}{L_w + L_\lambda}$$

In most practical cases, for both narrow-bandwidth and medium-bandwidth (i.e. *c.* 10 nm) interference filters, the colorimetric purity is approximately 100%, and the dominant wavelength is approximately the same as that for peak energy transmission, although the displacement of dominant wavelength for filters whose centre wavelengths are in the deep blue or above roughly 630 nm may be significant in some circumstances. Data from which calculations can be made of the dominant wavelengths and colorimetric purities of wide-band pigment filters (e.g. Kodak Wratten Filters),[461a] are usually given by the manufacturers.

The rigorous system of specifying colour by three numbers and the notion of the unit of colour-producing effect are thoroughly discussed by Wright[882] and by Graham.[334]

TERMS WHICH REFER TO THE STIMULUS AND THE CORRESPONDING TERMS WHICH REFER TO SENSATION (IN BRACKETS)

Wavelength or dominant wavelength (hue), purity (saturation), spectral energy distribution (both hue and saturation), chromaticity (hue and saturation), luminance (luminosity, subjective brightness).

PHOTOMETRIC UNITS: CONVERSION FACTORS

Units of luminance

Unit	Number of millilamberts
cd/m^2	0·314
cd/cm^2	3140
cd/ft^2	3·38
cd/in^2	487
ft-lambert	1·08
lambert	1000
International Apostilb	0·1

Units of illumination (illuminance)

Unit	Number of lumen/ft^2 (foot-candles)
lumen/m^2 (lux)	0·093
lumen/cm^2 (phot)	930
milliphot	0·93

5.1.2 *Maxwellian view versus 'free' view*

There are a number of advantages to the stimulation technique typified by projecting an image on to a screen. These advantages include: (*a*) the subject is not constrained; (*b*) binocular viewing is straightforward; (*c*) slide projectors are cheap and simple. Disadvantages include (*a*) the maximum stimulus luminance which can be achieved using simple projectors is low.* This means that narrow-band monochromatic stimuli which are sufficiently bright to fall well within the photopic range are difficult to generate with simple projectors. The resulting problems are especially severe in the red and blue. (*b*) Light sources of large dimensions are usually used in simple projectors, which means that there is no narrow focus at any point in the system. This may give rise to practical difficulties if it is required to use cheap devices either to change the stimulus intensity with a fast time course or to modulate stimulus intensity. A source of large dimensions is also unsuitable if monochromators or graded interference filters are to be included in the system.

MAXWELLIAN VIEW

Maxwellian view means that a lens or mirror throws an image of the light source into the plane of the pupil of the subject's eye (Fig. 5.1). The subject should see the lens L3 (Fig. 5.1) evenly illuminated, and giving the appearance of a patch of light. The stimulus field can be very bright since it is easily arranged that (almost) all the light which enters the optical system is projected into the subjects eye. The maximum theoretical luminance of a stimulus is equal to the luminance of the light source.[417] A Maxwellian view system can (ignoring losses in the optics) generate stimuli of this maximum theoretical luminance. This is the main reason for using Maxwellian view optics, and is of special importance in colour studies where narrow-band monochromation

* Reference 516, pp. 238–246 gives an account of the design of a projector system and a method of calculating the luminance of the projected image.

can cut down the available luminance to very low levels. This problem is especially serious in the blue where it is particularly important to ensure that stimuli are sufficiently bright to fall well into the photopic range. Note that the maximum field luminance does not depend on the power, nor on the luminous intensity of the source.

Lenses L1, L2 and L3 (Fig. 5.1) should be well-correlated achromats. The exit pupil should be comfortably smaller than the pupil of the subject's eye under the brightest viewing conditions, otherwise tiny head movements may cause the eye pupil to cut into the beam. If the exit pupil is made larger than the eye pupil, then less light enters the eye, and in addition any variations in pupilliary diameter may alter the retinal illumination. On the other hand, if the exit pupil is made too small, diffraction effects may become obtrusive.

A common way of minimising head movements is to use a bite bar. A suitable method of mounting a bite bar is on a lathe carriage or on a heavy optical bench slider which has micrometer adjustments in three dimensions. The bite bar itself can be made of the type of dental resin which softens in hot water, mounted on a piece of $\frac{1}{8}$ in. aluminium sheet. If the exit pupil is smaller than the eye pupil, centring may be accomplished by moving the eye until it is midway between the positions where the beam is cut off by the edge of the pupil.

If a bright stimulus is required, a source of high *luminance* must be selected. A physically-small source will give a narrow focus (Fig. 5.1) which enables the luminance of the beam to be chopped with a fast time course, and is also convenient for various types of light modulators.

The relation between object and image positions for Maxwellian view optics has been developed by Westheimer.[866] It is sometimes found that the lens L3 appears to be unevenly illuminated. Four common reasons for this

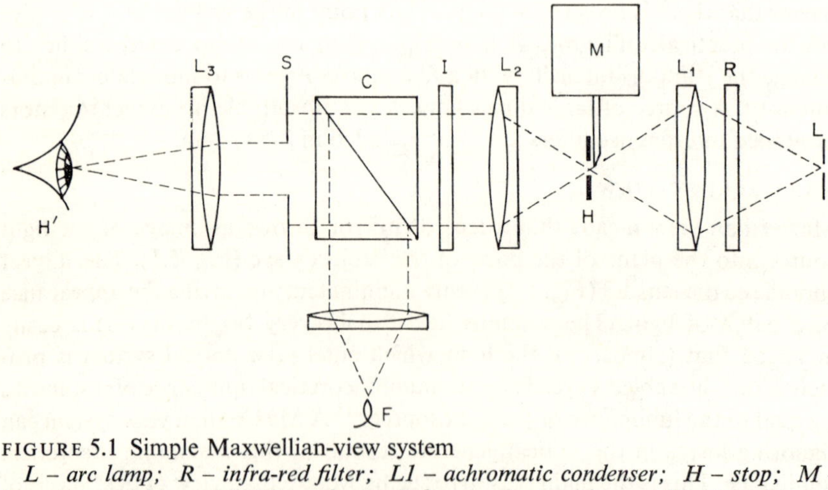

FIGURE 5.1 Simple Maxwellian-view system

L – arc lamp; R – infra-red filter; L1 – achromatic condenser; H – stop; M – intensity modulator; L2, L3 – achromatic lenses; I – interference filter in collimated beam; C – beam-splitting cube; S – field stop placed so that it will appear to be in sharp focus when the eye is relaxed; F – fixation light; H′ – image of H in plane of eye pupil (i.e. H′ is the exit pupil of the system).

are as follows (1) lens L3 is not of sufficiently good quality. A suitable lens for L3 is a well-corrected medium telephoto lens or an ex-military aero camera lens. Geometrical aberrations, particularly spherical, give characteristic darker patches in the field of view. The effect of aberrations is exaggerated when the eye pupil is off-centre. (2) The lenses in the system are either not on-axis or are tilted. (3) The source does not evenly illuminate lens L3. This may be due to inadequately corrected lenses in the early part of the system or merely due to their poor positioning. (4) The image of the source which falls on the cornea is small compared with the size of corneal irregularities.

A bite bar or chin rest is essential with Maxwellian view stimulation and this is the major disadvantage of the method.

By the use of a modified ophthalmoscope it is possible for the experimenter to view the retinal image of the stimulus during the stimulation procedure. Fixation and even accommodation can be monitored in this way.[731]

5.1.3 *Exit pupils*

The light flux incident on the retina depends not only on the luminance of the stimulus but also on the area of the eye pupil. The area of the pupil depends on a number of factors including the state of adaptation of the eye. Everyday changes in adaptation level can produce very considerable changes in pupilliary area (e.g. 15 : 1). It follows that a specification of stimulus intensity which does not include the effect of pupilliary area may be a very vague specification indeed. Some information of typical pupilliary diameters under differing adaptation levels is given by Walsh*[839] but the most satisfactory ways of controlling pupilliary diameter are (*a*) by viewing the stimulus through a hole placed in front of the eye, the hole being small enough to ensure that the cone of rays passing the eye pupil is narrower than the pupil (note the maximum hole diameter is determined by adaptation level, stimulus field subtense and the distance of the hole from the eye pupil); (*b*) by using a Maxwellian view system to image an exit pupil of appropriate diameter in the plane of the eye pupil (Fig. 5.1), and (*c*) by introducing an agent into the eye which causes the eye pupil to remain dilated. (Note: this manoeuvre also causes the stimulus to look brighter even though it is physically unchanged.)†

It is worth remembering here that light passing through the outer parts of the eye pupil is less effective in generating a brightness sensation than is light passing through the centre of the pupil (Stiles-Crawford effect).

The diameter of the exit pupil in a Maxwellian view system is best controlled by designing the optics so that it is clear which aperture is imaged to form the exit pupil. Works on practical optics[456, 516] include discussions on the correct placement of stops to determine the exit and entrance pupils of a system, to

* For example, very roughly 2 mm at 10,000 cd/m², 3 mm at 100 cd/m², 4 mm at 7 cd/m², 5 mm at 0·7 cd/m², 6 mm at 0·06 cd/m², 7 mm at 0·001 cd/m² and 7·7 mm in darkness.[839] However, pupil size tends to fall with increasing age.

† Fibre optic bundles have been used to transfer light to a small spot in front of the eye pupil.

delimit the stimulus field, to minimise lens aberrations and (in conjunction with clean optics and blackened lens holders) to minimise scattered light.

1.4 *Filters and monochromators*

It is difficult to vary the luminance of a white or broad-band stimulus without also changing the spectral energy distribution (i.e. the colour). Of course this difficulty does not exist with narrow-band monochromatic stimuli. The problem is due to the fact that so-called 'neutral density (ND) filters' are not really neutral, that is their transmission is not independent of wavelength. This means that separate calibrations of transmission of ND filters should be made at every wavelength used in experiments. It is often found in practice that the transmission of an ND filter depends on its location in the optical system. Neutral density filters should, therefore, be calibrated *in situ.*

Stimulus luminance may be varied in steps of 0·1 or even 0·05 log units by inserting ND filters. Since a little dirt or a thumbprint can seriously change the transmission of an ND filter they are better operated remotely. Stimulus luminance can be varied continuously by using an ND wedge. These are made in strip or circular form. A single wedge suffices if it can be placed at a point focus, but if the beam is of considerable area, either a compensating filter must be added, or two counterbalanced ND wedges used. These latter arrangements have the disadvantage that their maximum light transmission is considerably less than 100%.

If the stimulus colour is to be varied, a very suitable source would be a variable-wavelength laser which could be set to any wavelength within the visible range. Unfortunately such devices are not yet commercially available. Until then we are left with the inefficient method of filtering the light from a continuous-spectral or a line-spectral source. The major problem is to ensure that there is an adequate amount of light left to carry out the experiment after the beam has passed through the optics and the filters. Quite simple optical systems, *even when the optical surfaces are clean*, have an astonishingly low light transmittance. When faced with this problem, consider first a Maxwellian view system. If a Maxwellian view is chosen, then a source of high luminance is essential (but such a source may be of low power). A tungsten strip filament lamp or car headlamp bulb may be adequate, but if not, a hotter light source may be required. The higher the source temperature, the higher its luminance, and also the higher the luminance in the blue. The high-pressure Xenon arc is a convenient high-luminance source, although these lamps bring problems of power supply, cooling, handling, ultra-violet radiation, infra-red radiation, arc stability and ozone disposal.

Pigment (gelatine) filters transmit the greatest amount of light, but pass a correspondingly wide band of wavelength. Wratten (Kodak) filters are widely used; some of the range have sharp spectral cut-offs. Interference filters operate quite differently from pigment filters. Narrow-band filters may transmit a band of wavelengths whose half-width is only a few nm, but they consequently transmit very little light. Medium-bandwidth interference filters transmit more light but have half-widths of (typically) 10 nm. Interference filters must be used in a parallel light beam and must be placed accurately normal to the beam.

Before using an interference filter in any experiment it is worthwhile ensuring that it has no appreciable 'side peaks', and that the effects of the 'skirts' of the transmission curve can be neglected. If it is required to vary stimulus colour continuously, then a graded interference filter offers the advantage of simplicity. The light transmission is high but the bandwidth is unlikely to be less than 15 nm and the 'skirts' may be unacceptably wide. Furthermore, a light source of small dimensions is essential. Graded interference filters can be used to provide a stimulus whose *wavelength* can be modulated with a variety of temporal waveforms.[650] A monochromator provides a stimulus whose wavelength is continuously variable, and whose bandwidth can be small (e.g. 0·3 to 6 nm). However, the light transmission may be correspondingly low, the instrument may be expensive and a source of small dimensions is essential. Single monochromators are cheaper and transmit rather more light than double monochromators. However, the ratio of transmitted light to background scatter may be much inferior. For example, an amount of scatter of 'only' 1% may mean that when the monochromator is set to pass a wavelength to which the eye is unsensitive (for example in the blue or red) the scattered light may appear to be even brighter than the selected monochromatic beam. Boynton[90] points out that a useful trick for assessing the visual effect of scattered light is to view the transmitted beam through a cheap direct-view pocket spectroscope. An effective manoeuvre is to use a cheap single monochromator in conjunction with gelatine filters or broad-band interference filters. Prism monochromators may have higher transmittances than grating monochromators, but the bandwidth of the transmitted beam varies with mean wavelength for the prism type.

Monochromators give the maximum transmitted light energy for a given bandwidth when the entrance and exit slits are set to be of equal widths. Under these conditions the transmitted band has a triangular distribution whose half-height bandwidth is equal to the bandwidth equivalent to the setting of either the exit slit or the entrance slit alone. The energy distribution within the transmitted band can be modified by appropriate choices of the widths of the entrance and exit slits.[90]

5.1.5 *Stimulation by luminance changes: light sources of variable luminance*

Devices which produce changes in the luminance of a visual stimulus fall into two classes. These are (1) stimulators in which the luminance of the source varies and (2) stimulators in which the source luminance is constant and luminance modulation is achieved separately. In general, luminance modulation can be achieved more conveniently with stimulators of type (1), but the maximum luminance of the stimulus is lower than for stimulators of type (2). Type (2) includes the sources which are most suitable for colour work at the present time.

GLOW MODULATOR TUBE

Glow modulator tubes are cheap, and straightforward circuits have been designed to drive them.[524, 576] However, their luminous intensities are very low although their luminances are reasonably high so that they are suitable for Maxwellian view optics. Furthermore, their light changes in colour during the modulation cycle unless pulse-width modulation is used, a technique which may be physiologically undesirable.

FLOURESCENT TUBES

The domestic type of fluorescent tube makes an excellent light source. Such tubes may easily be driven by direct current from valve or transistor circuits, and if suitable photoelectric feedback is arranged, they can generate pulse, sinewave, triangle or ramp changes of stimulus luminance. The tubes are suitable for colour work if an appropriate phosphor is chosen. An array of small tubes placed behind a diffuser can serve as a panel source; a single large tube can be driven so that the illumination of a whole room is modulated.[506] Fluorescent tubes with appropriate phosphors can be electronically switched on and off with a time course which is sufficiently fast to allow the tubes to be used in tachistoscopes.[411]

XENON FLASH TUBES

Xenon-filled tubes can be designed for continuous operation (arcs) or for periodic flashing. Flash tubes require appropriate trigger circuits; suitable circuit designs are supplied by the tube manufacturers. The flash duration can be modified within wide limits by appropriately designing the trigger circuit. The maximum flash rates advised by the manufacturers for commonly-available tubes range from 3 per minute for the tubes used in photography to 300 per second for the tubes built into 'stroboflashes' intended for the examination of rotating machinery. In EP work it is essential to check that the total light flux does not vary from flash to flash, and that the mean light flux does not vary with frequency when different frequencies are used. In EP experiments it is important to guard against the effects of the clicks which accompany Xenon flashes. Even though the clicks produce no detectable EP when the light is occluded, it is still conceivable that they might influence the EP to the flash, or enhance the myogenic response to flash.

Very short Xenon flashes presented on a background of low adaptation level are likely to excite scotopic as well as photopic mechanisms. The very high percentage change of stimulus luminance during such a flash cycle can lead to unnecessary ('nonessential') distortions of the EP (Chapter III).

Xenon flashes have been widely used in EP work. This may have been due partly to the easy availability of stroboflash equipment, although a better choice might have been made on more rational criteria such as (*a*) physiological appropriateness (e.g. contour-rich stimuli) or (*b*) ease of describing the characteristics of the system (e.g. 'small signals', whether transient steps or sinewaves).

The advent of commercial frequency-modulated signal generators suggests that Stroboflash units could be used to generate modulated light stimuli, although this application does not seem to have been previously described. The F.M. signal generator could be set to drive the stroboflash, at a 'carrier frequency' of (say) 410 Hz, well above critical flicker fusion frequency. The desired modulation waveform (e.g. a 3 Hz triangular wave) would then drive the FM input of the FM signal generator via a potentiometer. The 3 Hz signal would vary the frequency of the stroboflash about the 410 Hz mean level. Modulation depth could be controlled by the potentiometer, and would be variable between 0% and roughly 60%.

ELECTROLUMINESCENT PANELS

Some materials emit light when placed in a sufficiently large electric field. The conversion of electrical energy to light is very efficient and does not involve the evolution of heat. However, the light levels available are so far very low and rather large voltages are required. Electroluminescent panels have been used as stimulators in EP work.[550]

PROJECTION TELEVISION TUBE

The television tubes which were originally designed for use in projection television sets give a very bright, small picture. By means of suitable circuits a bright area can be generated on the tube face in such a way that its luminance can be modulated by control signals. The tube face can be directly viewed, or a Maxwellian-view system can be arranged. Maximum luminances are fairly high but the device is of only limited use in colour work.

CRO STIMULATORS

Ordinary laboratory oscilloscopes can be used as stimulators (especially those with Z-mod, external X and external Y facilities). It is useful to have in addition a number of pulse generators and a waveform (ramp, triangle) generator.

Moving spot or moving bar stimuli are easily arranged.[542] If a sinewave signal (of say 10K Hz) is shifted in phase by 90°, and the 0°-phase and 90°-phase sinewaves are then fed to the X and Y inputs of the oscilloscope, a circular figure will appear on the screen (Lissajou figure). If now, the amplitude of the sinewave reaching the phase-shifting network is modulated by a signal S by means of an analogue multiplier, then the diameter of thz circular figure will vary with the time course of the signal S.

A de-tuned television set can be used to produce visual noise.[531]

By suitable circuitry a spatial sinewave grating can be generated on an oscilloscope screen.[118, 703] The luminance of the spatial sinewave grating can then be temporally modulated. Oscilloscope stimulators offer convenient electronic control of both the position and speed of movement of the stimulus, but maximum luminance is low and the control of luminance is quite non-linear.

TUNGSTEN FILAMENT LAMPS

The thermal capacity of small (2W) filament lamps is sufficiently low to allow their luminance to be modulated by changing the lamp current. The colour of the lamp varies with lamp current, and the luminance is related to lamp current in a very nonlinear manner. However, over a limited frequency range (very roughly 8 to 20 Hz), a sinewave variation in lamp current gives an approximately sinewave variation of luminance, and this may provide an adequate stimulus in some circumstances. It is possible to change the luminance of very small (pin) lamps with quite an abrupt time course.

5.1.6 *Stimulation by luminance changes: light sources of constant luminance, and luminance modulators*

TUNGSTEN FILAMENT LAMPS

As mentioned already, the brightest stimulus fields are produced by using Maxwellian view in conjunction with a light source of high luminance (the total power is immaterial). For light sources which operate by raising matter to a high temperature, the hotter the source, the higher the luminance. It is unfortunate that for tungsten filament lamps the hotter the filament the shorter the life of the lamp and the more rapidly its luminance changes with time. In tungsten-iodine lamps this ageing process is slower.

Tungsten lamps with a heavy strip filament are particularly suitable for illuminating slits, since they are of even luminance, and the large thermal capacity of the filament helps to minimise temperature fluctuations. Automobile headlamp bulbs or slide projector iodine-quartz lamps can also be used. These can be run from stabilized d.c. power supplies.

HIGH-PRESSURE XENON ARC LAMPS

The running temperatures of these lamps are very high (*c.* 5500°K), so that their luminances are very high, especially in the blue. Their emission spectrum is effectively continuous and, if care is taken, the position of the arc is reasonably stable.[219] The Xenon arc is very suitable for colour work. In animal experiments a Maxwellian-view Xenon arc stimulator has been described which allows the stimulated retina to be directly observed.[333]

Xenon arcs range in power from 75 W to water-cooled 6·5 kW lamps. All lamps must be handled cautiously because of the danger of explosion. When running, Xenon lamps emit dangerous ultra-violet and infra-red radiations. They have a negative resistance characteristic, and require special high-voltage igniting circuits. A Xenon lamp should be mounted inside a robust lamphouse made of nonmagnetic material. The smaller lamps (up to 150 W) can be cooled by natural convection, but larger lamps need extractor fans. The fan must not exhaust into the room, as poisonous ozone gas is generated by the ultra-violet radiation within the lamphouse. Once installed, however, a Xenon lamp powered by d.c. can be expected to provide roughly 1000 hours of trouble-free service.

ELECTROMECHANICAL LUMINANCE MODULATORS

The use of a light source of small dimensions allows the stimulating beam to be brought to a narrow focus. This is a requirement or an advantage in several types of luminance modulator.

An old method* of pulsing the luminance of a light beam is to cut a slot in an opaque disc, and then to rotate the disc in the path of the light beam. The rise- and fall-time of the pulse can be shortened by (*a*) reducing the diameter of the beam where it passes through the slot, and (*b*) increasing the linear speed of the slot by either using a larger disc or a faster rate of rotation. A rate of rotation sufficiently high to produce sharp pulses may produce the pulses too frequently. To overcome this problem a second slotted disc may be driven by gears from the first disc so that only (say) one pulse in ten reaches the subject's eye. Pulse duration may be varied by using a sectored disc with a variable aperture.

Isolated flashes of variable durations can be produced by a camera shutter. However, it is best not to rely too heavily on the accuracy of the exposure times engraved on the shutter, nor of the shot-to-shot constancy of a particular setting.

On-off switching of a light beam can be carried out with approximately a 3 msec rise time by means of a piece of card attached to a relay. A stepping motor can be used in a similar manner. Lower modulation depths can be achieved by replacing the card with an ND gelatine filter.

The devices described so far can be used so as to modulate rather than switch luminance by adding a second steady beam to the 'chopped' beam. However, they are restricted to pulses or square waves unless rather difficult stratagems are used.[406]

A number of electromechanical devices enable stimulus luminance to be modulated by anyone of a variety of waveforms in such a way that the modulation depth is continuously variable from 0 to 100%. Gubisch[344] described a device in which stimulus luminance was modulated by moving a blade in the focused image of the light source. A similar device was described by Van der Mark.[706] However, this latter device was originally designed to generate spots of light, and its adaptation to Maxwellian-view optics brings the problem that the subject may see a blurred image of the moving edge. At the expense of some light loss this can be avoided by appropriate positioning of lenses and by the use of a diffuser.[640]

Problems due to the subject's seeing movements of the modulator blade can be minimised by using an impressively simple device described by Smith.[743] This consists of no more than a small piece of polaroid attached to the arm of an EEG pen motor. A second piece of polaroid is placed in the beam immediately before the pen motor, and rotated until the luminance of the transmitted beam is half the maximum value. If, now, the small piece of polaroid is oscillated by the pen motor, the luminance of the beam can be modulated approximately linearly from a depth of 0% to roughly 60% with a

* Epicotister.

passband of (typically) d.c. to 70 Hz (−3 db). Squarewave, sinewave triangular and ramp modulations are possible. This device is cheap and reliable. The author has found that its simplicity has the advantage in EP work that problems of stimulus artifacts are minimised. The low impedance EEG pen motor can be driven by a simple transistor power amplifier.[231]

There are some devices which can modulate the luminance of an extended beam of light in such a way that luminance remains uniform over the whole area of the beam. A polaroid disc which is steadily rotated in a plane-polarised light beam will modulate the luminance of the light with a sinusoidal waveform whose frequency is equal to twice the rotation rate.[217] The modulation depth is almost 100% but may be varied by appropriately mixing the modulated beam with a second steady beam.[453] A 'pile of plates' replacing the fixed polaroid is another method which allows modulation depth to be varied.[642] The rotating polaroid method is restricted to sinusoidal modulation. Good-quality, clean polaroid is essential, as serious harmonic distortion can be produced by irregularities or thumbprints on the rotating disc. It should be noted that the introduction of extra polaroid or doubly-refracting media into the optics can lead to large waveform distortions. The rotating polaroid device has the disadvantages that rotating machinery is inconvenient, and its construction requires greater workshop skills than are demanded by the pen-motor modulator.

ELECTRO-OPTICAL LIGHT MODULATORS

The optical characteristics of certain liquid and solid media can be varied by the application of electric fields. In general, devices using these effects are either expensive to purchase or to maintain. Commonly, they can handle beams up to about $\frac{3}{4}$ in. diameter. Their particular features of enormously fast switching times is not an advantage for EP work. Solid-state devices based on Pockels' effect usually require high driving voltages, and consequently need expensive associated circuitry. The high driving voltages might bring interference problems to EP recording. Pockels' effect devices alter the spectral content of white light. Liquid cells (Varad) can be operated by lower voltages and can deal with wider beams but problems arising from the deterioration of the liquid cannot be ignored.

5.1.7 *Useful optical components*

Three useful optical devices are (*a*) Dove prism; rotation of the prism turns the entire visual world through any desired angle. (*b*) Corner cube prism, which returns light rays along their own path independently of their original direction. (*c*) Roof reflecting prism, which performs both left-to-right and upside-down transformations, on the visual world and (*d*) Beamsplitter, which either divides a beam or unites two beams. Double images can be avoided by using a beamsplitting cube, but semi-aluminised mirrors are cheaper.

When coloured patterns are used, the sharpness of the retinal image may be affected by the chromatic aberration of the eye. This blurring may be much reduced by viewing the stimulus through a lens whose chromatic aberration is approximately equal and opposite to that of the eye.[812, 882]

5.1.8 *Stimulation by spatially-structured (patterned) fields*

PATTERN APPEARANCE AND DISAPPEARANCE: PATTERN REVERSAL

The simplest way to generate a patterned stimulus is to illuminate a suitable pattern and view it either by reflection or transmission. A Xenon-flash can be used to evoked potentials to a brief flash-presented pattern, whereas if a steady beam is switched on and off the responses to stimulus-appearance and stimulus-disappearance may be recorded.

A disadvantage of the methods described above is that the appearance and disappearance of pattern is accompanied by luminance changes. Unless it is possible to show otherwise, potentials evoked by the luminance changes will be confounded with the pattern EPs, and it is also possible that before the EPs are generated there might be nonlinear interactions between the responses to luminance and pattern input. This problem has been countered by attempting to balance-out the associated change in stimulus luminance.

A tachistoscope allows one stimulus field to be rapidly replaced by one of several others. A patterned stimulus field can be replaced by an evenly illuminated field which has, for example, either the same total flux or the same maximum luminance as the patterned field. Multi-channel versions are available commercially but a satisfactory device can often be constructed in the laboratory.[411]

In one tachistoscope[411] the light sources are small, fast-phosphor fluorescent tubes which are placed behind diffusing panels. Patterned transparencies are placed in front of the panels, and superimposed by viewing them through half-reflecting mirrors. The light sources are switched electronically. The half-reflecting mirrors must be very uniform and colour-free. Some problems can arise in aligning the transparencies. In another version, superimposed images are thrown on to a screen by two or more projectors whose beams are electromechanically switched on and off.

A patterned-mirror method of generating patterned stimuli has the advantage that since only one pattern is used there are no problems of misalignment (Fig. 5.2). However, it is difficult to generate pattern-reversal signals whose modulation depth is much less than 2–5% without using an auxiliary adapting beam. The patterned-mirror method can be adapted to produce patterns in which chromatic contrast reverses at constant luminance (Fig. 5.2).

A patterned stimulator in which, again, one stimulus field is replaced by another, but which uses Maxwellian view, was developed in Riggs' laboratory.[674] Riggs' method is suitable for colour work. As it stands the method is restricted to a high modulation depth, and even with 3 mm monochromator slits there may be some problem with EP 'edge artifacts'. The author's experience is that edge artifacts which were prominently visible when a checkerboard mirror was observed in Maxwellian view could be much reduced (though with light loss) by placing sandblasted plexiglass (diffusing perspex) close to both sides of the mirror. This artifact seemed to be a diffraction effect, and might have been the result of the use of Maxwellian-view optics with a light source of small dimensions.

A checkerboard-patterned transparency mounted on a vibrator can generate pattern reversal stimuli when the excursion of the vibrator is exactly one square's width.[158] The transparency may be transilluminated and viewed

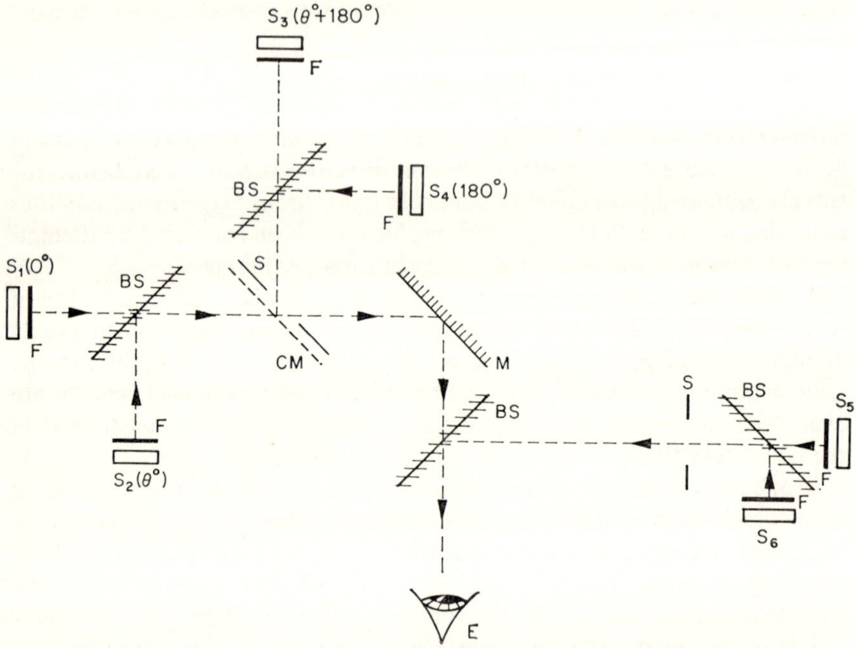

FIGURE 5.2 *Patterned-mirror method for generating chromatic or luminance contrast-reversal in a checkerboard stimulus pattern.* S_1, S_2, S_3, S_4 *– sources of modulated light;* S_5, S_6 *– sources of steady light; F – neutral density and colour filters; BS – beamsplitter; CM – checkerboard patterned mirror; S – field stop; M – mirror.*

directly, or alternatively may be projected on to a screen by a modified slide projector. A third arrangement is to leave the transparency stationary (e.g. in a slide projector) and to vary the position of the projected image by reflecting the beam with a rotatable mirror.[355] The mirror may be mounted on a pen motor. A zoom lens arrangement (mounted, for example, on an optical bench) can be used to vary the checkerboard square size of a projected stimulus.[649] As it stands the method is restricted to high modulation depths, but if a projector system is used a second projector can easily be arranged to reduce modulation depth by superimposing a uniform path of light on the image of the pattern. The time course of the pattern reversal stimulus is fixed and is equivalent to square-wave modulation in the checkerboard mirror system described above. Interesting motion effects can be observed when asymmetric waveforms are applied to the vibrator.

5.1.9 *Moving stimuli*

It has already been mentioned that moving spot, moving bar and expanding circle stimuli may conveniently be generated by means of an oscilloscope. Accelerated motion of more complex patterns can be arranged by placing an appropriate transparency in a modified slide projector and then moving the transparency by means of a velodyne motor or a vibrator.[542] Alternatively, the method used by Halliday of moving the projected image by rotating a mirror can be adopted.

5.1.10 *Evoked potentials triggered by eye movements*

When eye movements occur, the image of the outside world moves across the retina. Potentials evoked by eye movements while viewing patterned fields have been recorded both for large voluntary movements (Chapter 2, Section 2.6) and for involuntary movements of a few minutes of arc (Chapter 2, Section 2.4.7) by triggering an averaging computer by a (shaped) signal recorded from electrodes placed near the eye.

5.1.11 *Stereoscopic stimuli*

Julesz patterns have been used to evoke scalp potentials which are specific to changes in perceived depth under conditions where there was minimal change in the stimulation of either eye. Three projectors threw superimposed images on to a screen. Two images were of the reference pattern (1) and the third was of the comparison pattern (2). A mechanical chopper rhythmically exchanged pattern (2) for one of the reference patterns (1). By viewing through appropriate polaroids one eye saw an unvarying pattern (1) while the other eye saw patterns (1) and (2) alternately. The subject had the compelling illusion that the displaced part of the pattern rhythmically moved in depth. This technique as it stands has the disadvantage that correct alignment of the images is difficult, and that separate transparencies are required for each value of retinal disparity.[646, S53]

5.2 Methods of presenting odorous and taste stimuli

Allison and Goff described a method of inserting brief pulses of odorised air into a steady flow of clean air.[19] The timing of the odorous stimuli was sufficiently well defined to allow EPs to be recorded (Chapter 2, Section 2.2.5).

Plattig[610] described a method of electrically eliciting taste sensations, and of recording EPs to such stimuli.

5.2.1 *Somatosensory stimulators*

Somatosensory EPs have been studied using both electrical and mechanical stimulation. The general conditions under which EPs to mechanical and electrical stimulation are equivalent have not yet been clearly defined. In one specific case, that of electrical *versus* mechanical stimulation of a finger, some of the characteristics of the EPs obtained are quite different,[295, 811] although it should be mentioned that the same subjects were not used in both electrical and mechanical stimulation procedures.

Somatosensory electrical stimulators have been described by Uttal[811] and by Allison *et al.*[18]

Werner and Mountcastle[864] described a device which used a moving-coil vibrator for mechanically stimulating the skin. The relation between the mechanical displacement of the vibrator's coil and the driving voltage was made linear by feedback from a mechanoelectrical transducer fixed to the vibrator. Some method (such as feedback from a displacement sensor) for ensuring that a mechanical stimulator has, in effect, a very high stiffness is essential in order to minimise the effects of varying mechanical load during the stimulation cycle.

The separate problem of defining the way in which the skin surface follows the movements of the mechanical vibrator can be handled by sticking the vibrator's tip (which may be, for example, a 1 cm disc) to the surface of the skin.

Franzen and Offenloch[295] have described a mechanical stimulator which they have used in EP work.

5.3 Auditory Stimulators

DELIVERY

Auditory stimuli may be delivered either by a loudspeaker or by earphones. The use of a loudspeaker has the advantage that the subject is not restrained, but the disadvantages that the acoustic properties of the room may seriously affect the stimulus intensity *versus* frequency curve, and that the curve may be different in different parts of the room. Stereophonic, moving-coil earphones do not have this disadvantage. Furthermore, they allow each ear to be separately stimulated so that differences between the intensities, waveforms or timings of the stimuli to the two ears can be introduced as stimulus parameters. Earphones have the further advantage over loudspeakers that they minimise the time-lags due to the transmission between the sound transducer and the ear. Such time-lags can amount to several milliseconds and may not always be negligible in determining EP latencies.

GENERATION

In EP work the most commonly used forms of auditory stimuli are clicks, noise bursts, tone bursts, and changes in the frequency of a tone. Examples are given below of the many ways in which the electrical signals required to generate these stimuli may be generated.

Clicks of variable duration may be generated by driving either a loudspeaker or earphones by a pulse generator. The intensities of click stimuli may conveniently be varied by using a calibrated attenuator. If the source and load impedances are correctly matched to the attenuator, changes in stimulus intensity can be directly read off in decibels (db). Once the attenuator setting for which the subject can just detect the stimulus (absolute threshold) has been determined a calibrated attenuator allows subsequent stimulus levels (in db) relative to absolute threshold to be conveniently read off.

In EP audiometry it is usual to employ tables which give the sound pressure levels (expressed relatively to 2×20^{-4} dyne/cm^2) for the subjective hearing thresholds of a standard average subject. There are both international standard tables (ISO) and National Standard Tables.[633, 765] The sound pressure level at subjective threshold varies with the frequency of the stimulus tone; by using the tables of threshold pressure levels, the subjective thresholds of the standard subject can be taken as zero in expressing the patients' EP thresholds. The pressure levels for the patients' EP thresholds then give a direct indication of his hearing loss. Commercial noise generators provide an electrical noise signal whose amplitude *versus* frequency spectrum is accurately specified. Less stringent requirements may be satisfied by the noise generated by a high-gain amplifier of appropriate bandpass. Tone stimuli are conveniently generated by sinewave oscillators. An important point in generating tone bursts or noise bursts is that, if the stimulus is abruptly switched on or off, a switching transient will be present which may be so pronounced that it masks effects due to different tone frequencies. Switching transients may be specially important for stimuli of short durations. The effects of such transients may be minimised by devices (which are in effect multipliers) which shape the tone bursts so that their onsets and offsets are less abrupt. It is necessary to find a compromise between (*a*) an abrupt onset which may give a larger EP whose amplitude depends more on stimulus intensity but which spreads the energy of a tone burst to frequencies other than that of the tone, and (*b*) a too gradual onset which is unsuitable for eliciting time-locked EPs. If the energy of a tone burst is not restricted to a narrow frequency range it is difficult to detect losses which are restricted to narrow frequency bands in the sensitivity of the ear. One suggested compromise is a 15 msec rise and fall time.[547]

Although the frequency of a tone can be changed or modulated by mechanically moving the tuning dial of a sinewave oscillator, frequency changes are more precisely obtained by using a voltage-controlled signal generator. Tones whose frequencies follow, for example, a sinusoidal or a ramp waveform may be generated by feeding the sinusoidal or ramp outputs of a waveform generator to the input of a voltage-controlled signal generator.

CALIBRATION

One way of calibrating a sound field by the 'free field' method is to record the output of a calibrated microphone placed in the field at the site formerly occupied by the subject's ear.[633, 765] The free field method has the advantages that it can be carried out 'on-line' during an experiment, but has the disadvantages that the acoustic properties of the structures of the ear are not taken into account. An approximation to the sound pressure inside the subject's meatus may be found by using a calibrated microphone in conjunction with an *artificial ear*.[633] This method, however, does not allow 'on-line' monitoring of stimulus intensity.

5.4 Methods of recording and analysing evoked potentials

5.4.1 *Introduction. Evoked potentials and the EEG*

The first, and most basic obstacle to recording evoked potentials (EPs) from the scalp is that in almost all circumstances EPs cannot be recorded directly since they are between 2 and 100 times smaller than the 'biological noise' level.

In most subjects it is certainly straightforward enough to record some form of electrical activity from sites on the scalp. This activity (the EEG) often takes an oscillatory form, particularly when the eyes are closed with a predominant component in the region of 10 Hz (alpha activity). The EEG is 'spontaneous', although in only a limited sense, since the amplitude and frequency content of a subject's EEG can be modified by sensory stimulation. Nevertheless, it is a common practice to make a clear distinction between the 'spontaneous' EEG and scalp evoked potentials. Evoked potentials are commonly *defined* as scalp potentials which are locked in time (or in phase) to the sensory stimulus which evokes them; this definition may be forced upon an experimenter who uses equipment which is expressly designed to record potentials which are time-locked to the stimulus. Changes in the 'spontaneous' EEG which are triggered (directly or indirectly) by the sensory stimulus are sometimes regarded as being distinct from the evoked potential. Although this view may not be stated clearly, it is implicit in the procedures of an experimenter who ignores the changes (sometimes very marked) in the 'raw' EEG which are triggered by his stimuli. In general, the assumption that such EEG changes will necessarily 'average out' is not justified. One likely result of stimulus-dependent EEG changes is that the EPs recorded during low-alpha phases will appear to be less variable than the EPs recorded during high-alpha phases.* Such differences in variability can lead to problems of interpretation when certain statistical procedures are used to test whether two EPs are different (see Sections 5.4.11 and 5.4.12).

Clearly there is a problem in making a distinction between 'signal' and 'noise' if it is accepted that the brain may recognise as 'signals' electrical changes which are neither completely random, nor completely time-locked to the physical stimulus which they represent.

Scalp evoked potentials range in amplitude from approximately 0·3 to 20 μV; the amplitude of the 'spontaneous' EEG may reach 60–100 μV and its bandwidth overlaps with the bandwidth of the EP. Electrical activity from muscles may be at least as large especially for subjects who are tense or uncomfortable. These figures illustrate the degree to which evoked potentials

* Another possible result is discussed in supplementary footnote No. 21.

can be 'buried in noise', so much so that they are quite undetectable to visual inspection. In general, quantitative studies of EPs are impossible unless some method is used to enhance the signal-to-noise ratio of the 'raw' scalp record. Nonadaptive methods of enhancing signal-to-noise ratio (e.g. averaging) employ some *prior knowledge* or rigid working definition of the signal in order to 'recognise' the desired signal, in other words to progressively discriminate against activities which do not fit the definition of signal (i.e. 'nonsignals' or 'noise'). In contrast, adaptive methods of enhancing signal-to-noise ratio are capable of changing their working definitions of 'signal' in response to a developing clarification of the characteristics of the system under study.

When an averaging (summation) computer is used to enhance signal-to-noise ratio it is a temptation to visualise the waveform recorded by the computer as some sort of enlarged representation of an EP to a single stimulus. It is easy to forget that an averaging computer records the result of performing a certain statistical procedure on 'raw' EEG. On the other hand, it is certainly true that clear EPs to individual stimuli can be recorded from exposed cortex, and furthermore it is also true that (say) one hundred identical, individual EPs would be summed to give a summed EP identical in form to the individual EPs but one hundred times larger. In spite of all this it should not be assumed that a summed EP waveform made up of N sweeps *necessarily* represents the contributions of N identical individual EPs. One consequence of this uncertainty is that if the amplitude of summed EPs are found to differ in two stimulus situations, it is not immediately clear whether the difference reflects (*a*) a difference between the amplitudes of the individual EPs comprising the two samples, (*b*) a difference between the variability of the latencies of individual EPs in the two stimulus situations or (*c*) a spatial dispersion of the neural signal which is greater in one stimulus than in the other.

5.4.2 *Electrodes and amplifiers*

Thorough practical accounts of electrodes, electrode application and amplifiers are available.[316, 380] The most popular scalp electrodes are made of silver coated with silver chloride. Their major advantage is that a pair of such electrodes do not generate a large standing voltage when fixed to the scalp (i.e. they are 'reversible' or 'non-polarisable'). Even then, some care is necessary in order to minimise 'polarisation noise'.[287, 288, 867, 605 p. 84]

One method of applying electrodes is as follows: an area of scalp should first be cleaned by rubbing with cotton wool damped with alcohol, and then (locally) rubbed with electrode paste. The electrode may be mounted in a stiff framework which is held onto the scalp by an elastic band or by a strap. If more flexibility in placing electrodes is required they may be stuck to the scalp by means of quick-drying Collodion glue. The glue is squeezed or painted over the surface of the electrode; drying can be speeded by the use of a hair-drier or commercially-available air gun. In order to reduce contact resistance, a quantity of electrode jelly should be inserted underneath the electrode. Domed electrodes are supplied with holes so as to allow jelly to be injected through the blunted needle of a syringe. The blunted needle can also be used to abrade the skin in order to reduce interelectrode resistance to a suitably low value (less than 5000 to 10,000 ohms or so). Abrasion should be gentle for no other reason than the possibility that a subjcct might well refuse to participate in further experiments if he is subjected to painful jabbings. In any case an obstinately high interelectrode resistance is more likely to be due to a faulty or dirty electrode, or to inadequate cleaning of the scalp than to 'skin resistance'. Care in applying electrodes is worthwhile, if only to avoid the annoyance of having an electrode fall off at a crucial stage of an experiment. The likelihood of such a disaster can also be reduced by firmly clipping the electrode wires to the subject's collar. It is essential to keep electrode needles and syringes clean and sterilised since the over-enthusiastic use of dirty needles can lead to unpleasant local infections. If an earlobe reference is used, then some discomfort may be produced as the electrode glue gradually dries and contracts. This discomfort may be avoided by fixing earlobe electrodes by means of commercially-available sticky rings.

Even when no more than three or four electrodes are used, the process of attaching electrodes can take up an appreciable proportion of the subject's total available time; this wastage will be repeated in every experiment. It is therefore well worthwhile to ensure that the application of the electrodes is carried out as efficiently and as routinely as possible.

Scalp electrodes are potent sources of drift (i.e. noise) in d.c. recording. Specially-designed electrodes are commercially available for d.c. use.

The interelectrode impedance should be negligible in comparison with the input impedance of the amplifier, otherwise the voltage between the electrodes which is 'seen' by the amplifier is lower than the true 'open circuit' voltage. Furthermore unless interelectrode impedance is negligible, the 'open circuit' voltage depends to an important extent on the (arbitrary) relation between interelectrode impedance and the input impedance of the amplifier.

Differential amplifiers are generally used for EP recording because of their ability to reject noise signals (e.g. mains interference) which are common to the two input leads. Nevertheless, even when differential amplifiers are used, some initial problems with interference can confidently be anticipated when the experimenter's aim is to record microvolt signals (see Section 5.4.3).

5.4.3 *Noise*

It is noise (defined as undesired signal), and not the maximum available amplication factor which determines how small a signal can be detected. Methods of recording and measuring such very small signals as evoked potentials are basically procedures for minimising noise, and for circumventing its effects (Sections 5.4.1–5.4.14). In EP recording the three major sources of noise are (1) internal instrumental noise, (2) electrical magnetic and radiated interference and (3) biological noise (e.g. alpha activity).

Amplifier[67, 877] noise is generally of negligible importance when low resistance (i.e. a few kohm) scalp electrodes are used. On the other hand it is usually necessary in EP research to deal with problems due to interference. In practice, the investigator must make a compromise between flexibility and a 'once and for all' cure of interference problems. The principles of the systematic detective work required in tracking down sources of interference are discussed by Donaldson[237] (see also Reference 557). A source of electrical interference can often be located by soldering a 5 kohm resistor to the end of a pair of wires which are screened almost up to the resistor. If the screened lead is connected to a high-gain amplifier, then the resistor at its end can be used as a probe in order to assess the distributions of interfering electric fields.[237] A loop of wire can be used in a similar manner in order to track down a source of magnetic interference.[237]

Correct grounding and screening is essential. This point is discussed by Morrison (see also References 237 and 877). Ground loops are a potent cause of interference. It is therefore essential that the recording equipment should be grounded at only one point, and that the connection to ground is of low resistance. On occasion it is necessary to construct a low-resistance ground by connecting a thick wire to a buried, watered metal plate. If such a ground is used, then all connections to the mains ground should be broken (see References 237 and 877).

Radio frequency interference can often be identified by connecting a loudspeaker to the amplifier's output. Such interference can often be reduced by placing small inductors (e.g. a wire wrapped several times round a resistor) right at the input grids. Even though high-frequency interference may not appear to pass through the recording equipment, it can cause amplifiers to saturate and to produce spurious readings, so that efforts should be made to detect high-frequency interference and to prevent its reading the amplifier inputs. Electrical interference at mains frequency can be attenuated strongly by surrounding the subject with a grounded Faraday Cage made, for example, of chicken wire. Often it proves possible to obtain satisfactory screening while leaving large holes in the cage. Nevertheless it is good practice to remove electrical interference at source by using screened mains leads, and by enclosing electrical devices in grounded metal boxes. Magnetic interference can also be removed by screening – in this case with a number of layers of high-permeability metal. Unfortunately, this solution is generally impractical. Three ways of minimising magnetic interference are (*a*) to twist the electrode leads together so as to reduce the area of the pick-up loop, (*b*) to move the source of the interference as far away as possible and (*c*) to align the source so that it produces minimum interference.

ARTIFACTS

Artifacts fall into two classes (1) those which are not time-locked to the stimulus and (2) those which are time-locked to the stimulus.

If their amplitudes are sufficiently large, artifacts which are not locked to the stimulus, or even artifacts which occur only once or twice may be prominent in the averaged EP waveform. Examples of such artifacts are those due to mains pulses, eye blinks[S42] or movements of the subject. One way of guarding against such contamination is to monitor and record the EEG during the period of stimulation.

Even artifacts of very small amplitudes predominate in the averaged EP, if the time of occurrence of the artifact is locked to the averaging sweep. Time-locked artifacts may be both biological and instrumental. Although auditory EPs to the click of a stroboflash may be of small amplitude, the sound is best eliminated since it is difficult to ensure that the auditory stimulus does not affect either the EP or the myogenic response to the visual stimulus.

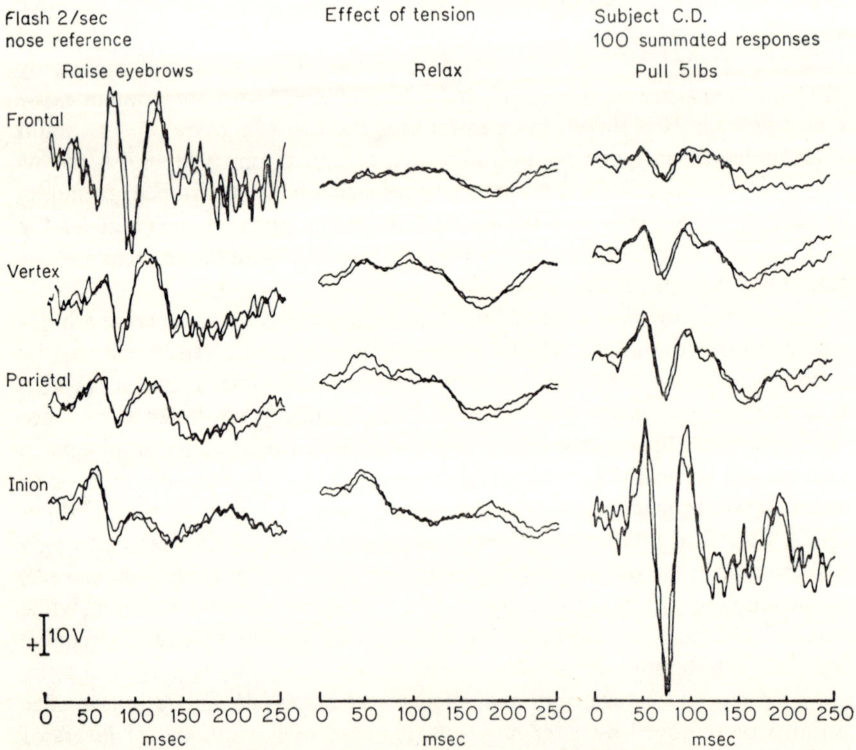

FIGURE 5.3 *Effect of muscle tension on photic-evoked myogenic responses. The centre section shows responses from midline electrodes for a relaxed subject. When the eyebrows are raised a new response with a latency comparable to an evoked cortical response appears in the frontal region and to a lesser extent at other electrodes (left section). The right section shows that, when the neck and posterior cranial muscles are tensed by having the subject support a weight, a large response appears which is maximal in the occipital regions and has latencies of N50, P75 and N100. The responses shown in the figure were produced by a stimulus of intensity 8 (Grass Photo – stimulator P2), although photic-myogenic responses can be obtained down to perceptual threshold. From R. G. Bickford (1969).* Average Evoked Potentials, *Ed. E. Donchin and D. B. Lindsley. NASA SP-191.*

The Bickford myogenic potential is, perhaps, the most notorious of biological artifacts. It is more serious for visual and auditory EPs than for somatosensory EPs.[225] The degree of myogenic contamination of an EP can be assessed by varying muscle tension,[77, 79] but perhaps the most satisfactory way of distinguishing myogenic from other potentials is to measure topographical distributions.[816] Topographical plots also offer a solution to the problem of recognising contamination of the EP due to the ERG, eyeblinks and the a.c. potentials due to changes in the direction of the d.c. corneoretinal field during eye movements.[816]

Visual EPs have been reported to be influenced by the phase of the cardiac cycle.[111, 177]

The reported influence of eye position on alpha activity[559, 560] has been attributed, not to changes in eye position *per se*, but rather to accompanying changes in visual input.[130, S46] The amplitude of 'averaged alpha' can be reduced by averaging only during periods of low alpha activity, although it is not clear whether this manoeuvre might bias the EPs to any serious extent.[S21]

When a particular stimulus is the subject's cue to make some sensory discrimination or to perform some motor action, then *if the time of occurrence of the stimulus is predictable* he may alert himself and prepare for mental or motor activity. If the EPs to such cueing stimuli are found to be different to EPs to control stimuli, then the differences may be due in part to the subject's stimulus-locked alerting reaction.[561] One way round this problem is to randomise the stimulus delivery so that the subject cannot anticipate the nature of the next stimulus.[561]

Photoelectric artifacts can occur if the stimulus light is allowed to reflect on to the electrodes. Acoustic or vibratory signals generate artifacts due to microphony in valve amplifiers. When shock stimuli are used (e.g. in order to generate phosphors) some care is necessary to ensure that electrical signals from the stimulus do not spread to the recording electrodes. Direct electrical coupling between stimulus circuits and the recording circuits must be eliminated by such tactics as using separate power supplies, avoiding earth loops, and by maintaining a generous distance between the stimulus and the recording leads and circuitry.

It is best to calibrate the recording system by feeding microvolt signals into the headboard from a source impedance which is comparable to that of the subject's electrodes. When recording EPs to stimuli of any modality it is essential to control for stimulus-locked artifacts by recording averages under 'stimulus-off' conditions. Since it is conceivable that the presence of a stimulus could alter the background EEG activity and the subject's psychological state, a useful control is to record averages while stimulating at a slightly different frequency to the averager sweep frequency *without previously warning the subject*. (Note: it is essential to ensure that the frequencies are sufficiently different that any averaged EP is of negligible amplitude.) This procedure gives an estimate of the noise level in the averaged EP; a knowledge of the noise level is essential before two waveforms can be judged to be different. By computing the ±Reference, the level of noise can be measured for runs during which EPs were actually recorded.[705] The ±Reference is obtained by alternately adding and subtracting successive samples of EEG, then finally dividing the result by N (N = the number of EEG samples).

When 'raw' EEG data is recorded on magnetic tape and subsequently analysed off-line, there are dangers of artifacts due to 'wow' and 'flutter' of the tape system. If the timing pulses are separated by intervals approximately equal to the sweep time, then some irregularities in triggering may result with consequent omissions of responses.

Digital computers introduce digitising errors which may be important when EPs of small amplitudes are recorded.

The methods of analogue-to-digital conversion of signal amplitude adopted in some special-purpose averagers may give problems if very small numbers of sweeps are used.

5.4.4 *Multi-channel recording*

Differences between the topographical distributions of EP components are important indicators of possible differences between their sites of origin (see Chapter 2, Section 2.10). Because of EP variability, topographical 'contour-maps' (i.e. equipotentials) must in practice be obtained by simultaneously recording responses from many electrodes. One way of achieving multi-channel EP recording with two-channel or four-channel averagers is to record on a multichannel FM (frequency-modulated) tape recorder raw EEGs from a number of sites [e.g. up to 14 sites with an 'ordinary' (i.e. very expensive) instrument, up to 32 or 64 sites with more advanced or larger devices]. On the other hand, if an FM tape recorder is required to enable no more than one or two channels of 'raw EEG' to be analysed off-line, then an FM attachment can be fitted to a domestic quarter-inch tape recorder. Such a device is very much cheaper per channel than even the cheapest 1 in. tape systems. Fairly cheap, quarter-inch four-channel FM systems are currently commercially available. A number of EEG channels can be recorded on a single track[484] by multiplexing. Extra channels can be added comparatively cheaply when an on-line Fourier analyser is used to analyse the raw EEG (see below, Section 5.4.9) but such a device has only restricted applications.

5.4.5 *The ten-twenty electrode system*[784]

The ten-twenty electrode system stems from an attempt to place particular electrodes over particular brain areas independently of skull size. The anterior-posterior measurements are based on the distance between the nasion and the inion as measured along the midline over the vertex (Fig. 5.4). Five points are marked along this line, designated Frontal pole (F_p), Frontal (F), Central (C), Parietal (P) and Occipital (O). Point F_p is 10% of the nasion-inion distance above the nasion. F is 20% of this distance back from point F_p, and so on in 20% steps for points C, P and O (hence the name

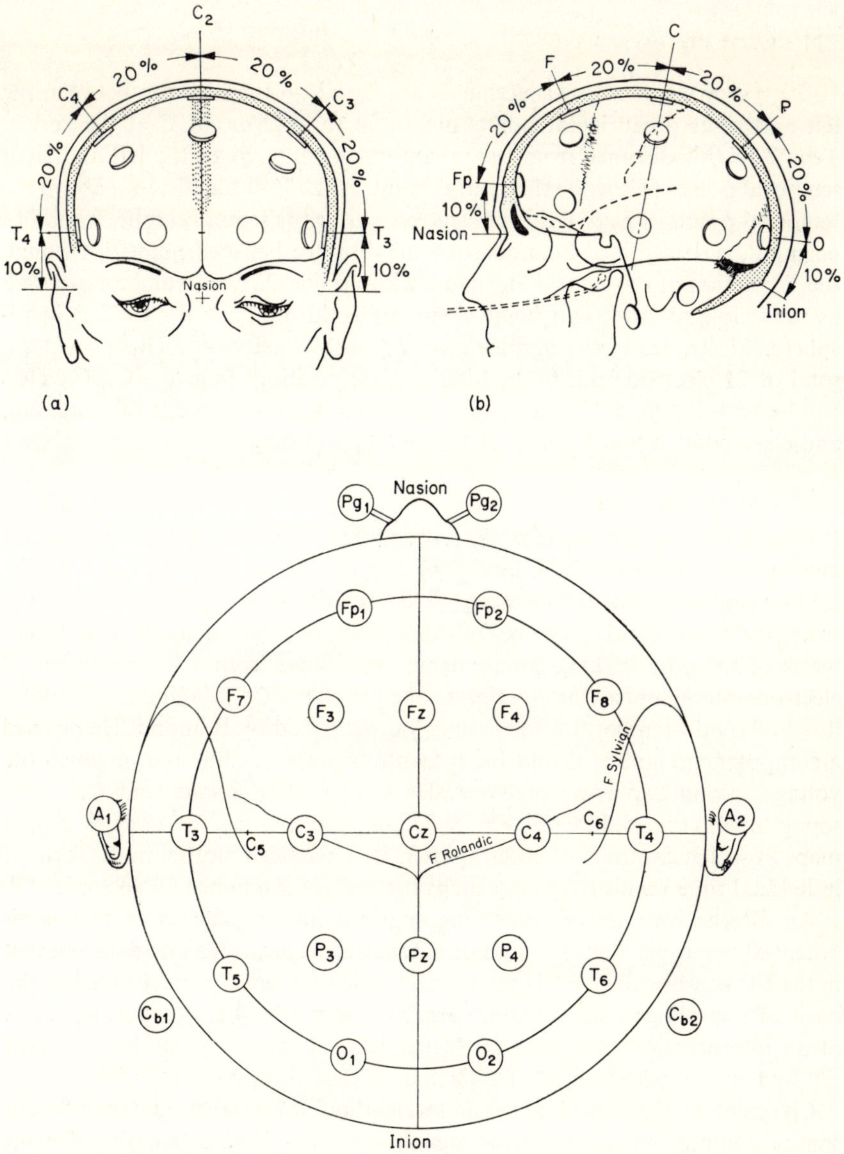

FIGURE 5.4 (a) *Frontal view of the skull showing the method of measurement for the central line of electrodes.* (b) *Lateral view of skull to show methods of measurement from nasion to inion at the midline. F_p is frontal pole position, F is the frontal line of electrodes, C is the central line of electrodes, P is the parietal line of electrodes and O is the occipital line. Percentages indicated represent proportions of the measured distance from the nasion to the inion. Note that the central line is 50% of this distance. The frontal pole and occipital electrodes are 10% from the nasion and inion respectively. Twice this distance, or 20%, separates the other line of electrodes.* (c) *A single-plane projection of the head, showing all standard positions and the location of the Rolandic and Sylvian fissures. The outer circle was drawn at the level of the nasion and inion. The inner circle represents the temporal line of electrodes. This diagram provides a useful stamp for the indication of electrode placement in routine recording. From H. H. Jasper (1958). 'The ten-twenty electrode system of the international federation',* Electroenceph. clin. Neurophysiol., ***10***, *371–375.*

10-20 system). Lateral measurements are based on the distance between the left and right preauricular points measured through point C at the vertex. Ten % of this distance from the preauricular points gives the left and right temporal points (T), while the central points lie 20 % of the distance above the temporal points. The A-P line of electrodes over the temporal lobe, frontal to occipital, is determined by measuring the distance between point F_p through the T position of the central line and back to point O. Even numbers are used as subscripts for the right hemisphere, and odd numbers for the left hemisphere. Electrodes in the midline have z (zero) as subscript. This provides a total of 21 electrode positions. Intermediate positions (e.g. F_2, C_2, C_6, etc.) can be added. Fig. 5.4 shows additional pharyngeal electrodes Pg_1 and Pg_2, and electrodes over the posterior fossae Cb_1 and Cb_2.

5.4.6 *Spatio-temporal maps*

It is clear that the EP waveforms recorded from a single electrode placement give at best only a partial impression, and sometimes may even give a misleading impression of the electrical field distribution over the surface of the scalp. Evoked potentials can be fully described, in terms of space as well as in terms of time, by making simultaneous recordings from a large number of electrode placements. One solution to the problem of displaying the resulting flood of spatio-temporal information was described by Rémond. He devised a computer method of displaying a 'contour map' of potential in which the voltages along two rows of electrodes were plotted *versus* time ('chronotopograms') (Fig. 5.5).[545, 651–656, 862] Digital filtering can be used to obtain maps in which contours of spectral intensity have been plotted in the form of individual time *versus* frequency maps for each of a number of electrodes.[843]

An alternative way of presenting spatio-temporal data is to plot equipotential 'contour' maps for a number of different peaks which are prominent in the EP waveform.[324, 816] Topographical field maps can be constructed on the basis of recordings taken from an array of only 4 by 4 electrodes by means of an interpolation procedure.[525] More detailed mapping has been carried out by Lehman with the aid of a 48-channel recording system.[484, 554]

Clynes[146, 151] developed a computer method for extracting the different spatial components of EPs from signals recorded from a 'rosette' of eight electrodes (see also Chapter 2, Section 2.9.1).

There can be no doubt that the more detailed of the mapping techniques described above are analytical techniques of great power. So far, however, they have been paired with comparatively weak stimulation procedures. With few exceptions[413, 536, 816] stimuli employed in the more detailed mapping experiments have not been chosen on the grounds of their physiological appropriateness. In some cases the only stimuli used have been Xenon flashes.

There are a number of other stimuli which seem likely to prove more physiologically revealing than Xenon flashes (see Chapter 2). Furthermore, although the visual stimuli used in most mapping studies have been exclusively symmetrical, centrally-viewed fields, it seems clear that a comparison of the

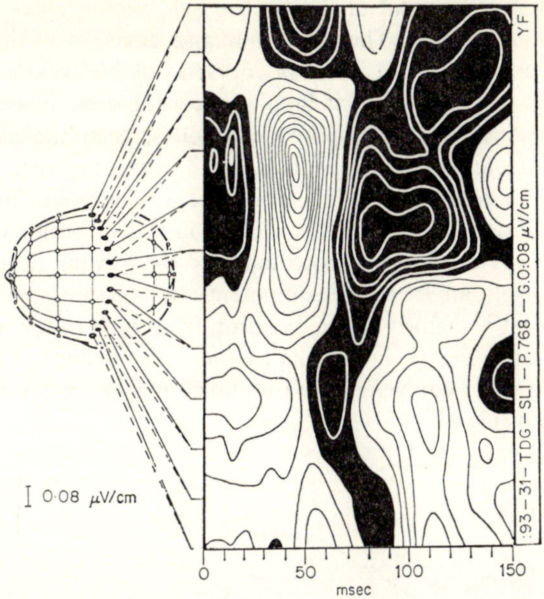

FIGURE 5.5 *Spatio-temporal map (Rémond) of scalp potential gradients along a transverse series of electrodes in a normal adult subject. Average central responses to 200 stimuli delivered at time zero to the left median nerve at the wrist. The potential gradient between adjacent lines is 0·08 µV/cm. Negative gradients appear in black and positive gradients in white backgrounds. The early potential source on the right hemisphere (components 2–3) is followed by a sink (component 4) located approximately on the midline. From I. Mézan, N. Lèsevre and A. Rémond (1968). 'Étude chrono-topographique de la réponse somesthésique évoquée moyen recueillie sur le scalp par stimulation électrique du nerf médian', in* Rev. Neurol., ***119**, 288–295. Masson and Cie, Paris.*

responses to focal stimulation of different retinal areas is a valuable adjunct to topographical mapping.[355, 413]

5.4.7 *Bipolar versus referential (i.e. 'monopolar') recording*

Contradictory statements are scattered throughout 'the literature' on the relative merits of bipolar *versus* 'monopolar' electrode placements: there is even disagreement on the differences which characterise bipolar and 'monopolar' recordings. At the one extreme Bergamini and Bergamasco[71] regarded bipolar and monopolar data as basically similar, while at the other extreme Vaughan[815, 816] considered most bipolar components to be artifactual. The core of this problem seems to be the awkward fact that in practice only a part of the distinction between bipolar and 'monopolar' recordings can be clarified on theoretical grounds: some points can be settled only by experiment.

It is clear that a bipolar electrode pair of separation δx cm (A and B in Fig. 5.6) records the potential *difference* δV volts ($\delta V = V_2 - V_3$) between the electrodes. If the electrodes are sufficiently close together the ratio $\delta V/\delta x$ volts per cm gives a reasonably close approximation to the magnitude at point M of that component of the electric field vector which lies along the line of the two electrodes. The magnitude and direction of the electric field vector E at the mid-point M is not of course available from a single bipolar recording (Fig. 5.6). However, if bipolar recordings are made from a large number of chains of closely-spaced electrodes, then the samples of δV measurements recorded at a single instant can be put together so as to give a 'contour map' of equipotential lines (i.e. lines joining points of equal potentials – shown dotted in Fig. 5.6). The electric field distribution can be derived from a sufficiently detailed equipotential map by drawing in lines which are everywhere at right angles to the equipotentials. The direction of the electric field at any point is defined as the direction from high to low potential. The descriptions of the electric field given by the scalar quantity V or the vector quantity E are quite equivalent, and a choice may be made merely on the grounds of convenience.

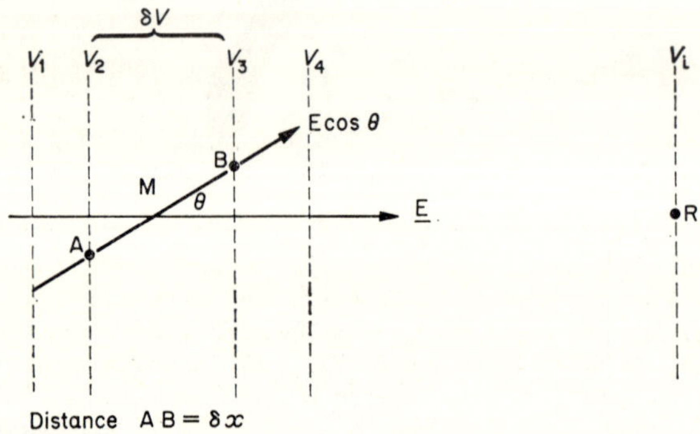

FIGURE 5.6 *V_1, V_2 – – – V_i are equipotentials; E is the electric field vector at point M; E cos θ is the component of the electric field at point M which is at an angle θ to the direction of E.*

Although the use of bipolar recording can give an adequate description of the distribution of either the electric or the potential field in any practical region of interest, it is clear from Fig. 5.6 that the procedure of measuring the *difference* between the potentials of different points ($\delta V = V_2 - V_1$) does reject information about the absolute values of potential V. The common approach to this problem is to aim at monopolar recording; that is to record the potential of one active electrode with respect to the unvarying potential of an electrically-distant 'reference' or 'indifferent' electrode. Electrical 'indifference' may be achieved in one of two ways (*a*) the reference electrode may be placed at a point which is (electrically) at infinity, that is a point which is at absolute zero potential. It should be emphasised that spatial distance and electrical distance are quite distinct notions, and that an infinite electrical distance need not be a long spatial distance. (*b*) The second way to achieve electrical indifference is to place the reference electrode at a point where the positive and negative potentials due to different sources cancel (for the subject being studied in the special circumstances of the experiment).* In practice there is no such thing as true monopolar recording, since a truly

* But see for example supplementary footnote No. 17.

indifferent electrode placement cannot be found. So-called monopolar records are therefore better called 'referential'. The reference electrode (R in Fig. 5.6) is, to a greater or lesser extent, an active electrode. The nearest approximation to an indifferent electrode seems to require intracerebral placements.[847] This apart, a working criterion for indifference is that the electrode should show no consistent time-locked activity with respect to any of a number of other sites.[324] On this basis the best extracerebral reference site for somatosensory, visual and auditory modalities has been reported to be the earlobe contralateral to the stimulus.[324 p.99] Halliday and Michael, however, find that the earlobe is not indifferent when pattern reversal stimuli are used (personal communication).[S17]

A practical point relating to the choice of bipolar *versus* monopolar recording is illustrated in Fig. 5.7 A. This figure illustrates potentials due to two separate sources (italic and boldface numbers); the net potential at any point is of course the algebraic sum of the potentials due to the two sources. If it is required to detect and separately measure the field due to the

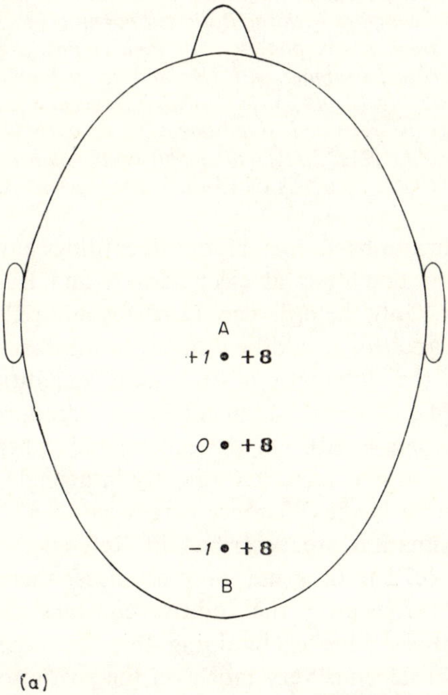

FIGURE 5.7 A: *Diagram of head showing at three points the instantaneous potential (in microvolts) due to two intracranial generators. The potentials due to one source are marked in italics and the potentials due to the other source are marked in boldface type. The net values of potential are (reading downwards)* $+9$, *8 and 7* μV. *Monopolar recordings at A and B would record potentials whose amplitudes differed by only roughly 20%, so that the contribution of the italicised source could be assessed only imprecisely. However, bipolar recordings made between A and B will cancel the contribution of the stronger boldface source and give a more precise measurement of the small italicised source.*

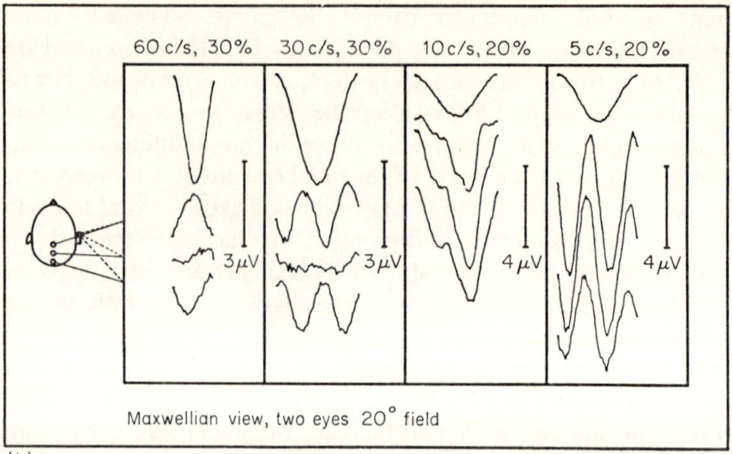

FIGURE 5.7 B: *A practical example of the hypothetical situations shown above. The traces on the far left show pure high-frequency EPs. Note the opposite polarity of the top and bottom traces; compare with the italicised potentials in A. The traces on the far right are pure low-frequency responses. Note their comparatively large amplitudes and the constant polarities; compare with the boldface potentials in A. At stimulus frequencies between roughly 13 and 25 Hz both high-frequency and low-or-medium-frequency responses may be recorded simultaneously at each electrode, but bipolar recordings between A and B (Fig. 5.7A) will emphasise the high-frequency components. From H. Spekreijse (1966).* Analysis of EEG Responses in Man. *Junk Publishers, The Hague.*

weaker source (italic numbers), then bipolar recordings have some advantage. The true monopolar potentials at electrodes A and B would be +9 and +7 μV respectively. Only the *difference* (2 μV) would reflect the presence of the weaker source, and this would be difficult to measure with precision if it were measured as the difference of two large quantities (since constant percentage errors of $x\%$ in measurement mean large absolute errors when large quantities are measured). On the other hand, when the difference in voltage between A and B is measured directly in a single bipolar recording, then the absolute error in the difference is reduced to $x\%$ of 2 μV (practical examples of this situation are described in References 636 and 748 and illustrated in Fig. 5.7 B). In some circumstances, therefore, it can be a positive benefit to throw away the additive constant included in absolute measures of potential. Whether in doing this the experimenter gains in physiological insight depends very much on the spatial organisation of the neuronal EP generators: at the present time this is a subject of *empirical* rather than *a priori* judgements. One example of a practical gain in using bipolar rather than monopolar placements is the measurement of the spectral sensitivity of certain EP components whose intrinsic interest is out of proportion to their relative amplitudes[639] (see Chapter 2, Section 2.9.3). Perhaps the safest practice is to routinely record all EEG channels on multichannel FM tape together with recordings from several reference sites. Either referential or bipolar averages may then be made off-line.

5.4.8 *Morphology of transient evoked potentials*

Sensory evoked potentials to transient stimuli (i.e. pulses, steps, ramps) are usually displayed as plots of voltage *versus* time (Fig. 5.8). The way in which the various features of the response (i.e. the peaks and humps) are labelled implies certain assumptions about the nature of the neural processes which determine the waveform.* If it is assumed that contiguous negative and positive deflections reflect a single neural process, then an analysis of the EP waveform into peak-to-peak deflections is indicated. On the other hand, if it is true that separate neural processes underlie positive and negative components,[21, 617] then a description of the EP waveform in terms of baseline-to-peak measurements would seem more likely to lead to physiological insights. The use of the baseline-to-peak measure does, however, bring problems (*a*) in defining the baseline and (*b*) in allowing for the fact that, for example, a negative-going peak may be displaced bodily into the positive region by a simultaneously-occurring positivity and (*c*) an apparently single peak may be composed of two separate components.

Fig. 5.8 illustrates three systems for describing transient EP waveforms.[136, 309, 324] The generality of all the classification systems so far proposed for visual EPs is limited by the fact that they are all based on EPs to diffuse flashes. It is clear that the waveform of the EP can be markedly influenced by a number of factors including the spatial structure of the stimulus, the colour of the stimulus, the instructions given to the subject and the electrode derivations. Ciganek classified the transient EP waveform into three regions (*a*) a 'primary response' up to 90 msec, (*b*) a secondary response (90–240 msec) and (*c*) an after-discharge. Ciganek[136] suggested that the scalp-recorded 'primary response' (to flash) is 'specifically evoked in area 17 by a stimulus following a specific pathway'. Although this notion has received support[241, 816] it has also been challenged (Chapters 2 and 5); in a later paper Ciganek has argued against the notion. Evidence from animal experiments[399] suggests that the evoked neural activities may be different when the stimulus is patterned rather than being a diffuse flash, and indeed the EP data in man do support the notion that an early (80 msec) component of the pattern-appearance EP is generated in primary visual cortex.[413]

Ciganek[136] suggested that his 'secondary response' was 'nonspecific'. The notion that late components of the EP and especially those late components recorded near the vertex are 'modality-nonspecific' is the subject of a controversy which is complicated by the fact that the term 'nonspecific' is used ambiguously in EP research. 'Modality-nonspecific' is sometimes used in the sense of 'a wave that is grossly similar in appearance when evoked by stimuli

* Fox and Rudell[293a] have shown that in cats an individual EP component can be selectively changed in amplitude by operant conditioning. They suggested that their finding implies that individual EP components reflect functions which are independent of each other. Rosenfeld *et al.*[684a] have reported evidence that the amplitudes of individual EP components can be altered by operant conditioning procedures in man, although the effect seemed less marked than in cat.

of different modalities'. In other cases the usage of the term seems to imply the existence of neural populations whose functioning is independent of the modality of the stimulus.

The neuroanatomical structures involved in the genesis of auditory and somatosensory EPs are discussed in Chapter 2.

Goff has pointed out that systems in which waves are numbered sequentially (Fig. 5.7) suffer from the following disadvantages (*a*) if additional components need to be labelled, all later components must either be renumbered or subscripts must be added to the existing subscripts, and (*b*) in any sequential

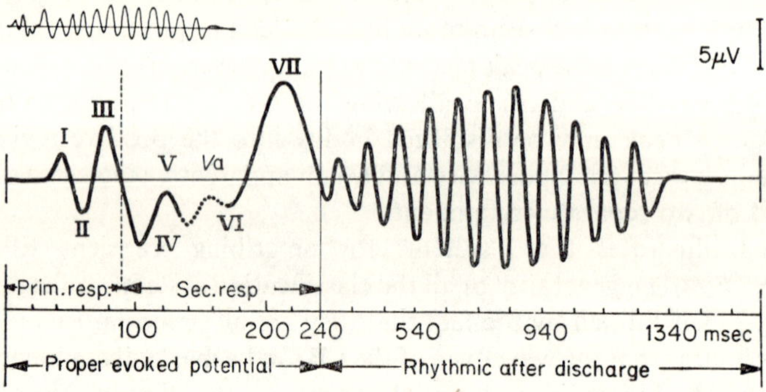

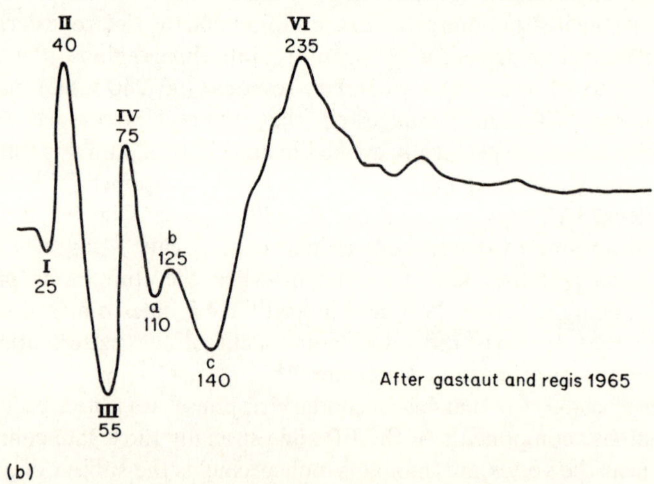

FIGURE 5.8 A: *Scheme for the human EEG response to light flashes recorded with the electrodes* O_z–P_z. *The mean values are used. Negativity at electrode* O_z *results in an upward deflection of the graph. Because the large disproportionality between the length of the normal-evoked potential and the rhythmic after-discharge, beginning from 240 msec after the stimulus, another scale is used. On the left at the top of the figure the scheme for the evoked potential with the real ratio of both constituents is reproduced. From L. Ciganek (1961).* Electroenceph. clin. Neurophysiol., *13, 165–172. Elsevier Publishing Co., Holland.*

B: *From N. W. Perry and D. G. Childers (1969).* The Human Visual Evoked Response. *Charles C. Thomas, Publishers, Illinois.*

system, identical components may have different labels at different electrode sites because not all components appear at all locations. As an alternative to sequential labelling, Goff has suggested that the waveform should be divided into a number of latency ranges, and that the polarity of each wave should be explicitly stated.[324] Goff's suggestion was based on the notion that certain potentials of roughly similar latencies, waveforms and topographical distributions might reflect the same underlying neural activities, regardless of the

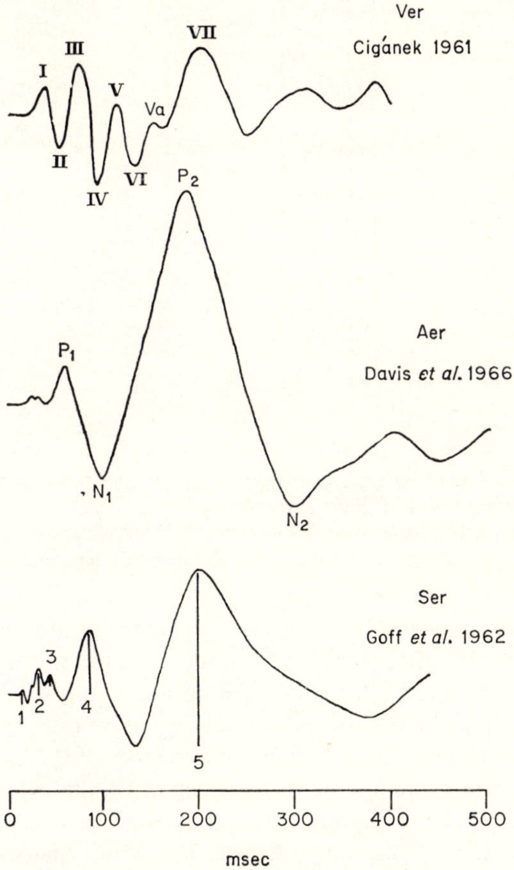

FIGURE 5.8 C: *Examples of different terminologies for AEP.*

modality of the stimulus. Donchin,[241, 242] however has challenged the validity of this notion.

Rémond has pointed out that a general obstacle to analysing waveforms on the basis of latency is that the variation of latency from one recording site to another makes it difficult to distinguish between a single component of variable latency, and a multiplicity of components each having a different latency.[536 p.240]

The 'after discharge' of the EP (Fig. 5.7) is not usually evident to visual

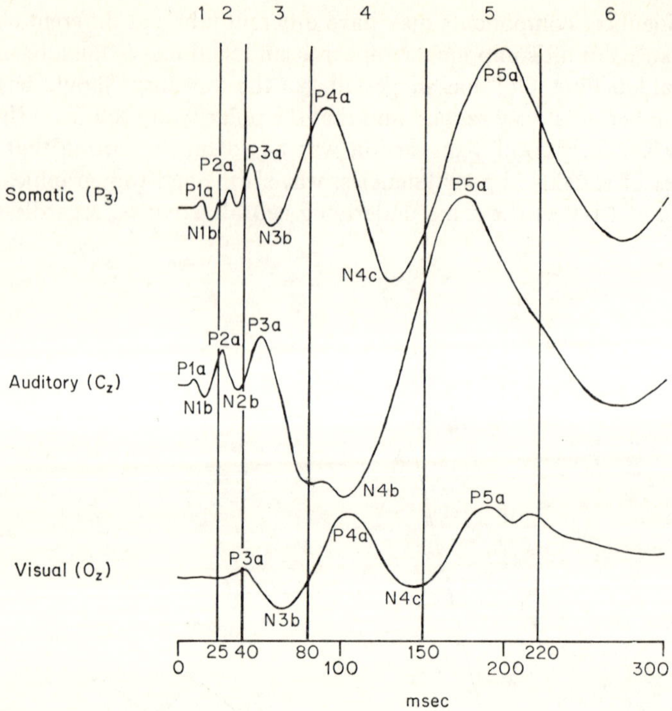

FIGURE 5.8 D: *Suggested system of nomenclature applicable to the three types of AEP indicated. The total AEP is divided into six latency ranges with limits as indicated by the vertical lines.* C *and* D *from W. R. Goff, Y. Matsumiya, T. Allison, G. D. Goff (1961). In* Average Evoked Potentials, *Ed. E. Donchin and D. B. Lindsley. NASA SP-191.*

inspection of the raw EEG, but is often apparent in averaged records.[47] It seems clear that the 'after discharge' cannot, in spite of its name, usefully be modelled in terms of the 'ringing' of a resonant R–C–L circuit.[168] There is disagreement on whether the 'after discharge' is an off-response.[262] Barlow has presented evidence that although the frequency of the 'after discharge' is generally close to the predominant frequency of the alpha activity, nevertheless the after discharge cannot entirely be explained as an instrumental sampling artifact.[44, 45, 47] Although Brazier has shown that some dissociation between the 'after discharge' and alpha activity can be achieved by the use of pharmacological agents, there is wide agreement that the two phenomena are closely related.[45, 47, 600, 847] By subtracting 'spontaneous' activity from EEG samples recorded after stimulation, Magnus and Ponson[513] obtained results which, they claimed, showed that the 'after discharge' was little affected by the phase of the alpha cycle at which stimulation took place. On the other hand, Rémond and Lesèvre have made a contradictory claim,[536] although van der Tweel[536 p.240] has suggested that Rémond's apparently disparate data might be due to the inclusion of appreciable background alpha activity in his summated responses. Peacock[600] has suggested that the 'after discharge' should be regarded as the averaged development of alpha regeneration following flash-induced blocking.*

5.4.9 *Steady-state evoked potentials: analysis in terms of frequency*[92, 844]

INTRODUCTION

In the following section analogue filters, digital filters and Fourier Analysers have been lumped together on the grounds that those individuals who have used Fourier Analysers in EP work have used them to perform frequency filtering. The author's experience has been that it can be more helpful to introduce Fourier Analysis by describing the way in which it is *used* rather than by introducing it as a special case of cross-correlation.

The signal-to-noise ratio of steady-state EPs can usefully be enhanced by means of narrow-band filtering.[335] The basis of this enhancement is closely related to the reasons why Fourier analysis can enhance the signal-to-noise ratio (see below). However, an important practical distinction should be made between (*a*) a narrow-bandwidth (e.g. 0·2 Hz) filter whose centre frequency is fully determined by the stimulus frequency, and (*b*) a filter whose bandwidth may be either quite broad (e.g. 5 Hz) or narrow, but whose centre frequency is not fully determined by the stimulus frequency. Filters of type (*a*) can provide both amplitude and phase information, either directly (as with Fourier Analysers) or with the aid of auxiliary equipment. In contrast, filters of type (*b*) can provide amplitude information only. With filters of type (*b*), some drift is liable to occur between the stimulating and filtering frequencies. This means that, even when a wide (e.g. 5 Hz) bandwidth is used, the phase shift produced by the filter varies with time. Small changes of signal frequency about the resonant frequency result in large changes in the amplitude and phase of the response of a sharply tuned circuit. More important, the rate of centre-frequency drift of a tuned filter sets a limit to the narrowest usable bandwidth, and hence to the practical signal-to-noise enhancement which can be provided by the filter. In addition, a resonant circuit's bandwidth may be sufficiently wide that it will accept more than one Fourier component at once. Furthermore, a filter whose resonant frequency is F Hz will respond to a signal of F Hz independently of whether F Hz is the fundamental component or any other harmonic component of the steady-state EP.

ANALYSIS IN TERMS OF FREQUENCY: MEDIUM BAND FILTERING

Banks of filters have long been used to reduce the information content of the 'raw' EEG. A number of methods have been described for displaying the EEG voltages measured within narrow frequency bands. These methods include displays of integrated voltage recorded over successive 10 second periods, and running-average displays.[336] A particularly convenient presentation of the running-average data has been described.[435] This display takes the form of a number of vertical bars on an oscilloscope. The height of each bar corresponds to the output of a particular filter. Between 2 and 15 Hz the

* For a description of the vertex (V) potential see Section 4.2.1.

filter bandwidth is 0·5 Hz, between 16 and 20 Hz the bandwidth is 1 Hz and between 20 and 30 Hz the bandwidth is 2 Hz.

ANALYSIS IN TERMS OF FREQUENCY: PHASE-LOCKED FILTERING

The filters described so far have been of the type whose centre frequency cannot be locked to an external reference frequency. This means that, although they may be excellent for the purpose of reducing the information-content of 'raw' EEG, and although they may even be useful indicators of the presence of steady-state EPs, such filters have limited value for measuring the amplitudes of steady-state EPs, and furthermore are not at all suitable for measuring phase. In order to overcome these limitations Fricker[297] designed a heterodyne filter whose centre frequency could be locked to an external reference signal. This facility allowed the narrow bandwidth of 0·1 Hz to be used in order to enhance the signal-to-noise ratio of steady-state EPs. Fricker claimed that signal-to-noise ratios could be enhanced by 20–28 db for visual stimulation, and by 15–19 db for electrical stimulation of the distal median nerve.[297]

When Fourier Analysis is used, it is a straightforward matter to obtain a precise description of the steady-state EP in both phase and amplitude terms. Provided that the steady-state EP can be regarded as being stationary (i.e. samples taken at any instant are equivalent), then for practical purposes its repetitive waveform can be described as a linear sum of elementary sinusoidal terms. These terms are called *Fourier Components*. The frequency F Hz at which the EP waveform repeats itself is equal to the frequency of the *fundamental* (or first harmonic) component, i.e. the Fourier component of lowest frequency. All other Fourier components have frequencies which are greater than F Hz and are multiples of F. For example, the *second harmonic* component has a frequency of $2F$ Hz, the *third harmonic* component has a frequency of $3F$ Hz, and so on. A practical point is that only a few Fourier components may be required in order to give an adequate description of a steady-state EP waveform. In many cases no more than the fundamental and second harmonic components may be needed to give a good description of a the waveform,[640] and in special cases either the fundamental or second harmonic only will suffice.[120] It should be noted that the phases as well as the amplitudes of the Fourier components are required for a full description of a signal waveform.

The signal-to-noise enhancement obtainable by means of Fourier Analysis is, for a given recording period, considerably greater than that possible by straightforward averaging (e.g. five to ten times greater). For example, with one-minute stimulations runs it is easy to record components whose amplitudes are no greater than 0·2 μV (Figs. 3 and 4 in Reference 639; also see Fig. 5.12 of this chapter). The reason why Fourier analysis can give greater signal resolution than straight averaging can be understood as follows. The salient point is that an assumption which underlies the application of Fourier Analysis to EP recording is similar to an assumption basic to the exclusive use of average waveforms. This assumption is that in any particular experiment it is safe to neglect EP components which may not be time-locked to the stimulus. If this is valid, and 'phase-locked' is substituted for 'time-locked', then all the power of the steady-state scalp EP to stimulation at *F* Hz will be found to be concentrated in the EEG at frequencies of *F* Hz, 2 *F* Hz, etc. The technique of Fourier Analysis is in effect a filtering process of extremely narrow bandwidth.* Its basis is to use the prior information (strictly, a prior definition in this case) that the signal is made up of frequencies of *exactly* *F* Hz, 2 *F* Hz, etc. in order to discriminate against all other electrical activities (i.e. to discriminate against 'noise').

The Fourier technique has the special advantage that phase information as well as amplitude information is available. The importance of this point is that phase information is an essential part of a full steady-state description of any system. For example, only if phase information is available can the waveform of the steady-state EP be obtained from the amplitudes of its various constituent harmonics. Furthermore, only if phase information is available can some estimate be made of the delay time (latency) for the various harmonic components.

The different bandwidths of a Fourier Analyser and of a summation device are the basis for their different signal-to-noise resolutions. By 'throwing away' bandwidth, the experimenter gains considerably in signal-to-noise enhancement. The investigator can choose whether to translate this gain into individual recordings 'runs' of shorter durations than are possible when conventional averaging is used, or whether he wishes to continue with experimental 'runs' of customary length, but instead to obtain precise measures of signals whose amplitudes are so small that they are inaccessible to conventional averaging techniques. The price that must be paid for these gains is, as has already been mentioned, a corresponding loss in the bandwidth of the recording equipment. This means that unless the experimenter has chosen to simultaneously analyse at a sufficient number of harmonic frequencies, his method may blind him to important, perhaps major, signal components which would have been clearly recorded by the simultaneous use of the wider-bandwidth averaging method.

A number of investigators who have used Fourier Analysis to study steady-state EPs conventionally describe the Fourier component at the

* The bandwidth of the Fourier analyser described in references 121a, 634, 644 whose performance is illustrated in Fig. 5.12 is roughly 0·001 Hz (half power). The system gives a tenfold attenuation of sinusoidal noise whose frequency differs by only 0·016 Hz from the signal frequency and a hundredfold attenuation of sinusoidal noise whose frequency differs from the signal frequency by only 0·05 Hz. In practical EP recording, however, the author's experience is that the device is not so effective as these bandwidth figures suggest when either (*a*) the analysis frequency is very close to the alpha frequency (in subjects with marked alpha activity) or (*b*) when the EP amplitude is very small (e.g. 0·1 μV). The reason for (*a*) is most likely to be frequency drift of alpha power. The reason for (*b*) may be an increased variability in the EP at very low EP amplitudes.

stimulus repetition frequency F as the fundamental component. In their terms, Fourier components whose frequencies were *lower* than F (e.g. $F/2$ Hz, $F/3$ Hz) would be called *subharmonics*. The reason for using this nomenclature is that linear systems do not generate subharmonics. Subharmonic generation is characteristic of certain classes of nonlinear systems (in fact the particular subharmonics generated can give clues to the type of nonlinearity within the system[365]). The little experimental evidence that is available suggests that subharmonics are uncommon in EPs.[506, 508, 642, 796]

When driven (e.g. stimulated) by a sinusoidal input of frequency F Hz the response of a linear system is a pure sinusoid of frequency F Hz. In other words *only* the fundamental component is generated by a linear system. For certain ('minimum phase') linear systems the steady-state description in terms of Fourier components (amplitude *versus* frequency plus phase *versus* frequency) is immediately equivalent to the description in terms of amplitude *versus* time (transient transfer function).[34, 83]* For such systems the 'steady-state' description can easily be transformed into the 'transient' description, and vice versa. In one class of non-minimum phase linear systems the departure from the minimum-phase description can be obtained by adding to the normal minimum phase a phase shift which is proportional to frequency (e.g. a system which includes a pure delay). A number of EP findings can be accounted for in this simple manner.[506, 636, 748]

In nonlinear systems the situation is quite different.[365, 549] There is no generally-valid relationship between the steady-state and transient descriptions of a nonlinear system. The two descriptions may therefore be *complementary* in that the transient description, for example, may contain information which cannot be obtained from the steady-state description, and *vice versa*. The discrepancies between the transient and steady-state descriptions of a nonlinear system may give clues to the type of nonlinearity involved but because of the difficulties this possibility has so far received little practical attention.

If the amplitudes of higher harmonics (relative to the amplitude of the fundamental component) can be made negligible by reducing the modulation depth of the stimulus, then the nonlinearity is called *analytic*, or *nonessential* (for example a saturation, logarithmic or power function nonlinearity). If the relative amplitudes of the higher harmonics are not reduced by this manoeuvre, then they are due to a *nonanalytic* or *essential* nonlinearity (for example a rectifier element). In spite of the absence of any general method for the analysis of nonlinear systems, an extension of the transfer function method of linear systems analysis has been successfully applied to the analysis of certain

* The transient responses of linear systems to slowly repeated stimuli can be imagined to overlap to an increasing extent as the stimulus repetition frequency is slowly increased until, in the steady-state regime, no response cycle can be attributed to any particular stimulus cycle. In a linear system, however, the overlapping of successive response would lead only to *linear superposition* and not to nonlinear interactions.

nonlinear elements.[196] Chapter 2, Section 2.8.8 discusses one method of analysing the rectifier-type of nonlinearity which has been identified in EP studies.

The terms 'entrainment' and 'photic driving' have been widely used to describe visual EPs to rhythmical stimulation. Entrainment is a term which implies the possibility of altering the natural (free-running) frequency of a self-oscillatory system to that of an externally imposed 'entraining' signal. If the self-oscillatory systems are envisaged as nonlinear oscillators (e.g. multivibrators) which are coupled to some degree, then the theoretical analysis of 'entrainment' presents severe difficulties. A preliminary study of a hardware model of 'photic driving' or 'entrainment' has shown that the apparent simplicity of such entrainment is deceptive, and that such a model has unexpected properties which are at variance with certain EP observations.[796]

A general point relating to time-domain *versus* frequency-domain analysis of EPs concerns the physiological basis for the analysis. All analysis of the EP consists of decomposing it into elements. In time-domain analysis the elements may be peaks (waves) of different latencies: but there is no compelling evidence that a classification of the EP into peaks has general physiological meaning. When methods of multivariate analysis are used to decompose the EP waveform, then the criteria for selecting the elementary functions are almost always entirely mathematical rather than physiological (see Section 5.4.12). The situation is similar in the frequency domain. There is no compelling evidence that an analysis of a waveform into sinusoidal Fourier components is physiologically meaningful *in itself* (although different frequency components may sometimes have quite different physiological properties,[639, 640] just as different transient components may have different physiological properties[413]). The reason why the choice of elementary functions for EP analyses has been arbitrary on physiological grounds in both the frequency domain and the time domain is, of course, that nobody has yet been able to suggest elementary functions which have a demonstrable physiological basis. The analysis of the EP into elementary functions selected on mathematical grounds can provide the experimenter with powerful, immediately-available analytic techniques. Studies initiated on such a basis have already led to a number of physiological insights. Hopefully they will lead to future analytical techniques whose bases are more closely related to physiology.

As has been mentioned already, a waveform which (indefinitely) repeats itself F times per second can be regarded as a linear sum of sinusoids of frequencies, F, $2F$, $3F$, etc. If the steady-state EP is equivalent to such a waveform, then the amplitude and phase of the fundamental component (of frequency F Hz) can be obtained by separately multiplying the EEG by $\sin(2\pi Ft)$ and $\cos(2\pi Ft)$ waveforms.[181] It can easily be verified that the product of two sinusoids which differ in phase by 0° or 180° maintains a constant sign, but that when the sinusoids differ in phase by 90° or 270° the product oscillates symmetrically about zero. After multiplication by sin $(2\pi Ft)$ or cos $(2\pi Ft)$ all frequency components of the EEG (other than that whose frequency is exactly F) result in an a.c. output but no mean d.c. output. Similar arguments apply to the second harmonic ($2F$ Hz) frequency component of the steady-state EP waveform. Only the second harmonic component gives a mean d.c. output after multiplication by sin $(2\pi[2F]t)$ or cos $(2\pi[2F]t)$ waveforms. The mean d.c. outputs resulting from multiplication of the EEG by the sin $(2\pi Ft)$ and cos $(2\pi Ft)$ pair can be used to calculate the amplitude and the phase of the fundamental component in the following way.[181] Let these mean d.c. outputs be A and B respectively. Then

$$S = C\sqrt{(A^2 + B^2)} \quad \text{and} \quad \phi = \tan^{-1}\left(\frac{A}{B}\right)$$

where S is the amplitude of the fundamental component, C is a constant which can be obtained by calibration, and ϕ is the phase of the fundamental component (relative to the zero of phase implicit in the sine or cosine term). The amplitude and phase of the second harmonic component can be similarly obtained from the mean d.c. products which result from multiplying the EEG by sin $(2\pi[2F]t)$ and cos $(2\pi[2F]t)$: and so on. Sub-harmonics can be extracted in an analogous manner.

Since 1965, to some enthusiasts 'the year of the Cooley-Tukey algorithm'[172] (i.e. the fast Fourier transform), it has been possible to carry out calculations of Fourier coefficients by digital computer in seconds rather than hours. Since that time, general-purpose digital computers have been increasingly used for Fourier analysis, and have indeed been used to Fourier analyse the EEG. Special-purpose, fixed-programme digital devices which will carry out on-line Fourier analysis by the fast Fourier transform are now commercially available, but these devices are still very expensive.

Phase-locked amplifiers can be used as Fourier analysers, but those which operate by multiplying the input by a square wave derived from the stimulus are in effect multiplying the EEG by the fundamental component of the stimulus frequency plus its odd harmonics. It is therefore possible to confuse the fundamental and odd harmonic components of the response, and furthermore, the device will be sensitive to noise located not only in the region of the stimulus repetition frequency but also at frequencies in the neighbourhoods of odd harmonics of the stimulus frequency. Also, a non-quadrature phase-locked amplifier may be inconvenient to use for the recording of evoked potentials when phase variability is marked (as, for example, at low signal levels), and when the phase of the EP component being recorded changes markedly from stimulus run to stimulus run (as, for example, when the luminance of a visual stimulus is changed from run to run). As a separate phase-locked amplifier is required for on-line analysis of each harmonic component of the EP from each electrode derivation it follows that the cost of such an on-line multi-channel analyser may be high.

Fig. 5.9 shows a fairly cheap analogue device which is capable of carrying out on-line multi-channel Fourier analysis at several component frequencies. An early version of this device allowed simultaneous on-line analysis of four EEG channels at one Fourier frequency, or one EEG channel at four harmonics, or any combination of harmonics and channels up to a total of four. The data were presented as a running average, so that the effects of a change in a stimulus parameter could be detected almost immediately on changing the parameter.[637] Analogue multiplication is a particularly appropriate method when carrying out Fourier analysis because of the ease with which a large rate of flow information may be handled.[S52]

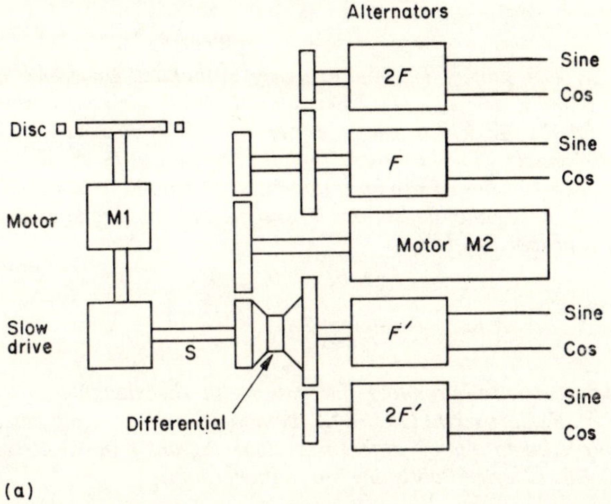

FIGURE 5.9 A: *Method of generating signals whose frequencies differ by a small variable, but stable, fraction. A high-stability, variable-speed motor (M2) drives some two-phase alternators directly, and some through a differential gear. The differential is rotated slowly at a frequency* $\pm(F^1 - F)$ *by a stabilised speed motor (M1) which drives through a 50:1 gearbox and shaft S. Holes are cut in a disc rotated by motor M1. These holes pass between lamp and photocell (not shown) to give pulses which are used to stabilise the speed of M1.*

A method of reducing the effect of EP variability by simultaneously stimulating and analysing at two slightly-different frequencies is illustrated in Figs. 5.9 and 5.10.[644] Results obtained by the use of this techniques are discussed in Chapter 2, Section 2.10.5.* The difference $\left(\frac{F' - F}{F}\right)$ between the two stimulus frequencies F' Hz and F Hz can be maintained constant to within roughly 0·1% over a period of 1 hour. This stability is sufficient to allow the two stimulus frequencies to be set so that the difference $\left(\frac{F' - F}{F}\right)$ is no more than 3%. It can be shown experimentally that such a small frequency difference *of itself* produces only negligible differences between the steady-state EPs to the F' and F stimuli. Any differences observed between the EPs to F' and F must therefore be due to factors other than the frequency difference such as, for example, different sites of stimulation (Fig. 5.10). The steady-state EPs which are phase-locked to the stimulus waveforms F'

* See also page 175.

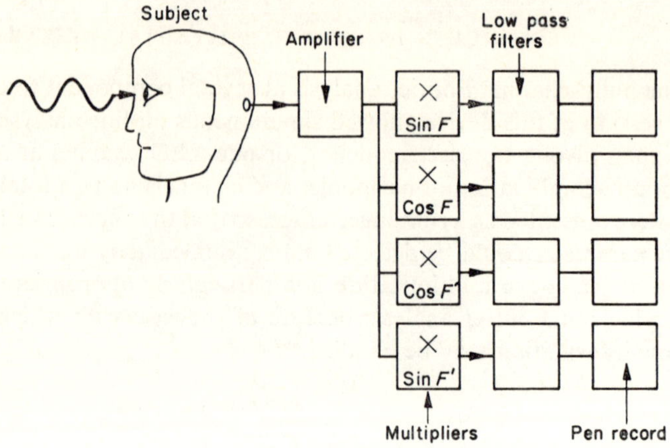

FIGURE 5.9 B: *The subject is simultaneously stimulated by visual signals whose frequencies are F and* F^1 *(Fig. 1). His EEG is multiplied by sine and cosine functions of frequencies F and* F^1, $2F^1$ *which are generated by the alternators (A). The resulting filtered products enable the phases and amplitudes of the fundamental and second harmonic components of the EPs to both the F and* F^1 *stimuli to be found. The outputs of a filter pair are steady d.c. deflections* θ_1 *and* θ_2. *The amplitude of the steady-state EP component is proportional to*

$$\sqrt{\theta_1{}^2 + \theta_2{}^2}$$

and the phase is given by

$$\tan^{-1}\left(\frac{\theta_1}{\theta_2}\right).$$

Noise (e.g. alpha activity) produces fluctuations in the steady d.c. outputs. From D. Regan and W. F. Cartwright (1970). 'A method of measuring the potentials evoked by simultaneous stimulation of different retinal regions', in Electroenceph. clin. Neurophysiol., ***28***. *Elsevier Publishing Co., Amsterdam.*

and *F* can be extracted from the EEG recorded at a single electrode by multiplying the EEG by sine and cosine waveforms locked to the *F′* and *F* waveforms respectively (Fig. 5.9). Second harmonic (Fig. 5.9), and other harmonic and sub-harmonic components can be obtained similarly. Average potentials evoked simultaneously by the *F′* and *F* stimuli can be computed off-line by recording on multi-channel magnetic tape the EEG plus two sets of trigger pulses, one of which is synchronous with the *F′* waveform and one with the *F* waveform. The effect of EP variability can be reduced by (very approximately) six times by the simultaneous stimulation procedure discussed above. There seems to be no reason why the method should not be extended to allow the recording of EPs to more than two simultaneous stimulations, and thus give even greater freedom from the effects of EP variability.* A proviso which should be mentioned is that the method assumes linear additivity and this has not yet been directly demonstrated.

5.4.10 *Time-domain analysis of evoked potentials*[844]

Although it is sometimes possible to make direct recordings of individual evoked potentials by placing electrodes directly on sensory cortex, in most

* A method of simultaneously stimulating four retinal quadrants and simultaneously analysing the resulting *four* EPs from each electrode has been used (Suppl. footnote No. 48).

circumstances an investigator's data are signals buried in overwhelming noise almost without trace. The methods he adopts in extracting the signals from the noise background reflect certain (possibly unexpressed) assumptions about the way in which the signals are generated.[213] By choosing some particular method of signal analysis an investigator may be, in effect, choosing

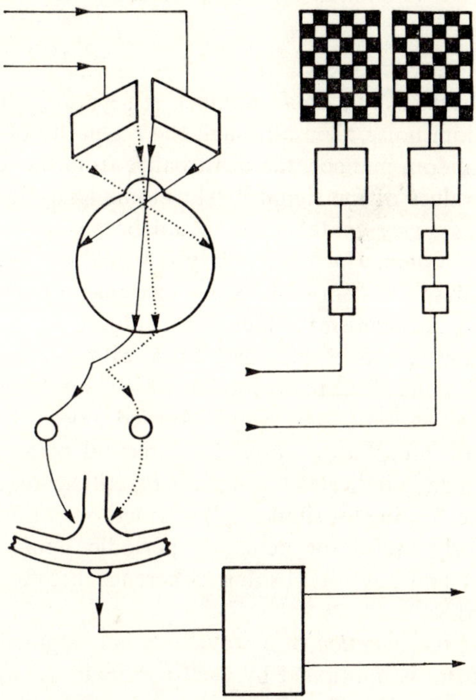

FIGURE 5.10 *Visual stimulators. Left half of figure shows two panels whose intensities are sinusoidally modulated at slightly different frequencies, F and F¹ (roughly 0·3 c/sec difference). Two Fourier analysers simultaneously analyse the EEG; one is locked to the F and the other to the F¹ input. The amplitudes and phases of the two potentials evoked by the F and F¹ stimuli are available on-line. The right half of the figure shows two chessboard patterns which are repetitively driven through one square's width. The left and right patterns alternate at slightly different frequencies; the two evoked potentials are measured by two Fourier analysers, as for the flicker stimulator. From D. Regan and R. F. Cartwright (1970). 'A method of measuring the potentials evoked by simultaneous stimulation of different retinal regions', in* Electroenceph. clin. Neurophysiol., ***28***. *Elsevier Publishing Co., Amsterdam.*

to test some hypothesis of the generation of the signals (see Section 5.4.12). It is true that different methods of analysis may do no more than present identical information in different formulations and with different emphases. Nevertheless, the ways in which an investigator can conveniently handle his data are to an important extent determined by his mode of data reduction (e.g. into the frequency domain *versus* into the time domain) so that his initial choice of mode of data reduction may exert an important influence on the subsequent interpretation of his data.* In the primitive state of neurophysiological understanding which obtains today, this consideration alone is a strong argument for reducing, analysing and displaying electrophysiological data in more than a single way.

In practice, of course, an investigator's reason for choosing a particular instrument may be dominated by such practical factors as the instrument's availability.

CORRELATION

If a signal is generated by a small number of separate harmonic oscillators with added random noise, then although the regularity of the signal will be disturbed in a random manner, the disturbance from the 'correct' value will not affect later values of the signal.[213] Harmonic analysis emphasises information about frequency content and would be an appropriate method of analysing such a system. Harmonic analysis would not be so revealing if it were used to analyse a system such as, for example, a freely-hung pendulum (with no driving mechanism) which was subject to occasional random impacts (e.g. from a crowd of small boys with peashooters).[213] Such a 'disturbed series' is one of the many models which have been suggested for the EEG. A revealing method of analysing disturbed series is by autocorrelation, which emphasises information about fundamental period. In other words autocorrelation mainly indicates the signal's repetition frequency.

Correlation (i.e. 'testing for similarity') is a method of time-domain analysis that is particularly useful for detecting periodic signals buried in noise (autocorrelation) and for establishing coherence between separate signals (crosscorrelation).[69, 466, 480, 481, 482]

The *autocorrelation function* of a waveform is computed in the following way: The waveform is multiplied by itself (ordinate by ordinate) with both waveforms starting at time zero. The ordinate-by-ordinate products are then summed to give y_0. One waveform is now shifted a distance τ along the time axis and the multiplication process is repeated, this time to give y_τ. A plot of y_τ *versus* τ for a series of values of τ is called the autocorrelation function of the waveform. The analogous function obtained when two separate waveforms are used is called the *crosscorrelation function.*

The use of autocorrelation techniques can reveal the presence of periodic components buried in noisy data even *when there is no prior knowledge of the signal* (Note: the length of the data sample must be large compared with the longest period of the signals to be detected). Particularly in the exploratory stage of an investigation this may be an important advantage. A disadvantage of autocorrelation is that the procedure does not retain information as to relative timing and phase.

* This point is perhaps more clearly evident in physics where a thoroughgoing change in fundamental concepts can be accelerated by describing old and well-known data in a new and suggestive way (e.g. Hamilton's reformulation of classical 'billiard ball' mechanics foreshadowed the radically different concepts underlying modern quantum mechanics).

Methods of analysing EEG data by crosscorrelation have appeared in a number of disguises. For example the 'summation' or 'averaging' computer is a crosscorrelator in which one waveform is an impulse function.[480, 481] A Fourier Analyser is a crosscorrelator in which the reference waveforms are sinusoids.

Each method of data reduction has its own 'blind spots'. By restricting his methods of data reduction to that of averaging, an investigator blinds himself to all signals other than those locked in time to his trigger pulses. By restricting himself to Fourier Analysis the experimenter blinds himself both to signals which are not phase-locked to his reference signals, and to frequency components other than those which his prior knowledge has led him to build into his apparatus. The limitations which result from allowing an incomplete prior knowledge of the signal to completely determine the design of a crosscorrelator can in principle be minimised by the use of *adaptive* crosscorrelators (see below). In principle, a notably powerful analytic technique is to crosscorrelate a random stimulus waveform with the system output. The stimulus waveform may be gaussian noise or (with some advantage) binary pseudorandom noise. The impulse transfer function of the linear part of a certain type of system can be derived from the resulting crosscorrelation function.[84, 481, 483] This procedure can be applied to systems which consist of a linear stage followed by a triggering or pulse-forming stage. In practice standard commercial averaging devices can be used in such a way as to give an acceptable crosscorrelation function between a noise-modulated stimulus and the physiological response. This approach has been used in EEG analysis.[506 p. 72]

SUMMATION OR SIGNAL AVERAGING

As mentioned already, signal averaging is a special case of crosscorrelation. The function of signal averaging is to extract a signal from an uncorrelated ('noisy') background by *defining* the signal as 'those data components which are time-locked to the stimulus'. An important advantage of signal averaging is that it enables the impulse response of a system to be determined with minimal disturbance of the system, though this point has often been ignored in EP studies.

Although the demands of radar in the 1939–45 war forced the most urgent development of techniques of signal-to-noise enhancement[854] it is nevertheless true, as Dawson pointed out,[214] that the underlying principle of signal averaging had been proposed as long ago as 1832 (by Laplace), and by 1847 had even been used (by Sabine) to detect the 'atmospheric tide'.*

* Dawson's intriguing introductory note should be quoted somewhere in this book. This is as good a place as any. '*A certain Dr. Brown, on being rebuked because he had failed to acknowledge some previous work on the subject of his writings replied: "I make no claim to originality for I have long since found that to consider oneself original one must read nothing at all. All I have done is to describe those methods which I have found to suit me best in practice.*" '

STATISTICAL TREATMENT OF SIGNAL AVERAGING[311]

Assume that the waveform $f(t)$ at the input to the summation device is the sum of two independent waveforms, the signal waveform $s(t)$ plus and added noise waveform $n(t)$. Assume further that the noise waveform is produced by a *stationary random process* with a mean $E(n)$ and a variance σ^2, whereas the variance of the signal term can be assumed to be zero.

Take N samples of the waveform $f(t)$, subject to the restriction that the sample instants must be time-locked to the periodic signal waveform and still give *uncorrelated samples of noise*. Such samples are indicated in Fig. 5.11a. The mean of these samples in the ith bin is

$$\bar{f_i} = \frac{1}{N}\sum_{k=1}^{N} f_{ik} = \frac{1}{N}\sum_{p=1}^{N}(S_{ik} + n_{ik})$$

$$\bar{f_i} = \frac{1}{N}\sum_{k=1}^{N} S_{ik} + \frac{1}{N}\sum_{p=1}^{N} n_{ik} = \bar{S_i} + \bar{n_i}$$

The bar indicates sample mean.

Since the sample mean $\bar{S_i} = S_i$, the equation may be rewritten in the form

$$\bar{f_i} = S_i + \bar{n_i}$$

The expected value (statistical average) of the sample mean is then given by

$$E(\bar{f_i}) = S_i + E(\bar{n_i}) = S_i + E(n)$$

If the *mean value of the noise is assumed to be zero*, then

$$E(\bar{f_i}) = S_i.$$

Now the variance of the sample mean in the ith bin can be obtained from the following definition

$$\sigma^2(\bar{f_i}) = \left|\frac{1}{N^2}\sum_{k=1}^{N}\sum_{p=1}^{N} E(f_{ik}f_{ip})\right| - E^2(\bar{f_i})$$

$$= \frac{1}{N^2}\sum_{k=1}^{N}\sum_{p=1}^{N}\left\{E(S_{ik}S_{ip}) + E(n_{ik}n_{ip})\right\} - S_i^2$$

Since the samples of $n(t)$ are noncorrelated

$$E(n_{ik}n_{ip}) = 0 \quad \text{for} \quad k \neq p$$

Therefore

$$\sigma^2(\bar{f_i}) = S_i^2 + \frac{1}{N}E(n_i^2) - S_i^2 = \frac{1}{N}\sigma^2(n_i) = \frac{1}{N}\sigma^2(n).$$

This means that after N samples have been taken, the expected value of the sample mean is equal to the amplitude of the signal, and that the variance of the sample mean is $1/N\,\sigma^2(n)$.

Thus that the expected values of the signal for one sample and for N samples are both s_i, but the variance about the mean is $\sigma^2(n)$ for one sample and $1/N\,\sigma^2(n)$ for N samples.

If the signal-to-noise ratio is defined to be the expected value of the signal divided by the standard deviation of the noise, then on this basis, the signal-

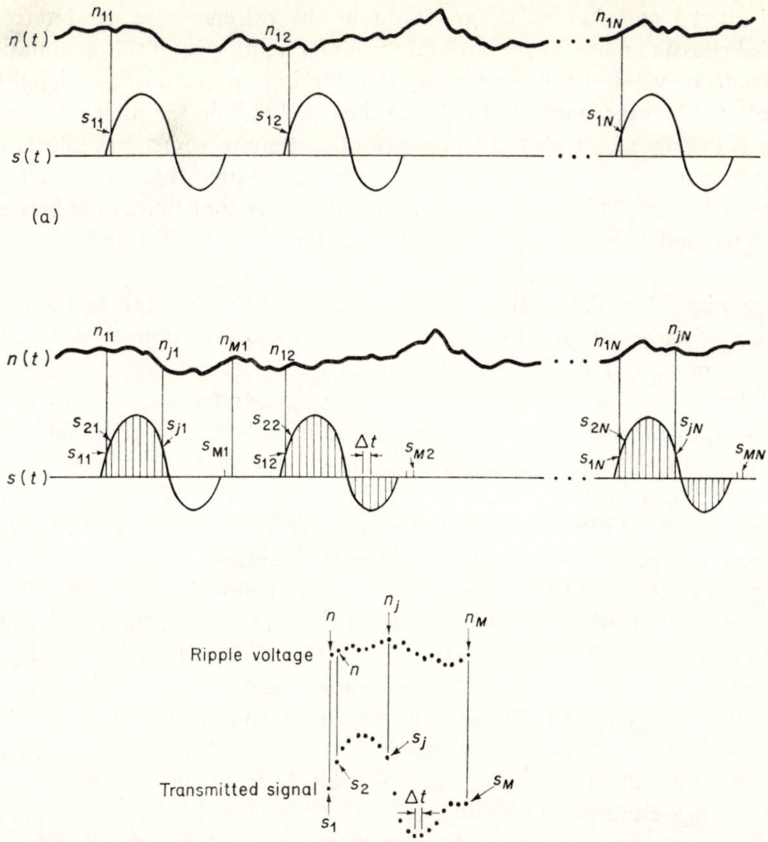

FIGURE 5.11 (a) *Component parts of the received waveform* f(t). *The received waveform* f(t) *is the sum of the random noise waveform* n(t), *and the transmitted waveform* s(t). *Samples* n_{1k}; k = 1, 2 . . . N *are uncorrelated, although time-locked to repetitions of the signal.* (b) *Sampling of the component parts of the received waveform* f(t). M *periodic samples, time-locked to the signal onset, are taken during each repetition of the signal.* (c) *Component parts of the average transmission. The average transmission is the sum of the ripple voltage and an individual transmitted signal. From C. D. Geisler (1960). 'Average responses to click in man recorded by scalp electrodes'. Massachusetts Inst. of Technol., Res. Lab. of Electronics, Tech. Rep. 380.*

to-noise ratio for one sample is $s_i/\sigma(n)$ and for the average of N samples is $s_i/\sqrt{N}\sigma(n)$. Subject to the assumptions and restrictions above in italics, (note especially the assumption that the various samples of noise are uncorrelated) this means that averaging N samples improves the signal-to-noise ratio by a factor $\sqrt{N}$. The simple analysis above has considered the extreme case of completely uncorrelated noise. Averaging, however, can still give some signal-to-noise enhancement even if this assumption is not valid. In the cases where a correlation exists between the noise samples, the improvement of the signal-to-noise ratio can be less than for the situation treated above. There is some agreement that spontaneous EEG may be considered as band-filtered gaussian noise, and even in the extreme case as selectively filtered gaussian noise (at and around the alpha frequency). If this assumption proves to be valid, it follows directly that the improvement of the signal-to-noise ratio by averaging EEG data reaches $\sqrt{N}$ only in the limit. However, there is evidence both that the presence of a stimulus sometimes affects the spontaneous EEG[750] and that phase may be retained between bursts of alpha activity.[328] This means that a correlation may sometimes exist between the signal and noise; in those circumstances the above derivation is not valid at all.

Ruchkin[690] has shown that contamination of EPs due both to the overlapping of successive responses and to certain forms of noise is reduced if stimulus presentations are aperiodic rather than periodic.

So far it has been assumed that both 'noise' and signal are *stationary processes*, in other words that a description of either noise or signal which is valid at any instant is equally valid some time later. In practice confusion may result from treating records of EEG noise and evoked potentials as though they were ideal stationary processes. This confusion may be serious. For example the signal-to-noise enhancement obtained in practice by summing a large number (N) of EEG samples may fall well below the predicted value of $\sqrt{N}$. Examples of situations where serious departures from stationarity may be observed are: (*a*) when N sweeps are summed during experimental procedures which are so taxing that the subject grows fatigued so that the EP either changes in amplitude or phase, or becomes increasingly variable; (*b*) summations of N sweeps during which the subject becomes so bored and sleepy that his alpha activity grows progressively more obtrusive.*

The comparison of EPs to different stimuli is often hindered by slow EP variations due to physiological changes. This is especially true for experiments which extend over several hours, and for experiments which are interrupted. *Order effects* may be introduced if stimulus parameters are varied in a regularly progressive manner (e.g. from dim to bright illumination). If regularity is unavoidable it is best to repeat the stimulus sequence in reverse order. An additional drawback to the progressive variation of stimulus parameters is that EPs may be affected by the subject's correct anticipation of stimuli (see Chapter 3). A method of minimising these problems by randomising the sequence of stimulus presentations has been described by Diamond.[229]

* Perry and Childers[605 p.16] show a rate of increase of average EP amplitude which is roughly proportional to N from a total of 120 to 960 flashes delivered at 4 flashes per second. Clearly, their subject's state remained effectively constant from 30 seconds to 240 seconds during the experiment. On the other hand, and quite apart from changes in the subject's state, for auditory stimuli it seems that stimulus repetition rate in itself may affect the way in which EP amplitude grows with an increasing number of stimuli. Milner[547] Fig. 9.5 shows that EP amplitude rises roughly proportional to N for repetition rates slower than one stimulus in 7·5 secs. For rates faster than one in 3 secs, however, the higher the stimulus rate the greater is the departure from proportionability to N. At a rate of 2 stimuli per second, the amplitude of the EP rises roughly proportional to $\sqrt{N}$.

A practical point is that, even after enhancement by signal averaging, the contamination of the signal by noise can often not be neglected. In many EP experiments the signal-to-noise ratio *after summation* is likely to range between 2 : 1 and 4 : 1.[605 p.90]

Commercial summation devices almost all use digital integration (i.e. memory)[145, 148, 171, 261, 354] though averaging devices have been made which are based on the integrating properties of capacitors[212, 214] barrier grid tubes,[174] magnetic tape,[539] photographic emulsions,[114, 115, 357, 737] or CRO tubes.[103, 469]

Commercial averaging (or summation) devices fall into two categories. These are (*a*) general purpose computers, and (*b*) special purpose averaging (or summation) devices. The general purpose device has the advantage of flexibility, so that if additional or alternative data processing is demanded as experiments progress, then this can be arranged if appropriate programmes are available. Special purpose averagers, although generally faster in operation than general purpose machines, have the disadvantage of inflexibility. In many instruments, however, inflexibility has been alleviated to some extent by incorporating a number of optional fixed programmes. The costs of most special purpose machines are not enormously less than the cost of the cheapest general purpose computer plus the necessary peripherals, but have important advantages in greater convenience in operation and higher speed.

The averaging computer's capacity for detecting minute electrical signals should be employed with some caution. Such exquisite sensitivity brings with it an enhanced susceptibility to artifacts, both instrumental and biological. Even when an averager is used it is best to ensure that the raw EEG is not seriously contaminated by mains hum or that the sweep frequency either drifts with respect to the mains frequency or is locked to the mains in such a way that alternate sweeps fall in amplifiers with respect to the mains cycle. There is some advantage in matching the effective bandpass of the averaging device *as a whole* to the amplifiers by a little cautious pre-filtering of the EEG input. As mentioned earlier it is tempting, but dangerous, to interpret the waveform displayed by an averaging computer as if it were necessarily the result of summing N identical single-stimulus EPs.

Although some averaging computers do in fact display an average which is normalised for N, most commercial devices actually compute the simple sum of each N sweep samples. This distinction is generally of little importance, except when the investigator wishes to compare summated responses in which different numbers of sweeps have been used, or when he falls foul of the change of instrumental scale which in some devices accompanies a change in sweep time.

Averaged waveforms may be recorded permanently by photographing a CRO face or by writing out the data with an X-Y plotter or strip chart recorder. Some care is needed to ensure that the write-out speed is not so rapid that details of the waveform are lost due to the sluggishness (i.e. poor high-frequency response) of the penwriter.

The *boxcar integrator* is a device which can be used to measure the amplitude of the signal at a single point in time even when the signal is buried in noise. Its operation can be compared to that of an averaging computer which is restricted to only a single address. The post-stimulus delay of this single 'address' can be varied over a wide range so that, given a repetitive signal, the boxcar integrator can extract a complete signal waveform. This procedure would be very inefficient. For example a boxcar integrator would take some 100 times longer than a 100-address averager to extract an equivalent waveform. Although boxcar integrators do not appear to have been used in EP work they might find some application in drastically reducing EP data to a measure of amplitude which refers to some narrow latency range. Such data reduction is within the scope of boxcar integrators in which both the latency of the post-stimulus delay and the duration of the sampling time are variable. The boxcar integrator has the advantages that (*a*) it is cheaper than an averaging device, (*b*) a boxcar integrator may be able to operate effectively at lower initial signal-to-noise ratios than an averaging computer (e.g. 10,000 : 1 for a boxcar integrator which will also accept signals 10 times full scale without overloading; 100 : 1 for a digital averaging device) and (*c*) commercially available boxcar integrators can be used to examine sections of a waveform with greater time resolution than is possible with commercially available averaging devices.

ZERO CROSSING ANALYSIS

Evoked potentials can be detected by analysing the zero crossing distribution in the EEG.[277, 471] The equipment required need not be expensive. One version of this technique[277] has the disadvantage that the waveform of the evoked potential cannot be obtained. A later version[278] does not have this disadvantage. In this later method the oscillations of the 'raw' EEG are represented as pulses which coincide with the zero-crossings of the EEG. These pulses are then used to generate equal-amplitude square waves whose zero crossings coincide with the original tape-recorded pulses. Ertl claimed that the averaged waveform obtained by summing 130 samples of these square waves was indistinguishable from the average waveform obtained by summing 130 samples of 'raw' EEG.

A form of zero crossing analysis can be performed by some of the commercial averaging devices currently available (though in some cases an accessory unit is required). The CAT, for example, operates by generating a pulse every time the EEG crosses the baseline. The interval between two successive zero crossings (one ascending, one descending) determines which memory address is incremented. After incrementing the memory, the CAT immediately starts to measure the interval between the next two zero crossings – and so on.

Zero crossing analysis does not necessarily provide a convenient alternative to frequency-filtering in determining the frequency spectrum of the EEG. Only in a restricted case has a relationship been found between frequency spectra and zero crossing analysis.[660]

THE DAWSON SUPERIMPOSITION TECHNIQUE

It was the practical problem of recording reliable somatosensory EPs in myoclonic epilepsy that led Dawson[209, 210] to use the superimposition technique of signal-to-noise enhancement in EP recording. The technique had previously been developed for less peaceful purpose.[824]* The procedure is to trigger the sweep of a CRO synchronously with the stimulus, so that samples of the EEG which occur in the 500 msec or so following successive stimuli are displayed on the face of the CRO tube. The waveforms which are successively displayed on the face of the CRO are then superimposed on a single photographic frame by leaving the CRO camera shutter open throughout the stimulation procedure. The superimposition technique offers some useful enhancement of the signal-to-noise ratio by virtue of the integrating properties of photographic emulsions. Features of the response which occur at a constant time after the stimulus grow to be more clearly defined after a number of sweeps, while those features which are not regularly related to the stimulus produce no more than a thickening of the baseline.

The superimposition technique does not lend itself to precise quantitative measurement of the EP. On the other hand it does offer direct visual indication of the variability of 'raw' individual traces. In view of the considerable dangers of grossly misinterpreting his data, and the exposure to a rich variety of artifacts which confront the investigator who relies *exclusively* on the results of his computer's powerful data-reduction procedures, the superimposition technique might still seem to have a useful place in EP research as a routine monitoring procedure.

5.4.11 *Variability*

When the signal-to-noise ratio *after summation* is no more than, say, 2 : 1 or the 4 : 1 of an 'acceptable' transient averaged EP, then even quite major features of the waveform can only be unequivocally identified as signal after comparing a number of average waveforms. It is therefore almost pointless to attempt to make conclusions as to whether two average waveforms are similar or different without careful consideration of waveform variability.[93, 105, 138, 430, 463, 865; 249 pp. 230, 231] A common practice is to superpose several examples of each average waveform in order to give some impression of variability. Another method of assessing variability due to noise is to subtract and add successive samples of EEG.[705] Computer programmes are available for calculating the variance of individual response samples.[36a] Some special-purpose computers display variance information as well as average waveforms.

In recording EPs from the human scalp it is in general a severe problem to distinguish between the intrinsic variability of EPs and the contribution to variability of background (EEG) activity. Aside from this there is an underlying question whether it is possible, even in principle, to distinguish

* A. M. Halliday has drawn my attention to an even earlier application – that of Galton in the nineteenth century in attempting to detect common features in the faces of murderers and other criminals by superimposing photographs of their faces.

between the EP and stimulus-locked changes in background activity. Another way of framing this question is to ask whether the averaged EP reflects some form of reorganisation or partial synchronisation of neural activity, or whether quite different cortical events underlie 'spontaneous' activity and the averaged EP.

When introducing the automatic averaging computer into neurophysiology, Dawson pointed out that the averaging process necessarily rejected variability in the amplitudes and variability in the time courses of EPs. Although automatic averaging eased the difficulties of measuring EPs with reliability, Dawson drew attention to the possibility that the variabilities rejected by averaging might *in themselves* be of physiological significance. This point has been made by a number of writers since Dawson, and some supporting evidence has accumulated. For example, a reduction in the variability of EP amplitude which is unaccompanied by any associated changes is average amplitude has been reported to be produced (in rabbit) by either LSD-25[461]; or plasma protein fraction of schizophrenics.[75a]

Axford[36a] finds that the variance of human EPs to pattern stimulation is reduced for approximately the duration of the prominent components of the response (Axford, J. personal communication). The question arises whether the reduction in variance is related to the amplitude of the response. This question is difficult to answer, since mutual cancellation of scalp potentials arising from different cortical sources may result in small net scalp responses, even when there would seem to be marked stimulus-locked cortical activity. For example, full-field pattern stimulation may give only small resultant scalp EPs due to mutual cancellation of comparatively large (but opposing) responses to upper and lower half-field stimulations (Chapter 2, Section 2.10.2). Axford suggests that his finding could be explained if the patterned stimulus attenuates spontaneous brain activity more markedly during the occurrence of the prominent response components than at other latencies. Barlow[42, 46] and Ciganek[138] earlier reported similar findings for flash EPs.

Zerlin and Davis [884a] were able to measure the amplitudes of individual vertex EPs to auditory stimuli in a human subject who gave very large potentials (100 μV on average). They claimed that the background EEG made only minor contributions to the measured variability of their subject's vertex responses. The variability of the N1–P2 wave's amplitude was gaussian. In cats which were paralysed, but anaesthetised with local and not general anaesthesia, Horvarth[393a] claimed that the variability of individual EPs was roughly six times larger than the contribution to net variability made by 'spontaneous' brain activity. In other words Horvarth claimed that individual EPs had an important intrinsic variability. It should be noted, however, that in Horvarth's experimental preparation the amplitudes of the EPs relative to the biological noise was much greater than is usually found in human scalp recording. Horvarth reported that, provided short-term and medium-term habituation effects were ignored by discarding both the first few runs of an experiment and the first few responses of any run, then the statistical distribution of the amplitudes of the initial positive wave of the EP (roughly 12 msec latency to peak) was both gaussian and stationary over a period of several minutes. Horvarth confirmed previous findings that when certain general anaesthetics were used, an increase in the depth of anaesthesia (measured roughly by anaesthetic dose) produced a reduction of EP variability. Horvarth found that (in cat) increasing the stimulus intensity to high levels could produce a decrease in the *normalised* variance (variance divided by square of mean amplitude). He attributed this to a saturation or threshold effect. Horvarth reported suggestive evidence that (in cat) the variability of individual EPs was independent of stimulus repetition rate for rates less than 1 Hz, but that variability increased when stimulus repetition rate was increased above 1 to 2 Hz. He attributed this increase in variability to the increasing effect of intrinsically variable neural recovery processes.

It seems clear that the presence of the poor signal-to-noise ratios usually encountered when recording EPs from the human scalp, causes the variability of the recordings to depend markedly on the effective band width of the recording apparatus (note: not only the band width of the amplifier but also the band widths of the averaging or correlation device plus the data write-out-device are involved. For example an X-Y plotter, when used at the higher writing speeds available with some averaging computers, can seriously limit the high-frequency response of the whole recording system). Fig. 5.12 illustrates this point. The figure shows running averages of EPs to similar visual stimuli recorded from similar electrode placements in the same subject (J. A.). Briefly, part A of the figure illustrates the running average of the EP computed by an averaging programme (written for a digital computer by J. Axford), while part B of the figure shows the running average of the EP computed by Regan's on-line Fourier analyser. Part A of the figure covers a 320 sec stimulation period, while part B covers a 420 sec stimulation period. It is clear from the figure that the response computed by the Fourier Analyser is much less variable than the response computed by the averaging programme. The reason for this is almost certainly mainly due to the fact that the effective bandwidth of the Fourier Analyser (half power point 0·001 Hz, tenfold attenuation 0·05 Hz, Fig. 5.12 part D) was very much narrower than the effective bandwidth of the averaging system. Under the particular stimulation conditions used, almost all the energy of the EP was precisely restricted to a frequency of 6 Hz. This energy passed through the Fourier Analyser, but because of the device's very narrow bandwidth comparatively little noise accompanied the signal. The signal also passed through the averaging system, but was accompanied by relatively more noise power, since the averaging system's bandwidth was comparatively wide. The Fourier Analyser made less information available than the averaging system, but in particular stimulus situations such as that of Fig. 5.12 where the power of the response is almost entirely restricted to one or two frequencies this can be a real advantage. On the other hand, the capacity of the averaging process for displaying a large amount of information is, of course, essential when transient EPs are recorded.

5.4.12 *Multivariate statistical analysis*

This section discusses how methods of comparing EPs by simply cross-correlating the *average* waveforms may sometimes give misleading results because of their blindness to the variabilities of the groups of the single stimulus samples which make up the average waveform. A number of alternative methods of analysis which can take single-trial variability into account fall under the general heading of *multivariate statistics* (general references: introductory [712], more advanced [455]). These methods attempt to describe EP waveforms quantitatively as linear sums of a number of elementary measures or factors. *Principal Factor Analysis* sets the number of independent factors at the minimum required to describe the given waveforms. Slightly differently, in *Discriminant Analysis* the factors are chosen so as to give maximum discrimination between different waveforms.

A popular method of estimating the difference between two average EP waveforms is to calculate their *Pearson Product Moment Correlation Coefficient*.[112, 254, 694] Donchin has pointed out that one weakness of the product–moment measure is that its use assumes independence of all the dimensions in which the EP is measured, although this has been shown to be an invalid assumption.[241] A further limitation is that the coefficient takes no note of the variability of the individual data samples which, when summed, constitute the EP. As a result, there can be confusion between differences in variability and genuine differences in EPs (Chapter 4, Section 4.2.4).

An alternative method of judging whether two EP waveforms are different is to analyse (decompose) the waveforms into 'waves' (i.e. components) of different latencies. Two waveforms may then be said to differ in terms either of the amplitudes or of the latencies of particular components so that for example any effects exerted on the EP by changing stimulus parameters can be described as changes of amplitudes and changes of latencies. There is widespread hope and some basis for optimism that the various peaks of EP waveforms will eventually prove to reflect discrete neural activities. It is unfortunately true, however, that there is as yet no general agreement on the physiological bases for the various peaks of the EP. More practically, there is still no agreement on an objective, non-arbitrary method for decomposing the EP waveform into separate 'waves'. This state of confusion led to a number of attempts to use multivariate statistics in order to analyse the EP waveform into a number of orthogonal (i.e. independent) vectors or waveforms.

One method of using multivariate statistics in EP analysis is to describe the EP waveform in terms of m values of amplitude measured at m different instants of time. Each waveform can then be described as a vector in an m-dimensional space.[238, 420, 712] If two different waveforms are represented by two such vectors, then the angle between the vectors provides a measure of the similarity of the waveforms. Continuing this line of argument, the two sets of N single-stimulus samples of EEG which, when summed, constitute two summed EPs, can be represented as two swarms of points in m-dimensional space. Whether the two EPs differ significantly can then be assessed by relating the separation of the centres of gravity of the swarms to the volumes of m-space occupied by the swarms (in other words by deciding whether the swarms overlap to so great an extent that they cannot be resolved).

Another way of putting this is to say that, in contrast with the Product Moment method of assessing the difference between two waveforms, the method of multivariate analysis takes into account the variability of the individual samples which make up each average waveform (but on the other hand assumes stationarity). A related point is that several different subsequences of individual samples may be lumped together in a single EP waveform. This possibility may be investigated by means of a method due to Ruchkin.[691]

According to Donchin the use of those techniques of *Multivariate Spectral Analysis* which stress the frequency content of the data[842, 843] are likely to be less applicable to EP analysis than to EEG analysis.[238] His view was based on the hypothesis that the various temporal features of the EP waveform reflect discrete neural events which have characteristic latencies and follow each other in an orderly sequence.[238]

An earlier section describes how the differences between a number of EP waveforms can be expressed in a quantitative form by describing each waveform as a linear sum of the Fourier Components. Further compression of data is possible if certain clusters of Fourier terms are found to be common to the several EP waveforms.[694] If this is so, then the EP waveforms can be described not only in terms of sinusoids, but also as a linear sum of a smaller number of elementary waveforms, not all of which waveforms are sinusoids.[694] When the elementary waveforms are chosen on the basis that there should be as few as possible then the procedure is called *Principal Factor Analysis* (or Principal Component Analysis). The resulting description can be two to four times more concise than the comparable description in Fourier terms. As few as three to six dimensions have been reported to be sufficient for an adequate description of the EP.[241] A drawback of Principal Factor Analysis is that the various factors do not necessarily have either anatomical nor physiological significance. One example of a way in which the physiological significance of Principal Factor Analysis can be enhanced was described by Ruchkin *et al.*[694] They defined their Principal Factors to be the various evoked potential waveshapes observed in different anatomical regions, so that the resulting Principal Factor description would take the form of a linear combination of the electrical waveforms arising in a small number of specified anatomical locations.

All the methods of multivariate analysis described above fall down in their handling of the situation that a change in some experimental variable has the effect of shifting the latencies of EP components.[241] Such shifts may create ambiguities in describing the EP, and may even call into question the definition of 'EP component'.

Loève-Karhumen (LK) analysis which has been applied to EP data[687, 773] can be regarded as a more generalised and economical descendent of Fourier Analysis, in which the component waveforms are not limited to sinusoids. Donchin has pointed out[241] that LK analysis bridges the gap between classical Principal Component Analysis and the analysis of EP data into different frequency components.

In most cases it is not immediately clear which of the many techniques of multivariate analysis would be most fruitful in any given experimental situation. Ruchkin's method of choosing waveforms which are characteristic of certain neuroanatomical sites as the basic elements does mean that these elements are no longer orthogonal[241] (i.e. mathematically independent or uncorrelated). On the other hand, the orthogonality of the 'elements' in Principal Component Analysis does not necessarily imply that they correspond to independent physiological generators, since the orthogonality is determined by mathematical rather than physiological factors.

The dimensions of Principal Component Analysis are chosen so that there shall be as few components as can possibly account for the variances within individual groups of single-trial samples. In contrast, the dimensions of *Discriminant Analysis* are chosen so as to account for the variance between different groups of single-trial samples.[240, 241, 243] In other words, the user of Discriminant Analysis selects his independent elementary components on the basis that they provide the maximum discrimination between the different averaged EPs. Discrimination Analysis can provide not only a judgement of whether two groups of single-trial samples are different but also information as to how the significance of the difference varies at points along the waveform of the averaged EP.[241, 242] *Stepwise Discriminant Analysis* is a particularly economical procedure. Ruchkin has used a *Cluster Analysis* technique in order to assess differences between EP waveforms.[248, pp.229–230 and p. 234]

5.4.13 *Adaptive filters**

Almost all the devices in common use for recording EPs are of the non-adaptive type. Non-adaptive filters 'recognise' the signal by some prior knowledge such as, for example, the signal is time-locked to the stimulus, or that the signal has a certain waveform (e.g. sinusoidal). As a consequence it is difficult to make a nonarbitrary distinction between signal and noise, and in practice an experimenter may often surrender his privilege to define what he means by 'signal'. This is because most investigators are restricted to a working definition of 'signal' such as 'what my averaging device records'. Nevertheless it is conceivable that the brain recognises as 'signals' neural activities which either are not locked to the stimulus or have variable waveforms. Averaging computers are inefficient at recognising such activity as 'signals'. A number of attempts have been made to overcome this limitation of inflexible 'prior-knowledge' filters by designing adaptive filters which are

* 'Filter' is often used in the sense of some procedure for emphasising (extracting) some desired waveform (signal). The filtering for example may be carried out entirely by digital computer.[844, 871]

capable of a progressive development of their criterion for recognising 'signal'.

Woody has described a method of adaptive filtering which is based on interative correlation and averaging of the data.[358, 880] Woody's method allows signals to be extracted from noise, even when the characteristic waveshapes of the signals are not known in advance. Woody's procedure is to crosscorrelate each data sample with some 'template' waveform. The correlation coefficient will be maximal for the time shift at which the template and any data sample are most similar. By knowing these different time shifts, the various data samples can be 'lined up' in time prior to averaging. Further resolution of the signal can then be achieved by replacing the template with this average and subsequently repeating the whole procedure time and again until the 'template' and the 'average' are no longer different. The process converges (i.e. is workable) almost regardless of the initial choice of template, but the more accurate the first guess, the shorter the filtering procedure. It is clear from this description that Woody's operational definition of 'signal' is 'the continuous waveshape of highest mutual correlation among all the data blocks examined at all possible shifts of time'.[880] His treatment is limited to waveforms which can be regarded as stationary and ergodic, so that the practical performance of such a filter with real EEG can only be assessed empirically.

Freeman[296] has used adaptive filters which also involve a crosscorrelation procedure. His method is to select some 'elementary waveforms' (e.g. damped sinusoids) which are then added in suitable proportions by an adaptive procedure until a waveform has been synthesised which replicates the experimentally-observed waveform. The end result of Freeman's procedure is to reduce the original flood of experimental data to a few numbers. The value of his method of data-reduction is likely to be determined by the physiological validity of his 'elementary waveforms'.

Adaptive filter techniques based on crosscorrelation should be carefully distinguished from non-adaptive crosscorrelation techniques.[48, 122, 634]

Other adaptive filter techniques have been described which do not employ correlation.[207, 339] Davisson's method[207] involves no stationarity assumptions. Groginsky *et al.*[339] described an adaptive filter technique which was based on comparing the signals from two receivers only one of which contained a 'signal' at any given instant. No other prior knowledge of the signal was required, and the noise was not required to be stationary, but signals weaker than a certain critical threshold could not be detected, regardless of the amount of data available.

5.4.14 *Pre-filtering of EEG data*

Pre-filtering of EEG data can be discussed under two headings. These are (1) filtering which rejects frequency components outside the signal pass band, and (2) filtering which attenuates selected frequency regions within the signal pass band.

FIGURE 5.12 *This figure illustrates the way in which the variability of averaged EPs is influenced by the bandwidth of the recording apparatus. The figure compares the moment-to-moment variability of the running averages of the amplitudes of the major component of an averaged EP (A) and the moment-to-moment variability of the amplitude of the major frequency component of an EP computed by Fourier Analysis (B). In both A and B the stimulus was a reversing pattern of 13′ checks whose total angular subtense was 4°. There were 6 reversals per second. The surround was dark. Monopolar recordings were made relative to one ear from an electrode 6 cm. in front of the inion along the midline. Both A and B apply to the same subject. The recording period in A was 320 seconds and in B 430 seconds.*

A. A digital computer integrated the EEG for a 50 msec period centred on a latency of 90 msec after each stimulus shown by black bars in C. A running average was formed of a block of 16 successive responses. The calibration mark in A shows the step response to a square 10 μV pulse. The horizontal dotted line is zero amplitude.

B. Output of Fourier Analyser. The stimulation conditions were similar as for A. The checkerboard made 6 reversals per second and the Fourier Analyser was locked to this 6 Hz wave. The figure shows the running average of the EEG multiplied by a sinewave locked to the stimulus waveform. (The cosine product was of negligible amplitude in this case.) The moment-to-moment variability can be seen to be much less than for the method of analysis shown in A.

C. The upper part shows two averaged EPs in which 200 sweeps were summed. The summations were made from the same recording which gave the running average in A. The horizontal black bar in A shows the length of record to obtain 200 sweeps. The usual way of employing an averaging computer would be to place the black bar (200 sweeps) at an arbitrary position along the time axis in A. The amplitude of the summated EP (between 65 and 115 msec) would then be given by the area under the trace encompassed by the black bar. It can be seen from A that the resulting EP would be of variable amplitude, depending on where the bar was placed. The two 'typical' traces in C illustrate this variability and the lines give the standard deviation of the mean amplitude. Note that roughly one-third of all readings would be expected to fall outside *even these limits. For this subject the standard deviation was independent of latency. The horizontal black bars above the averaged EPs shows the periods during which the computer integrated the EPs to form the running average in A (this shows how some of the variability in A could therefore be due to latency variability).*

D. Description of Fourier Analyser as a frequency filter, showing the extremely narrow effective bandwidth. The signal was a 7 μV(pk–pk) sinusoid of frequency 6·00 Hz. A sinusoidal interfering signal ('noise') was added to the 6·00 Hz signal. The 'noise' sinusoid was also of 7 μV(pk–pk) amplitude, but had a frequency of $(6{\cdot}00 + \Delta f)$ Hz. The value of Δf was varied from 0·0019 Hz (i.e. 1 cycle in 8 mins 20 secs) to 0·122 Hz. The result of adding the 'noise' sinusoid of frequency $(6{\cdot}00 + \Delta f)$ Hz to the 6·00 Hz signal was to cause beating of ΔF Hz at the output of the Fourier Analyser (shown in E for $\Delta F = 0{\cdot}075$, 0·042, 0·016, 0·009 and 0·0021 Hz (this last is 1 cycle in 7 minutes 20 secs). For an analysis period of 1 minute (often used by the author in EP experiments) the worst error in estimating the d.c. output of the Fourier Analyser would be when ΔF was such as to give one half cycle (or less) of beats during the one-minute analysis period. For higher values of ΔF (i.e. when the signal and 'noise' frequencies were further apart) the net d.c. error due to an integral number of beat cycles would be zero. The d.c. error due to any residual half-cycle would be less than when only one half-cycle of beats occupied the total 1 minute analysis period. This can be seen by regarding the estimation of the mean d.c. level of the Fourier Analysers output as a process of integrating the area under the trace (hatched in E) then dividing this area by the length of 1 minute analysis period. When several beat cycles occur during the analysis period E (lower half) the fractional error due to the area under the odd half cycle (black in E, upper half) is clearly less than when a single half-cycle occupies the whole integration period.

The filter characteristic of D was drawn by experimentally measuring the amplitude of the ΔF beats (as in E) for a series of values of ΔF, and then calculating the most probable error in the estimation of the mean d.c. level along the lines described above. (The mean d.c. level of the Fourier Analyser's output is shown dotted in E.)

The half-power bandwidth of the Fourier Analyser was found to be 0·002 Hz. The analyser attenuated the 'noise' relative to the signal by a factor of 10 when the noise differed from the signal by only 0·016 Hz, by a factor of 100 when the noise differed from the signal by 0·05 Hz and by a factor of 1000 when the noise differed from the signal by 0·122 Hz. The performance of the Fourier Analyser in practical EP recording is described in the text (Chapter 2, Sections 2.8.2, 2.8.3, 2.8.4, 2.9.3, 2.9.4; Chapter 4, Sections 4.2.2, 4.2.5, 4.3.3). Fourier analysis and

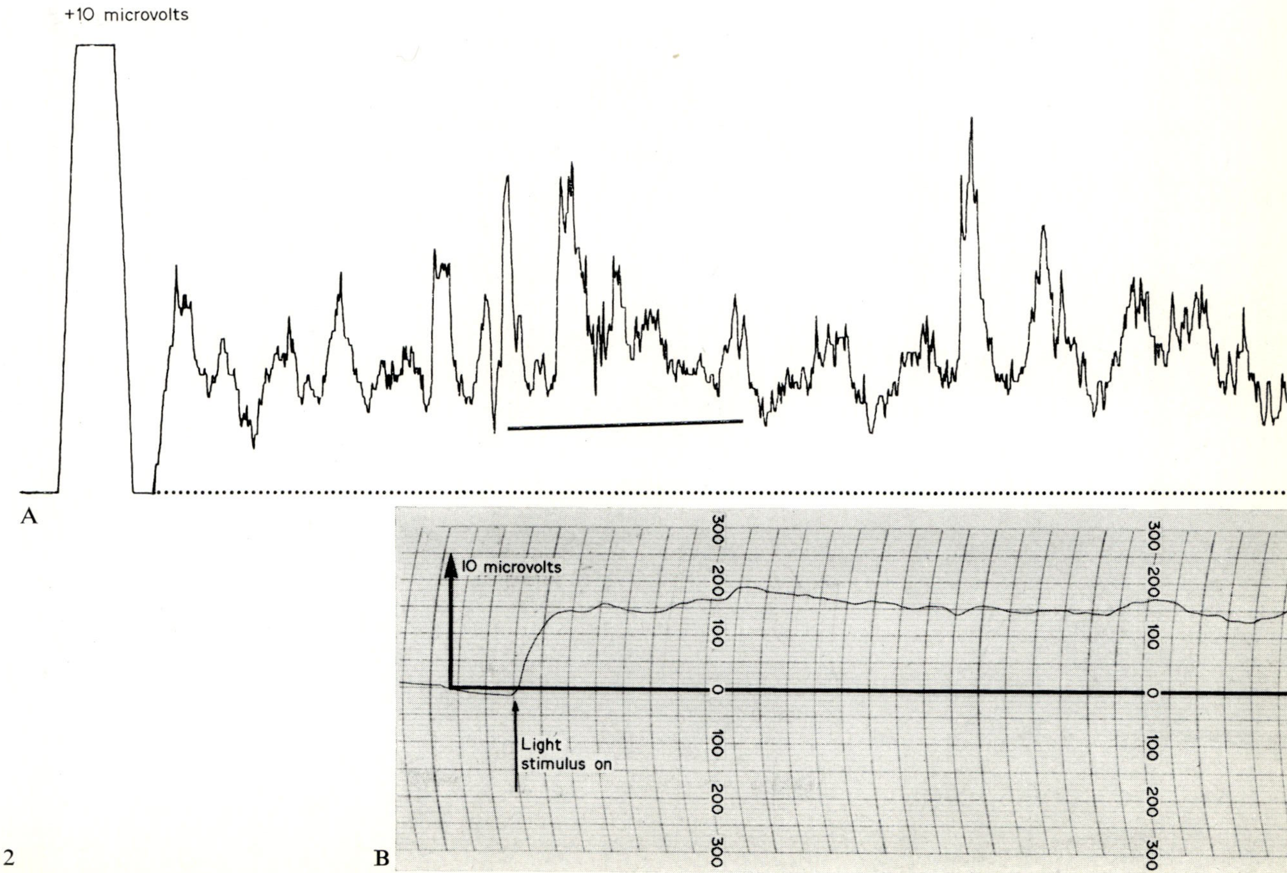
+10 microvolts
A
10 microvolts
Light stimulus on
300 200 100 0 100 200 300
300 200 100 0 100 200 300
B

FIGURE 5.12

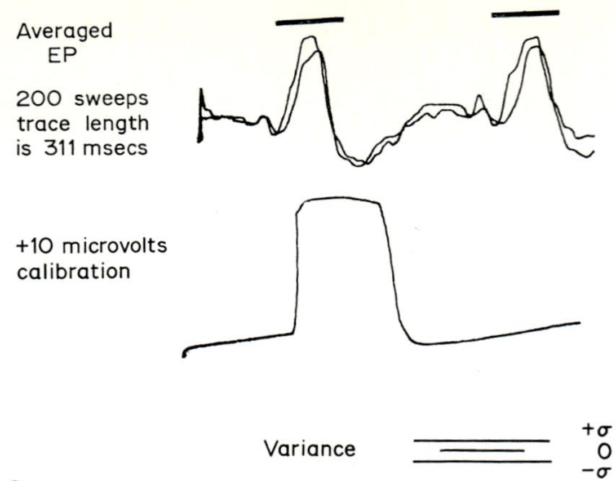

C

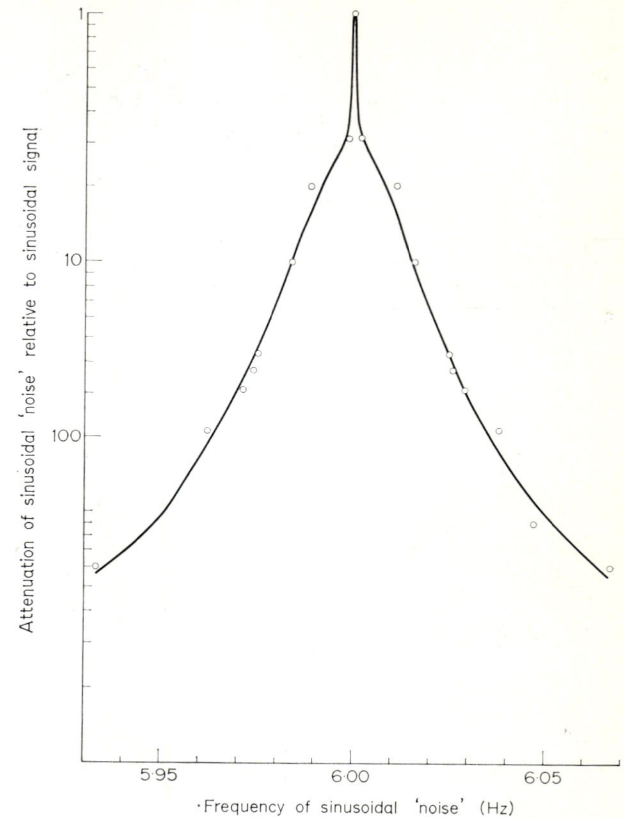

D

FIGURE 5.12 *cont'd*

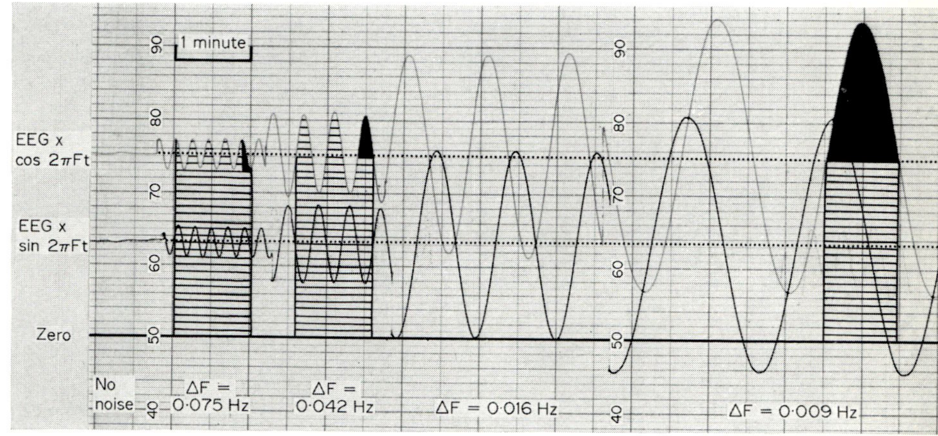

E

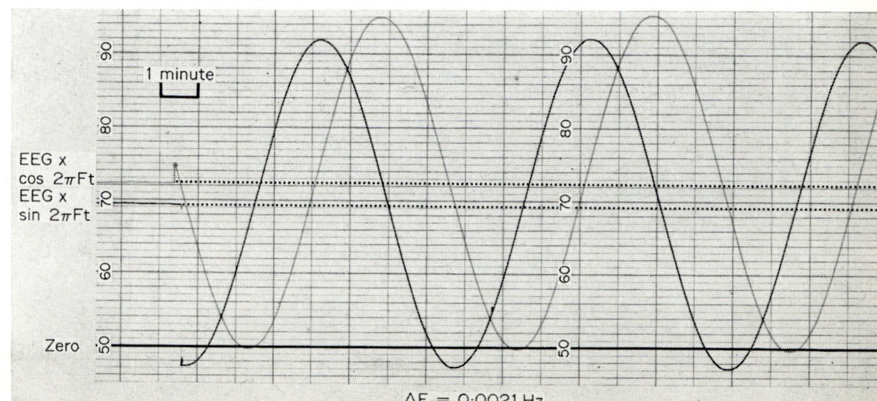

FIGURE 5.12 *cont'd*

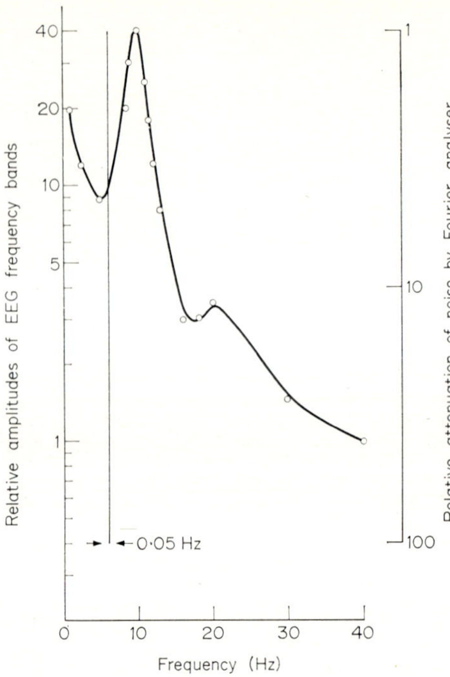

F

FIGURE 5.12 *cont'd*

averaging are described and their roles and relative merits in EP recording discussed in Chapter 5, Sections 5.4.9, 5.4.10 and 5.4.11.

E. The steady d.c. outputs of the Fourier Analyser corresponding to a 6·00 Hz input sinusoidal signal of 7 μV (pk–pk) is shown by the dotted lines. The beats were caused by adding at the input to the Fourier Analyser sinusoidal 'noise' signals whose frequencies were 0·075 Hz, 0·042 Hz, 0·016 Hz and 0·009 Hz (this last frequency is 1 cycle in 1 minute 53 secs). The lower part of the figure shows a similar experiment carried out on a different occasion in which the frequency difference was 1 cycle in 7 minutes 50 seconds. The phases of the 6·00 signal are different in the upper and lower parts of E; this is immaterial. Note the increasing attenuation of the beats as the noise frequency differs more and more from the signal frequency. Note also that by adding the difference *ΔF between the signal and noise frequencies directly, rather than by attempting to beat two independently-generated frequencies a frequency difference even as low as 1 cycle in 20 minutes can be maintained steadily even when a cheap unstabilised toy motor is used to introduce the difference ΔF. The method of introducing ΔF is described in Fig. 5.9, and Chapter 5, Section 5.4.9. For clarity the integrations, and odd half-cycles are shown for the cosine product only.*

F. The amplitude spectrum of the spontaneous EEG of a subject with prominent alpha activity. While the subject viewed a uniformly-illuminated diffuse field, his EEG was passed through a series of selective filters whose outputs were rectified and averaged over 100 second periods. (Replotted on log-linear paper from Spekreijse, Ref. 748, p. 47.) In order to illustrate the narrow bandwidth of the Fourier Analyser, the filter characteristic of D is replotted on F. This appears as a vertical narrow line. Compare the frequency scales in D and F. The base of the filter characteristic in F, which has a frequency width corresponding to a 100-fold attenuation of noise, is only 0·05 Hz wide and therefore cannot be adequately represented on a figure of this size.

The computer programme used to obtain records A and C was written by J. Axford who also made the recording A and C.

Conventional bandpass filtering to eliminate noise outside the signal passband will improve the signal-to-noise ratio of the input, and so reduce the signal averaging time. Cautious high-frequency filtering is required in any case since components of both noise and signal whose frequencies are greater than half the sampling frequency (Nyquist frequency) may be 'folded back' on to the low-frequency noise. Such 'folding back' can reduce the signal-to-noise ratio at the input and can also result in some distortion of the averaged waveform. As an example, if 100 samples were taken during a 1 second sweep, then the removal of EEG components whose frequencies were greater than 50 Hz would be required. Bandpass filtering pre-supposes a knowledge of the effective bandwidth of the signal. This can only be obtained by trial and error.

The purpose of the second type of pre-filtering is to increase the input signal-to-noise ratio so as to improve the sensitivity or speed of averaging. The general approach is to use Wiener's technique for separating signal from noise (*Wiener filtering*).[841] The method is to utilise one's prior knowledge of both the frequency spectrum of the signal and the frequency spectrum of the noise. If there are frequency bands in which the signal is weak but the noise is very strong, then these may be suppressed. On the other hand, if there is a frequency band where the stimulus is strong and the noise is weak, this should be allowed to pass unattenuated. This prior knowledge must be obtained empirically, for example by the following procedure (*a*) record EEG on magnetic tape, (*b*) compute the Fourier transform of each individual

EEG sample and average these Fourier transforms, (*c*) construct a frequency spectrum from the averaged Fourier transform, (*d*) now make a frequency spectrum of each individual EEG sample and average the spectra. The two spectra obtained [(*c*) and (*d*)] will be reasonable approximations to the spectra of the 'real response' and the 'real response'-plus-noise respectively. The ratio of these two functions is the transfer function of the optimum time-invariant linear filter for separating signal ('real response') from noise so as to obtain individual responses from the original tape-recorded EEG.[841] The optimum filter function for improving the resolution of the average EP is slightly different from that describe above.[841] As an example of the performance of such a filter Walter quoted a mean-square difference between the conventional average and the average 'real response' of 1·02 while that between Wiener-filtered average and the latter was 0·37.[841] In practice, Childers *et al.* experimentally confirmed Walter's prediction that for the average EP Wiener filtering would have little effect;[143] Wiener filtering, however, does not yet seem to have been thoroughly investigated in its more interesting application to the extraction of individual responses from 'raw' EEG.

References

The numbers which occur in the text as superscripts refer to the general references listed below. However, superscripts prefixed by a capital S refer to the supplementary footnotes added in proof and listed between pages 305 and 318.

1. ABRAHAM, K. and AJMONE MARSAN, C. (1958). Patterns of cortical discharges and their relation to routine scalp electroencephalography. *Electroenceph. clin. Neurophysiol.*, **10**, 447–461.
2. ABRAHAMIAN, H. A., ALLISON, T., GOFF, W. R. and ROSNER, B. S. (1963). Effects of thiopental on human cerebral evoked responses. *Anesthesiology*, **24**, 650–657.
3. ADEY, W. R. (1963). Discussion. In Brazier, M. A. B. (Ed.) 'Brain Function' Vol. 1, pp. 154–155. University of California Press, Berkeley, California.
4. ADEY, W. R. (1964). Data acquisition and analysis techniques in the Brain Research Institute. *Ann. N.Y. Acad. Sci.*, **115**, 844–866.
5. ADEY, W. R. (Ed.). Slow electrical phenomena in the central nervous system. *Neurosciences Res. Prog. Bull.*, **7**, 2.
6. ADEY, W. R., WALTER, D. O. and HENDRIX, C. E. (1961). Computer techniques in correlation and spectral analysis of cerebral slow waves during discriminative behaviour. *Exptl. Neurol.*, **3**, 501–524.
7. ADEY, W. R. and WALTER, D. O. (1963). Application of phase detection and averaging techniques in computer analysis of EEG records in the cat. *Exptl. Neurol.*, **7**, 186.
8. ADRIAN, E. D. and BUYTENDIJK, F. J. J. (1931). Potential changes in the isolated brain stem of the goldfish. *J. Physiol.*, **71**, 121–135.
9. ADRIAN, E. D. and MATTHEWS, B. H. C. (1934). The Berger rhythm Potential changes from the occipital lobes of man. *Brain*, **57**, 355–385.
10. ADRIAN, E. D. and MATTHEWS, B. H. C. (1934). The interpretation of potential waves in the cortex. *J. Physiol.*, **81**, 440.
11. ADRIAN, E. D. and MATTHEWS, B. H. C. (1936). The spread of activity in the cerebral cortex. *J. Physiol.*, **88**, 127.
12. ALAJOUANINE, T., SCHERRER, J., BARBIZET, J., CALVET, J. and VERLEY, R. (1958). Potentiels évoqués corticaux chez des sujets attenints de troubles somesthétiques. *Rev. Neurol.* (Paris), **98**, 757–761.
13. ALBE-FESSARD, D., ARFEL, G. and GUIOT, G. (1963). Activités électriques caractéristiques de quelques structures cérébrales chez l'homme. *Ann. de Chirugie*, **17**, 1185–1214.
14. ALBE-FESSARD, D., ARFEL, G., GUIOT, G., ALEONARD, P., DE LA HERRAN, J. and TRIGO, J. C. (1966). Electrophysiological studies of some deep cerebral structures in man. *J. Neurol. Sci.*, **3**, 37–51.
15. ALBE-FESSARD, D., ARFEL, G., DEROME, P. and DONDEY, M. (1970). Electrophysiology of the human thalamus with special reference to trigeminal pain. In Hassler, R. and Earl Walker, A. (Eds.) 'Trigeminal Neuralgia', Thieme, Stuttgart.
16. ALLISON, T. (1962). Recovery functions of somatosensory evoked responses in man. *Electroenceph. clin. Neurophysiol.*, **14**, 331–343.
17. ALLISON, T., GOFF, W. R., ABRAHAMIAN, H. A. and ROSNER, B. S. (1963). The effects of barbiturate anaesthesia upon human somatosensory evoked responses. *Electroenceph. clin. Neurophysiol., Suppl.*, **24**, 68–75.

18. ALLISON, T., GOFF, W. R. and BREY, J. H. (1967). An isolated constant-current stimulator for use with man. *J. Appl. Physiol.*, **22**, 612–613.
19. ALLISON, T. and GOFF, W. R. (1967). Human cerebral evoked responses to odorous stimuli. *Electroenceph. clin. Neurophysiol.*, **23**, 558–560.
20. AKIYAMA, Y., SCHULTE, F. J., SCHULTZ, M. A. and PARMELEE, A. H., JR. (1969). Acoustically evoked responses in premature and full-term newborn infants. *Electroenceph. clin. Neurophysiol.*, **26**, 371–380.
21. AMASSIAN, V. E., WALLER, H. J. and MACEY, J., JR. (1964). Neural mechanisms of the primary somatosensory evoked potential. *Ann. N.Y. Acad. Sci.*, **112**, 5–32.
22. ANDERSEN, P. and ANDERSSON, S. A. (1968). Physiological basis of the alpha rhythm. Appleton–Century–Crofts, New York, pp. 235.
23. ANDREWS, D. P. (1967). Perception of contour orientation in the central fovea. Parts I and II. *Vision Res.*, **7**, 975–997, 999–1013.
24. AOKI, Y. (1969). A clinical–electroencephalographic study on photo-sensitive epilepsy, with special reference to visual evoked potentials. *Folia Psychiatrica et Neurologica Jap.*, **23**, 103–119.
25. ARAKAWA, T., MIZUNO, T., CHIBRA, F., SAKAI, K., WATANABE, S., TAMURA, T., TATSUMI, S. and COURSIN, D. B. (1968). Frequency analysis of electro-encephalograms and latency of photically induced averaged evoked responses in children with ariboflavinosis. *Tokohu. J. Exp. Med.*, **94**, 327–335.
26. ARAKAWA, T., MIZUNO, T., HONDA, Y., TAMURA, T., SAKAI, K., TATSUMI, S., CHIBA, F. and COURSIN, D. B. (1969). Brain function of infants fed on milk from mothers with low serum folate levels. *Tokohu. J. Exp. Med.*, **97**, 391–397.
27. *Arch. Neurol.*, **11**, 435–443.
28. ARMINGTON, J. Personal communication.
29. ARMINGTON, J. C. (1964). Relations between electroretinograms and occipital potentials elicited by flickering stimuli. *Docum. Ophthal.*, **18**, 194–206.
30. ARMINGTON, J. C. (1964). Adaptational changes in the human electroretinogram and occipital response. *Vision Res.*, **4**, 179–192.
31. ARMINGTON, J. C. (1966). Spectral sensitivity of simultaneous electroretinograms and occipital responses. *Vision Res.*, *Suppl.* **1**, 225–233.
32. ARMINGTON, J. C. (1968). The electroretinogram, the visual evoked potential, and the area-luminance relation. *Vision Res.*, **8**, 263–276.
33. ARMINGTON, J. C., GAARDER, K. and SCHICK, A. M. L. (1967). Variation of spontaneous ocular and occipital responses with stimulus patterns. *J. Opt. Soc. Amer.*, **57**, 1534–1539.
34. ASELTINE, J. A. (1958). 'Transform Methods in Linear Systems Analysis', McGraw-Hill, London, p. 300.
35. AUERBACH, E. and ROWE, H. (1966). Electroretinogram and occipital response in congenital hemeralopia and rod-monochromatism. In *Clinical Electroretinography*, Suppl. to *Vision Res.*, 281–288.
36. AUERBACH, E. and ROWE, H. (1968). The 'good' eye in unilateral retinosis pigmentosa. *Ophthalmologica*, **155**, 98–116.
36a. AXFORD, J. (1971). Computerised methods of recording visually evoked scalp potentials. Thesis, University of Keele.
37. BAKER, J. B., LARSON, S. J., SANCES, A. and WHITE, P. J. (1968). Evoked potentials as an aid to the diagnosis of multiple sclerosis. *Neurology* (Minn), **18**, 286.
38. BAKER, J. B., SANCES, A. and LARSON, S. J. (1966). Neurophysiological evaluation of patients with multiple sclerosis. *Marquette Medical Review*, **32**, 37.
39. BALEN, A. T. VAN (1964). The influence of suppression on the flicker ERG. *Docum. Ophthal.* (Den Haag), **18**, 440–446.

40. BANCAUD, J., BLOCH, V. et PAILLARD, J. (1953). Contribution EEG a l'étude des potentiels évoqués chez l'homme au niveau du vertex. *Rev. Neurol.*, **89**, 399–418.
41. BARLOW, J. S. (1958). Relation to intrinsic alpha activity to rhythmic activity induced by photic stimulation in man. *Quart. Prog. Rep. M.I.T. Res. Lab. Electron.*, **48**, 128–133, Cambridge, Mass.
42. BARLOW, J. S. (1960). A small electronic analogue averager and variance computer for evoked potentials of the brain. In Smyth, C. N. (Ed.) 'Medical Electronics', Springfield, Thomas, 113–119.
42. BARLOW, J. S. A small electronic analogue averager and variance computer for evoked potentials of the brain. In Smyth, C. N. (Ed.) 'Medical Electronics', Springfield, Thomas, 1960, 113–119.
43. BARLOW, J. S. (1963). Some statistical characteristics of electrocortical activity in relation to visual-oculomotor tracking in man. *Bol. Inst. Estud. med. biol.* (Méx), **21**, 497–518.
44. BARLOW, J. S. (1964). Evoked responses in relation to visual perception and oculomotor reaction times in man. *Ann. N.Y. Acad. Sci.*, **112**, 432–467.
45. BARLOW, J. S. (1964). Discussion. *Ann. N.Y. Acad. Sci.*, **112**, 219–223.
46. BARLOW, J. S. (1966). Electronic simulation as an aid in evaluating computer-analysed data. *Electroenceph. clin. Neurophysiol.*, **22**, 109–117.
47. BARLOW, J. S. (1964). Rhythmic after discharge to flashes. *Quart. Prog. Rep. M.I.T. Res. Lab. Electron.*, **75**, 149–155, Cambridge, Mass.
48. BARLOW, J. S. and BROWN, R. M. (1955). An analog correlator for brain potentials. *Tech. Rep. M.I.T. Res. Lab. Electron.*, **41**, Cambridge, Mass.
49. BARLOW, J. S. and CIGÁNEK, L. (1969). Lambda responses in relation to visual evoked responses in man. *Electroenceph. clin. Neurophysiol.*, **26**, 183–192.
50. BARLOW, H. B. and HILL, R. M. (1963). Evidence for a physiological explanation of the waterfall phenomenon and figural after-effects. *Nature*, **200**, 1345–1347.
51. BARLOW, H. B., HILL, R. M. and LEVICK, W. R. (1964). Retinal ganglion cells responding selectively to direction and speed of image motion in the rabbit. *J. Physiol.*, **173**, 377–407.
BARLOW, H. B. and LEVICK, W. R. (1965). The mechanism of directionally selective units in the rabbit's retina. *J. Physiol.*, **178**, 477–504.
52. BARNET, A. B., BAZELON, M. and ZAPPELLA, M. (1966). Visual and auditory function in a hydranencephalic infant. *Brain Res.*, **2**, 351–360.
53. BARNET, A. B. and GOODWIN, R. S. (1966). Averaged evoked electroencephalographic responses to clicks in the human newborn. *Electroenceph. clin. Neurophysiol.*, **18**, 441.
54. BARNET, A. B. and LODGE, A. (1966). Diagnosis of deafness in infants with the use of computer-averaged electroencephalographic responses to sound. *J. Pediat.* (St. Louis), **69**, 753–758.
55. BARNET, A. B. and LODGE, A. (1967). Click evoked EEG responses in normal and developmentally retarded infants. *Nature*, **214**, 252–255.
56. BARNET, A. B., MANSON, J. I. and WILNER, E. (1970). Acute cerebral blindness in childhood. *Neurology* (Minn.), **20**, 1147–1156.
57. BARR, R. C., PILKINGTON, T. C., BOINEAU, J. P. and SPACH, M. S. (1966). Determining surface potentials from current dipoles with application to electrocardiography. *IEEE Trans. Bio. Med. Engng.*, **BME-13**, 88–92.
58. BARTLETT, F. and JOHN, E. R. (1970). Means and variances of average-response waveforms. *Science*, **169**, 304–305.
59. BARTLETT, N. R. and WHITE, C. T. (1968). Cortical potentials evoked by the onset and the termination of foveal stimulation. *Psychonom. Sci.*, **11**, 357.
60. BALEN, A. TH. VAN and TWEEL, L. H. VAN DER (1962). Aspects électro-encéphalographiques de l'amblyopie et de la suppression. In *ERG et Champ Visuel.*

61. BAYLOR, D. A. and NICHOLLS, J. G. (1969). Changes in extracellular potassium concentration produced by neuronal activity in the central nervous system of the leech. *J. Physiol.*, **203**, 555–569.
62. BEATTY, J. and UTTAL, W. R. (1968). The effects of grouping visual stimuli on the cortical evoked potential. *Psychophys.*, **4**, 214–215.
63. BEATTY, J. (1969). Some further studies on the effect of grouping elements of a visual stimulus on the cortical evoked potential. *Percept. Psychophys.*, **6**, 373–378.
64. BECHTEREVA, N. P., VVEDENSKAIA, I. V., DUBIKAITIS, Y. V., STEPANOVA, T. S., OVNATANOVE, B. S. and USOV, V. V. (1963). Localisation of focal brain lesions by electroencephalography. *Electroenceph. clin. Neurophysiol.*, **15**, 177–196.
65. BECK, C. and ROSNER, B. S. (1968). Magnitude scales and somatic evoked potentials to percutaneous electrical stimulation. *Physiology and Behaviour*, **3**, 947–953.
66. BEGLEITER, H. and PLATZ, A. (1969). Cortical evoked potentials to semantic stimuli. *Psychophysiology*, **6**, 91–100.
67. BELL, D. A. (1960). 'Electrical Noise', Van Nostrand, London.
68. BENDAT, J. S. (1958). 'Principles and Applications of Random Noise Theory', Wiley, New York.
69. BENDAT, J. S. and PIERSOL, A. G. (1966). 'Measurement and Analysis of Random Data', Wiley, New York.
70. BENNET-CLARK, H. C. and EVANS, C. R. (1963). Fragmentation of patterned targets when viewed as prolonged after-images. *Nature*, **199**, 1215–1216.
71. BERGAMINI, L. and BERGAMASCO, B. (1967). 'Cortical Evoked Potentials in Man', Thomas, Springfield, pp. 116.
72. BERGAMINI, L., BERGAMASCO, B., MOMBELLI, A. M. and GANDIGLIO, G. (1965). Visual evoked potentials in subjects with congenital aniridia. *Electroenceph. clin. Neurophysiol.*, **19**, 394–397.
73. BERGAMINI, L., BERGAMASCO, B. and MOMBELLI, A. M. (1966). Étude sur les elements qui influencent la variabilité des responses corticales évoquées visuelles chez l'homme. *Electrodiagnostic-Electrotherapie*, **1**, 22–33.
74. BERGAMINI, L., BERGAMASCO, B., MUTANI, R., POSTIR, A. and RICCO, A. (1966). Comportamento dell'attivatà corticale evocata in soggetti portatori di processi endocranici occupanti spazio. *Minerva Neurochir.*, **10**, 250–254.
75. BERGAMINI, L., BERGAMASCO, B., FRA, L., GANDIGLIO, G. and MUTANI, R. (1967). Diagnostic recording of somato-sensory cortical evoked potentials in man. *Electroenceph. clin. Neurophysiol.*, **22**, 260–262.
75a. BERGEN, J. R., CZIGMAN, J. S. and KOELLA, W. P. (1963). Influence of a plasma protein fraction from schizophrenic patients upon the optic evoked response in the rabbit. *J. Neuropsychiat.*, **4**, 219–223.
76. BERNHEIMER, S. (1899). Die wurzelgebiete der Augennerven ihre Verbindungen und ihr Anschluss an die Gehirnrinde. In 'Handbuch der Gesamten Augenheilkunde', Vol. 1, Part 2, pp. 1–115. Ed. Graefe, A. G. und Saemisch, T. S., Springerm, Berlin.
77. BICKFORD, R. G. (1964). The interaction of averaged multisensory responses recorded at the inion. *Electroenceph. clin. Neurophysiol.*, **17**, 713.
78. BICKFORD, R. G. (1969). In 'Average Evoked Potentials', Donchin, E. and Lindsley, D. B. (Eds.), Washington, NASA SP–191, 279–281.
79. BICKFORD, R. G., JACOBSON, J. L. and CODY, D. T. R. (1964). Nature of average evoked potentials to sound and other stimuli in man. *Ann. N.Y. Acad. Sci.*, **112**, 204–223.
80. BISHOP, G. H. (1936). *Cold Spring Harbor Symposium Quant. Biol.*, **4**, 305.
81. BISHOP, G. H. (1956). Natural history of the nerve impulse. *Physiol. Rev.*, **36**, 376.

82. BLACK, S. and WALTER, W. GREY. (1965). Effects on anterior brain responses of variation in the probability of association between stimuli. *J. Psychosom. Res.*, **9**, 33–43.

83. BODE, H. W. (1945). 'Network Analysis and Feedback Amplifier Design', Van Nostrand, New York, p. 551.

84. BOER, E. D. and KUYPER, P. (1968). Triggered correlation. *IEEE Trans. Bio. Med. Engng.*, **BME-15**, 169–179.

85. BOGACZ, J., VANZULLI, A., HANDLER, P. and GARCIA-AUSTT, E. (1960). Evoked responses in man. II. Habituation of visual evoked response. *Acta Neurol. Latinoamer*, **6**, 353–362.

86. BONIN, G. VON (1950). 'Essay on the Cerebral Cortex', Thomas, Springfield, Illinois.

87. BORING, E. G. (1942). 'Sensation and Perception in the History of Experimental Psychology', Appleton, New York.

88. BOSTOCK, H. and JARVIS, M. J. (1970). Changes in the form of the cerebral evoked response related to the speed of simple reaction time. *Electroenceph. clin. Neurophysiol.*, **29**, 137–145.

89. BOUGH, E. W. (1970). Stereoscopic vision in the macaque monkey: a behavioural demonstration. *Nature*, **225**, 42–44.

90. BOYNTON, R. M. (1966). In Sidowski, J. B. (Ed.) 'Experimental Methods and Instrumentation in Psychology', McGraw-Hill, New York, p. 803.

91. BRAZIER, M. A. B. (1949). A study of the electrical fields at the surface of the head. *Electroenceph. clin. Neurophysiol., Suppl.* **2**, 38–52.

92. BRAZIER, M. A. B. (Ed.) (1961). 'Computer Techniques in EEG Analysis'. *Electroenceph. clin. Neurophysiol., Suppl.* **20**.

93. BRAZIER, M. A. B. (1964). A study of the variability of responses to flicker: the influence of other sensory stimuli. *Docum. Ophthal.*, **18**, 221–236.

94. BREMER, F. (1958). Cerebral and cerebellar potentials. *Physiol. Rev.*, **38**, 357.

95. BREZNY, I. (1965). Visual EEG responses in neurological patients. 6th Internat. EEG. Congr., Vienna, EEG, abstracta, EMG 385.

96. BRINDLEY, G. S. (1960). 'Physiology of the Retina and the Visual Pathway', Arnold, London, p. 298.

97. BRINDLEY, G. S. and LEWIN, W. S. (1968). The sensations produced by electrical stimulation of the visual cortex. *J. Physiol.*, **196**, 479–493.

98. BRINDLEY, G. S., GAUTIER-SMITH, P. C. and LEWIN, W. (1969). Cortical blindness and the functions of the non-geniculate fibres of the optic tracts. *J. Neurol. Neurosurg. Psychiat.*, **32**, 259–264.

99. BRODY, D. A. (1968). The inverse determination of simple generator configurations from equivalent dipole and multipole information. *IEEE Trans. Bio. Med. Engng.*, **BME-15**, 106–110.

100. BORG, G., DIAMANT, H., STRÖM, L. and ZOTTERMAN, Y. (1967). The relation between neural and perceptual intensity. A comparative study on the neural and psychophysical response to taste stimuli. *J. Physiol.*, **192**, 13–20 (London)

101. BROWN, J. C. N., SHAGASS, C. and SCHWARTZ, M. (1965). Cerebral evoked potential changes associated with the ditran delerium and its reversal in man. In *Recent Advances in Biological Psychiatry*, Ed. J. Wortis, **7**, 223–234.

102. BUCHSBAUM, M. and FEDIO, P. (1969). Visual information and evoked responses from the left and right hemispheres. *Electroenceph. clin. Neurophysiol.*, **26**, 266–272.

103. BULLOCK, T. H. (1951). Facilitation of conduction rate in nerve fibres. *J. Physiol.* (Lond.), **114**, 89–97.

104. BURKHARDT, D. A. and RIGGS, L. A. (1967). Modification of the human visual evoked potential by monochromatic backgrounds. *Vision Res.*, **7**, 453–459.

105. BURNS, S. K. and MELSACK, R. (1966). A method for analysing variations in evoked responses. *Electroenceph. clin. Neurophysiol.*, **20**, 407–409.
106. BUTLER, B. V. and ENGEL, R. (1969). Mental and motor scores at 8 months in relation to neonatal photic response. *Develop. Med. Child. Neurol.*, **11**, 77–82.
106a. BUTLER, S. R. and GLASS, A. (1970). Alpha rhythm and fine eye movement. *Nature*, **228**, 1110–1112.
107. BUTLER, R. A., KEIDEL, W. D. and SPRENG, M. (1969). An investigation of the human cortical evoked potential under conditions of monaural and binaural stimulation. *Acta Otolaryng.* **68**, 317–326.
108. CALLAWAY, E. (1966). Averaged evoked potentials in psychiatry. *J. Nerv. Ment. Dis.*, **143**, 80–94.
109. CALLAWAY, E. (1968). Evoked responses for the study of complex cognitive functioning in children. Paper presented to American Psychological Assoc., San Francisco.
110. CALLAWAY, E. (1969). Diagnostic uses of the averaged evoked potentials. In Donchin, E. and Lindsley, D. B. (Eds.) 'Average Evoked Potentials'. NASA SP–191, Washington, D.C., pp. 299–311.
111. CALLAWAY, E. and LAYNE, R. S. (1964). Interactions between the visual evoked response and two spontaneous biological rhythms: the EEG alpha cycle and the cardiac arousal cycle. *Ann. N.Y. Acad. Sci.*, **112**, 421–431.
112. CALLAWAY, E., JONES, R. T. and LAYNE, R. S. (1965). Evoked responses and segmental set in schizophrenia. *Arch. Gen. Psychiat.*, **12**, 83–89.
113. CALLAWAY, E., JONES, R. T. and DONCHIN, E. (1970). Auditory evoked potential variability in schizophrenia. *Electroenceph. clin. Neurophysiol.*, **29**, 421–428.
114. CALVET, J. and SCHERRER, J. (1955). De certaines limites et possibilités nouvelles en électrophysiologie – Actes des Journées 'Measure et Connaissance'. *Rev. Métrologie*, 289–293.
115. CALVET, J., CALVET, M. C. and SCHERRER, J. (1964). Étude stratiagraphique corticale de l'activité EEG spontanée. *Electroenceph. clin. Neurophysiol.*, **17**, 109–125.
116. CAMP, W. A. and WOLFF, H. G. (1961). Studies on headache. Electroercephalographic abnormalities in patients with vascular headache of the migraine type. *Arch. Neurol. Chicago*, **4**, 475–485.
117. CAMPBELL, F. W. (1957). Depth. of field of the human eye. *Optica. Acta.*, **4**, 157–164.
118. CAMPBELL, F. W. and GREEN, D. G. (1965). Optical and retinal factors affecting visual resolution. *J. Physiol.*, **181**, 576–593.
119. CAMPBELL, F. W. and KULIKOWSKI, J. J. (1966). Orientational selectivity of the human visual system. *J. Physiol.*, **187**, 437–445.
120. CAMPBELL, F. W. and MAFFEI, L. (1970). Electrophysiological evidence for the existence of orientation and size detectors in the human visual system. *J. Physiol.*, **207**, 635–652.
121. CAMPBELL, F. W. and KULIKOWSKI, J. J. The use of the evoked potential to determine the visual contrast threshold. In press.
121a. CARTWRIGHT, R. F. and REGAN, D. Semiautomatic, off-line Fourier analysis of multichannel, steady-state EP data for clinical purposes. In preparation.
122. CASBY, J. V., SIMINOFF, R. and HOUSEKNECHT, T. R. (1963). An analogue cross-correlator to study naturally induced activity in intact nerve trunks. *J. Neurophysiol.*, **26**, 432–448.
123. CASTELLUCCI, V. F. and GOLDRING, S. (1970). Contribution to steady potential shifts of slow depolarization in cells presumed to be glia. *Electroenceph. clin. Neurophysiol.*, **28**, 109–118.
124. CAVONIUS, C. R. (1965). Evoked response of the human visual cortex: spectral sensitivity. *Psychon. Sci.*, **2**, 185–186.
125. CHALKE, F. C. R. and ERTL, J. (1965). Evoked potentials and intelligence. *Life Sci.*, **4**, 1319–1322.

126. CHANDLER, P. J. and PARSONS, O. A. (1965). EEG abnormalities and visual field deficits in flicker perception. *Electroenceph. clin. Neurophysiol.*, **19**, 481–483.
127. CHANG, H.-T. (1955). Cortical response to stimulation of medullary pyramid in rabbit. *J. Neurophysiol.*, **18**, 332–352.
128. CHAPMAN, R. M. (1969). In Donchin, E. and Lindsley, D. B. (Eds.) 'Average Evoked Potentials'. NASA SP–191, Washington, D.C.
129. CHAPMAN, R. M. and BRAGDON, H. R. (1964). Evoked responses to numerical and non-numerical stimuli while problem solving. *Nature* (Lond.), **203**, 1155–1157.
130 CHAPMAN, R. M., SHELBURNE, S. A., JR. and BRAGDON, H. R. (1970). EEG alpha activity influenced by visual input and not by eye position. *Electroenceph. clin. Neurophysiol.*, **28**, 183–189.
131. CHASE, R. and KALIL, R. (1968). Visual evoked responses to flashes and pattern shifts during voluntary eye movements. EPA Meeting, Washington.
132. CHATRIAN, C. E., BICKFORD, R. G., PETERSON, H. C. and DODGE, H. W., JR. (1960). Lambda waves with depth electrodes in humans. In 'Electrical Studies of the Unanaesthetised Brain', Hoeber, New York.
133. CHEATHAM, P. G. and WHITE, C. T. (1952). Temporal numerosity: I. Perceived number as a function of flash number and rate. *J. Exp. Psychol.*, **44**, 447–451.
134. CHILDERS, D. G., ROSS, J. J. and PERRY, N. W. (1970). Dyslexia and cortical correlates. ISCERG Symposium, Pisa.
135. CHOUDHURY, B. P., WHITTERIDGE, D. and WILSON, M. E. (1965). The function of the callosal connections of the visual cortex. *Quart. J. exp. Physiol.*, **50**, 214–219.
136. CIGÁNEK, L. (1961). The EEG response (evoked potential) to light stimulus in man. *Electroenceph. clin. Neurophysiol.*, **13**, 165–172.
137. CIGÁNEK, L. (1964). Excitability cycle of the visual cortex in man. *Ann. N.Y. Acad. Sci.*, **112**, 241–253.
138. CIGÁNEK, L. (1969). Variability of the human visual evoked potential; normative data. *Electroenceph. clin. Neurophysiol.*, **27**, 35–42.
139. CIGÁNEK, L. and INGVAR, D. H. (1969). Colour specific features of visual cortical responses in man evoked by monochromatic flashes. *Acta Physiol. Scand.*, **76**, 82–92.
140. CIGÁNEK, L. and ZALCIK, J. (1965). Application of the exponential time-base phase in the recording of evoked responses in man. *Electroenceph. clin. Neurophysiol.*, **18**, 190–191.
141. CIUREA, E. and CRIGHEL, E. (1967). Neurogenic mechanisms in the evolution of cerebral circulatory insufficiency. Investigations on the role of the brain stem reticular formation. *Confin. Neurol.*, **29**, 351–359.
142. CLARE, M. H. and BISHOP, G. H. (1956). *EEG Clin. Neurophysiol.*, **8**, 583.
143. CLARK, D. L., BUTLER, R. A. and ROSNER, B. S. (1969). Dissociation of sensation and evoked response by a general anaesthetic in man. *J. Comp. Physiol. Psych.*, **68**, 315–319.
144. CLARK, F. J. J. (1960). A study of Troxler's effect. *Optica Acta*, **3**, 219–236.
CLARK, F. J. J. and BELCHER, S. J. (1962). On the localisation of Troxler's effect in the visual pathway. *Vision Res.*, **2**, 53–68.
145. CLARK, W. A., BROWN, R. M., GOLDSTEIN, M. H., JR., MOLNAR, C. E., O'BRIEN, D. F. and ZIEMAN, H. E. (1961). The average response computer (ARC): a digital device for computing averages and amplitude and time histograms of electrophysiological responses. *IRE Trans. Biomed. Electron.*, **BME-8**, 46.
146. CLYNES, M. (1965). Brain space analysis of evoked potential components applied to chromaticity waves. Sixth Internat. Conf. Med. Electron. and Biol., Tokyo, Japan.

147. CLYNES, M. Personal communication.
148. CLYNES, M. and KOHN, M. (1961). In Frommer, P. L. (Ed.) 'Digest of the 1961 International Conference on Medical Electronics', New York, R.C.A. Labs. Princeton, New Jersey, p. 28.
149. CLYNES, M. and KOHN, M. (1964). Specific responses of the brain to colour stimuli. *Proc.* 17th Ann. Conf. Eng. Med. and Biol.
150. CLYNES, M. and KOHN, M. (1967). Spatial VEPs as physiologic language elements for colour and field structure. *EEG Journal*, *Suppl.* 1, **26**, 82–96.
151. CLYNES, M. and KOHN, M. (1968). Recognition of visual stimuli from the electric responses of the brain. In Kline, N. S. and Laska, E. (Eds.) 'Computers and Electronic Devices in Psychiatry', Grune, New York, pp. 206–237.
152. CLYNES, M., KOHN, M. and LIFSHITZ, K. (1964). Dynamics and spatial behaviour of light evoked potentials, their modification under hypnosis, and on-line correlation in relation to rhythmic components. *Ann. N.Y. Acad. Sci.*, **112**, 468–509.
153. CLYNES, M., KOHN, M. and LITCHFIELD, D. (1965). Chromaticity waves of evoked human brain potentials in normal and colour-blind vision. *Proc. Amer. Soc. for Exper. Biol.*
154. CLYNES, M., KOHN, M. and GRADIJAN, J. (1967). Computer recognition of the brain's visual perception through learning the brain's physiologic language. IEEE Int. Conf. Rec., Pt. 9, pp. 125–142.
155. COBB, W. A. and DAWSON, G. D. (1960). The latency and form in man of the occipital potentials evoked by bright flashes. *J. Physiol.*, **152**, 108–121.
156. COBB, W. A., ETTLINGER, G. and MORTON, H. B. (1967). Visual evoked potentials in binocular rivalry. *Electroenceph. clin. Neurophysiol.*, *Suppl.* **26**, 100–107.
157. COBB, W. A., MORTON, H. B. and ETTLINGER, G. (1967). Cerebral potentials evoked by pattern reversal and their suppression in visual rivalry. *Nature*, **216**, 1123–1125.
159. COBB, W. A. and MORTON, H. (1970). Evoked potentials from the human scalp to visual half-field stimulation. *J. Physiol.*, **208**, 39–40P.
160. COBB, W. A. and PAMPLIGNIONE, G. (1952). Occipital sharp waves responsive to visual stimuli. *Electroenceph. clin. Neurophysiol.*, **4**, 110 P.
161. CODY, D. T. R. and BICKFORD, R. G. (1965). Cortical audiometry; an objective method of evaluating auditory acuity in man. *Proc. Mayo Clinic*, **40**, 273–287.
162. CODY, D. T. R., JACOBSON, J. C., WALKER, J. C. and BICKFORD, R. G. (1964). Averaged evoked myogenic and cortical potentials to sound in man. *Ann. Otol.*, **73**, 763–777.
163. COHEN, J. (1969). Very slow potentials relating to expectancy: the CNV. In Donchin, E. and Lindsley, D. B. (Eds.) 'Average Evoked Potentials', NASA SP–191, Washington, D.C. pp, 143–163.
164. COHEN, M. W. (1970). The contribution by glial cells to surface recordings from the optic nerve of an amphibian. *J. Physiol.*, **210**, 565–580.
165. COHEN, J. and WALTER, W. G. (1966). The interaction of responses in the brain to semantic stimuli. *Psychophysiol.*, **2**, 187–196.
166. COHN, R. (1949). 'Clinical Electroencephalography', McGraw-Hill, New York.
167. COHN, R. (1963). Evoked visual cortical responses in homonymous hemianopic defects in man. *Electroenceph. clin. Neurophysiol.*, **15**, 922.
168. COHN, R. (1964). Rhythmic after-activity in visual evoked responses. *Ann. N.Y. Acad. Sci.*, **112**, 281–291.
169. COHN, R. (1969). Visual evoked responses in the brain injured monkey. *Arch. Neurol.*, **21**, 321–329.

170. COHN, R. Personal communication.
171. COMMUNICATIONS BIOPHYSICS GROUP and SIEBERT, W. M. (1959). 'Processing Neurolectric Data', Technology Press, Cambridge, Mass., Technical Report 351.
172. COOLEY, V. W. and TUKEY, J. W. (1965). An algorithm for the machine calculation of complex Fourier series. *Math. Comp.*, **19**, 297–301.
173. COOPER, R., OSSELTON, J. W. and SHAW, J. C. (1969). 'EEG Technology', Butterworths, London, p. 186.
174. COOPER, R. and WARREN, W. J. (1961). The use of barrier grid storage tubes 9511A for extraction of average evoked responses from the EEG. *J. Physiol.*, **157**, 38. P.
175. COOPER, R., WINTER, A. L., CROW, H. J. and WALTER, W. G. (1965). Comparison of subcortical, cortical and scalp activity using chronically indwelling electrodes in man. *Electroenceph. clin. Neurophysiol.*, **18**, 217–228.
176. COPENHAVER, R. M. and BEINHOCKER, G. D. (1963). Evoked occipital potentials recorded from scalp electrodes in response to focal visual illumination. *Invest. Ophthal.*, **2**, 393–406.
177. COPENHAVER, R. M., EISENBERG, M. F. and PERRY, N. W., JR. (1966). Visual evoked retinal and cortical potentials time locked to the electrocardiogram. Proc. 4th ISCERG Symposium, Tokyo, JJO Vol. 10, Suppl.
178. COPENHAVER, R. M. and PERRY, N. M., JR. (1964). Factors affecting visually evoked cortical potentials such as impaired vision of varying etiology. *Invest. Ophthal.*, **3**, 665–675.
179. CORCELLE, L., ROZIER, J., DEDIEU, E., VINCENT, J.-D. and FAURÉ, J.-M.-A. (1968). Variations in the cortical potentials evoked in accordance with the modality of sensory stimulation in the dyslexic child. *Rev. Laryng.* (Bordeaux), **89**, 458–468 (French, English summary).
180. CORLETTO, F., GENTILOMO, A., ROSADINI, G., ROSSIG, F. and ZATTONI, J. (1967). Visual evoked potentials as recorded from the scalp and from the visual cortex before and after surgical removal of the occipital pole in man. *Electroenceph. clin. Neurophysiol.*, **22**, 378–380.
181. COURANT, R. (1937). 'Differential and Integral Calculus', Vol. 1, Blackie, London.
182. COWEY, A. and WEISKRANTZ, L. (1962). *Quart. J. Exp. Psychol.*, **15**, 91.
183. COWEY, A. (1967). *Quart. J. Exp. Psychol.*, **19**, 232.
184. CREUTZFELDT, O. D. (1965). The human visual evoked potential (VEP) with special reference to its ontogenesis and pathology. Sixth Internat. EEG Congr. Vienna. EEG abstract – EMG. 10.
185. CREUTZFELDT, O. D., FUSTER, J. M., LUX, H. D. and NACIMIENTO, A. C. (1964). Experimenteller Nachweis von Beziehungen zwischen EEG-Wellen und Aktivität corticaler Nervenzellen. *Naturwissenschaften*, **51**, 166–167.
186. CREUTZFELDT, O. D. and JUNG, R. (1961). Neuronal discharge in the cat's motor cortex during sleep and arousal. In Wolstenholme, G. E. W. and O'Connor, M. (Eds.) 'The Nature of Sleep'. Churchill, London, pp. 131–170.
187. CREUTZFELDT, O. D., KUGLER, J., MOROCUTTI, C. and SOMMER-SMITH, J. A. (1966). Visual evoked potentials in normal human subjects and neurological patients. *Electroenceph. clin. Neurophysiol.*, **20**, 98–106.
188. CREUTZFELDT, O. D. and KUHNT, U. (1967). The visual evoked potential: Physiological, developmental and clinical aspects. *Electroenceph. clin. Neurophysiol., Suppl.* **26**, 29–41.
189. CREUTZFELDT, O. D., WATANABE, S. and LUX, H. D. (1966). Relations between EEG phenomena and potentials of single cortical cells. I. Evoked responses after thalamic and epicortical stimulation. *Electroenceph. clin. Neurophysiol.*,

20, 1–18. II. Spontaneous and convulsoid activity. *Electroenceph. clin. Neurophysiol.*, **20**, 19–37.

190. CRIGHEL, E. (1965). Flash evoked potentials, recovery cycle and seizure discharges induced by intermittent photic stimulation. *Excerpta Medica Int. Cong. Ser.*, **124**, 277–282.

191. CRIGHEL, E. and BOTEZ, M. I. (1966). Photic evoked potentials in man in lesions of the occipital lobes. *Brain*, **89**, 311–316.

192. CRIGHEL, E. and POILICI, I. (1968). Photic evoked responses in patients with thalamic and brain stem lesions. *Confin. Neurol.*, **30**, 301–312.

193. CRIGHEL, E., POILICI, I. and MARINCHESCU, C. (1966). The influence of hyperoxia on flash evoked potentials in normals and in patients with cerebral circulatory insufficiency. *Confin. Neurol.*, **28**, 348–354.

194. CRIGHEL, E., POILICI, I. and MARINCHESCU, C. (1968). Moderate hypercapnia and photic evoked responses in man. *Revue Roumaine de Neurologie*, **5**, 15–21.

195. CULVER, C. M., TANLEY, J. C. and EASON, R. G. (1970). Evoked cortical potentials: relation to hand dominance and eye dominance. *Percept. Mot. Skills.*, **30**, 407–414.

196. DAVENPORT, W. B. and ROOT, W. L. (1958). 'Random Signals and Noise', McGraw-Hill, New York.

197. DAVIS, H. (1964). Enhancement of evoked cortical potential in humans related to a task requiring a decision. *Science*, **145**, 182–183.

198. DAVIS, H. (Ed.) (1965). The Young Deaf Child: Identification and Management. *Acta. Otolaryng.* (Stockholm), Suppl. 206.

199. DAVIS, H. (1966). Validation of evoked-response audiometry (ERA) in deaf children. *Internat. Audiol.*, **5**, 77–81.

200. DAVIS, H. (1969). Comment on Callaway's paper. In Donchin, E. and Lindsley, D. B. (Eds.) 'Average Evoked Potentials', NASA SP–191, Washington, D.C., pp. 321–323.

201. DAVIS, H., DAVIS, P. A., LOOMIS, A. L., HARVEY, N. and HOBART, G. A. (1939). Electrical reactions of the brain to auditory stimulation during sleep. *J. Neurophysiol.*, **2**, 500–514.

202. DAVIS, H., HIRSCH, S. K., SHELNUTT, J. and BOWERS, C. (1967). Further validation of evoked response audiometry (ERA). *J. Speech Hearing Res.*, **10**, 717–732.

203. DAVIS, H., MAST, T., YOSHIE, N. and ZERLIN, S. (1966). The slow response of the human cortex to auditory stimuli: recovery processes. *Electroenceph. clin. Neurophysiol.*, **21**, 105–113.

204. DAVIS, H. and ONISHI, S. Maturation of the auditory evoked potentials. Presented to Ninth International Congress on Audiology 1968.

205. DAVIS, H. and ZERLIN, S. (1966). Acoustic relations of the human vertex potential. *J. Acoust. Soc. Amer.*, **39**, 109–116.

206. DAVIS, P. A. (1939). Effects of acoustic stimuli on the waking human brain. *J. Neurophysiol.*, **2**, 494–499.

207. DAVISSON, L. D. (1966). A theory of adaptive filtering. *IEEE Trans. Info. Theory*, **IT-12**, 97–102.

208. DAWSON, G. D. (1946). The relation between the electroencephalogram and muscle action potentials in certain convulsive states. *J. Neurol. Neurosurg. Psychiat.*, **9**, 5–22.

209. DAWSON, G. D. (1947). Cerebral responses to electrical stimulation of peripheral nerve in man. *J. Neurol. Neurosurg. Psychiat.*, **10**, 134–140.

210. DAWSON, G. D. (1947). Investigations on a patient subject to myoclonic seizures after sensory stimulation. *J. Neurol. Neurosurg. Psychiat.*, **10**, 141–162.

211. DAWSON, G. D. (1950). Cerebral responses to nerve stimulation in man. *Brit. med. Bull.*, **6**, 326–329.

212. DAWSON, G. D. (1951). A summation technique for detecting small signals in a large irregular background. *J. Physiol.*, **115**, 2–3.
213. DAWSON, G. D. (1953). Autocorrelation and automatic integration. *Electroenceph. clin. Neurophysiol., Suppl.* **4**, 26–37.
214. DAWSON, G. D. (1954). A summation technique for the detection of small evoked potentials. *Electroenceph. clin. Neurophysiol.*, **6**, 65–84.
215. DAWSON, G. D. (1954). A multiple scalp electrode for plotting evoked potentials. *Electroenceph. clin. Neurophysiol.*, **6**, 153–154.
216. DAWSON, G. D. and PITMAN, J. R. (1958). *J. Physiol.*, **140**, 34.
217. DE LANGE, H. DZN. (1957). Attenuation characteristics and phase-shift characteristics of the human fovea-cortex systems in relation to flicker fusion phenomena. Thesis, Technical University, Delft, The Netherlands.
218. DE LUCCHI, M. R., GAROUTTE, B. and AIRD, R. B. (1962). The scalp as an electroencephalographic averager. *Electroenceph. clin. Neurophysiol.*, **14**, 191–196.
219. DE VOE, R. D., SMALL, R. J. W. and ZVARGULIS, J. E. (1969). Spectral sensitivities of wolf spider eyes. *J. Gen. Physiol.*, **54**, 1–32.
220. DE VOE, R. G., RIPPS, H. and VAUGHAN, H. G., JR. (1968). Cortical responses to stimulation of the human fovea. *Vision Res.*, **8**, 135–147.
221. DEBECKER, J. and DESMEDT, J. E. (1964). Les potentiels évoqués cérébraux et les potentiels de nerf sensible chez l'homme et l'utilisation de l'ordinateur numérique Mnemetron 400-B. *Acta Neurol. Psychiat. Belg.*, **64**, 1212–1248.
222. DEBECKER, J. and DESMEDT, J. E. (1965). Sur la relation entre le seuil de perception tactile et les potentials évoqués de l'écorce cérébrale somatosensible chez l'homme. *Compt. Rend.*, **260**, 687.
223. DEBECKER, J. and DESMEDT, J. E. (1966). Rate of intermodulity switching disclosed by sensory evoked potentials averaged during signal detection tests. *J. Physiol.* (Lond.), **185**, 52–53.
224. DEECKE, L., SCHEID, P. and KORNHUBER, H. H. (1969). Distribution of readiness potential, pre-motion positivity and motor potential of the human cerebral cortex preceding voluntary finger movements. *Exp. Brain Res.*, **7**, 158–168.
225. DESMEDT, J. E. (19??). Somatosensory cerebral evoked potentials in man.
226. DESMEDT, J. E., MANIL, J., CHORAZYNA, H. and DEBECKER, J. (1967). Potential évoqué cérèbral et conduction corticipéte pour une volée d'influx somesthèsique chez le nouveau-né normal. *C.R. Soc. Biol.* (Paris), **161**, 205–208.
227. DESMEDT, J. E. and MANIL, J. (1970). Somatosensory EPs of the normal human neonate in REM sleep, in slow wave sleep and in waking. *Electroenceph. clin. Neurophysio.*, **29**, 113–126.
228. DIAMOND, S. P. (1964). Input-output relations. *Ann. N.Y. Acad. Sci.*, **112**, 160–171.
229. DIAMOND, S. P. (1964). A simple programming technique for comparing average responses. *Electroenceph. clin. Neurophysiol.*, **16**, 305–307.
230. DILL, R. C., VALLECALLE, E. and VERZEANO, M. (1968). Evoked potentials, neuronal activity and stimulus intensity in the visual system. *Physiol. and Behaviour*, **3**, 797–801.
231. DINSDALE, J. (1965 Jan.). Transistor high quality audio amplifier. *Wireless World*, pp. 2–9.
232. DODGE, R. (1900). Visual perception during eye movement. *Psychol. Rev.*, **7**, 454–465.
233. DOMINO, E. F., MATSUOKA, S., WALTZ, J. and COOPER, I. (1964). Simultaneous recordings of scalp and epidural somatosensory evoked responses in man. *Science*, **145**, 1199–1200.

234. DOMINO, E. F., MATSUOKA, S., WALTZ, J. and COOPER, I. S. (1965). Effects of cryogenic thalamic lesions on the somesthetic evoked response in man. *Electroenceph. clin. Neurophysiol.*, **19**, 127–138.
235. DONALD, M. W. (1970). Direct-current potentials in the human brain evoked during timed cognitive performance. *Nature*, **227**, 1057–1058.
236. DONALD, M. W. (1970). The P300 effect: dissociation from direct-current potentials in the human cortex. Presented to American EEG Soc., September 1970, Washington, D.C.
237. DONALDSON, P. E. K. (1958). 'Electrical Apparatus for Biological Research', London, Butterworth, 718 P.
238. DONCHIN, E. (1966). A multivariate approach to the analysis of averaged evoked potentials. *IEEE Trans. Bio. Med. Engng.*, **BME-13**, 131–139.
239. DONCHIN, E. (1968). Averaged evoked potentials and uncertainty resolution. *Psychon. Sci.*, **12**, 103.
240. DONCHIN, E. (1969). Discriminant analysis in average evoked response studies: the study of single trial data. *Electroenceph. clin. Neurophysiol.*, **27**, 311–314.
241. DONCHIN, E. (1969). Data analysis techniques in averaged evoked potential research. In Donchin, E. and Lindsley, D. B. (Eds.) 'Average Evoked Potentials', NASA SP–191, Washington, D.C., pp. 199–217.
242. DONCHIN, E. (1969). Discussion of Goff's paper. In Donchin, E. and Lindsley, D. B. (Eds.) 'Average Evoked Potentials', NASA SP–191, Washington, D.C., p. 132.
243. DONCHIN, E. (1971). Evoked potentials to stimuli presented to the suppressed eye in a binocular rivalry experiment. *Vision Res.* In press.
244. DONCHIN, E., CALLAWAY, E. and JONES, R. T. (1970). AEP variability in schizophrenia. The application of discriminant analysis. *Electroenceph. clin. Neurophysiol.*, **29**, 429–440.
245. DONCHIN, E. and COHEN, L. (1967). Average evoked potentials and intramodality selective attention. *Electroenceph. clin. Neurophysiol.*, **22**, 537–546.
246. DONCHIN, E. and COHEN, L. (1970). Evoked potentials to stimuli presented to the suppressed eye in a binocular rivalry experiment. *Vision Res.*, **10**, 103–106.
247. DONCHIN, E. and LINDSLEY, D. B. (1966). Average evoked potentials and reaction times to visual stimuli. *Electroenceph. clin. Neurophysiol.*, **20**, 217–223.
248. DONCHIN, E. and LINDSLEY, D. B. (Eds.) (1966). 'Average Evoked Potentials', NASA SP–191, Washington, D.C.
249. DONCHIN, E. and SMITH, D. B. D. (1970). The CNV and late positive wave of the average evoked potential. *Electroenceph. clin. Neurophysiol.*, **29**, 201–203.
250. DONCHIN, E. and SUTTON, S. (1971). The 'psychological significance' of evoked responses: a comment on Clark, Butler and Rosner. *Communications in Behavioural Biol.* In press.
251. DOW, D. J. and WHITTY, C. W. M. (1947). Electroencephalographic changes in migraine; review of 51 cases. *Lancet*, **II**, 52–54.
252. DUANE, T. D. and BEHRENDT, T. (1965). Extrasensory electroencephalic induction between indentical twins. *Science*, **150**, 367.
253. DUFFY, F. H. and LOMBROSO, C. T. (1968). Electrophysiological evidence for visual suppression prior to the onset of a voluntary saccadic eye movement. *Nature*, **218**, 1074–1075.
254. DUSTMAN, R. E. and BECK, E. C. (1966). Visually evoked potentials. *Science*, **151**, 1013–1015.
255. DUSTMAN, R. E. and BECK, E. C. (1969). The effects of maturation and aging on the waveform of visually evoked potentials. *Electroenceph. clin. Neurophysiol.*, **26**, 2–1.

256. EASON, R. G. and WHITE, C. T. (1967). Averaged occipital responses to stimulation of sites in the nasal and temporal halves of the retina. *Psychon. Sci.*, **7**, 309–310.

257. EASON, R. G., WHITE, C. T. and ODEN, D. (1967). Averaged occipital responses to stimulation of sites in the upper and lower halves of the retina. *Perception and Psychophysics*, **2**, 423–425.

258. EASON, R. G., GROVES, P., WHITE, C. T. and ODEN, D. (1967). Evoked cortical potentials relation to visual field and handedness. *Science*, **156**, 1643–1646.

259. EASON, R. G., WHITE, C. T. and BARTLETT, N. (1970). Effects of checkerboard pattern stimulations on evoked cortical responses in relation to check size and visual field. *Psychon. Sci.*, **2**, 113–115.

260. ECCLES, J. C. (1957). 'The Physiology of Nerve Cells', Johns Hopkins Press, Baltimore.

261. EDWARDS, D. B. G. and ASPINALL, D. (1965). *World Med. Electron.*, **3**, 276.

262. EFRON, R. (1964). Artificial synthesis of evoked responses to light flash. *Ann. N.Y. Acad. Sci.*, **112**, 292–304.

263. EHRENBERGER, K., FINKENZELLER, P., KEIDEL, W. D. and PLATTIG, K. H. (1966). Elektrophysiologische Korrolation der Stevensschen Potenzfunction und Objective Schwellenmessung am Vibrationssiun des Menschen. *Pflügers Archiv.*, **290**, 114–123.

264. ELLINGSON, R. J. (1964). Cerebral electrical responses to auditory and visual stimuli in the infant (human and subhuman studies). In Kellaway, P., "Neurological and Electroencephalographic Correlative Studies in Infancy". Grune and Stratton, New York, pp. 78–114.

265. ELLINGSON, R. J. (1966). Development of visual evoked responses in human infants recorded by a response averager. *Electroenceph. clin. Neurophysiol.*, **21**, 403–404.

266. ELUL, R. (1962). Dipoles of spontaneous activity in the cerebral cortex. *Exptl. Neurol.*, **6**, 285.

267. ELUL, R. (1969). Gaussian behaviour of the electroencephalogram: changes during performance of mental task. *Science*, **164**, 328–331.

268. ELUL, R. (1967). Statistical mechanisms in generation of the EEG. In 'Progress in Biomedical Engineering', Vol. 1, Spartan Books, Washington, D.C.

269. ELUL, R. (1968). Brain waves: intracellular recording and statistical analysis help clarify their physiological significance. In 'Data Acquisition and Processing in Biology and Medicine', Vol. 5, pp. 93–115, Pergamon, Oxford and New York.

270. ELUL, R. and ADEY, W. R. (1966). Instability of firing threshold and 'remote' activation in cortical neurones. *Nature*, **212**, 1424–1425.

271. ENGEL, G. L., FERRIS, E. B., JR. and ROMANO, J. (1945). *Am. J. Med. Sci.*, **209**, 650.

272. ENGEL, R. (1965). Maturational changes and abnormalities in the newborn electroencephalogram. *Develop. Med. Child Neurol.*, **7**, 498–506.

273. ENGEL, R., CROWELL, D. and NISHIJIMA, S. (1968). Visual and auditory response latencies in neonates. In 'In Honour of C. C. De Silva', Kularatne, Ceylon, pp. 1–10.

274. ENGEL, R. and YOUNG, N. B. (1969). Calibrated pure tone audiograms in normal neonates based on evoked electroencephalographic responses. *Neuropadiätrie*, **1**, 149–160.

275. ENNEVER, J., GARTSIDE, I. B., LIPPOLD, O. C. J., NOVOTNY, G. and SHAGASS, C. (1967). Contamination of the human cortical evoked response with potentials of intra-orbital origin. *J. Physiol.*, **191**, 5 P.

276. ENROTH-CUGELL, C. and ROBSON, J. G. (1966). The contrast sensitivity of retinal ganglion cells of the cat. *J. Physiol.*, **187**, 517–522.

277. ERTL, J. P. (1965). Detection of evoked potentials by zero crossing analysis. *Electroenceph. clin. Neurophysiol.*, **18**, 630–631.

278. ERTL, J. P. (1967). Evoked potential recovery from tape recorded zero crossings of the EEG. *Electroenceph. clin. Neurophysiol.*, **22**, 387–388.

279. ERTL, J. (1968). Evoked potentials, neural efficiency and I.Q. Paper presented at International Symposium for Biocybernetics, Washington, D.C.

280. ERTL, J. P. and SCHAFER, E. W. P. (1969). Brain response correlates of psychometric intelligence. *Nature*, **223**, 421–422.

281. EVANS, C. C. (1952). Comments on 'Occipital sharp waves responsive to visual stimuli'. *Electroenceph. clin. Neurophysiol.*, **4**, 111P.

282. EVANS, C. C. (1952). Some further observations on occipital sharp waves (lambda waves). *Electroenceph. clin. Neurophysiol.*, **4**, 371.

283. EVANS, E. F. (1968). Cortical Representation. In 'Hearing Mechanisms in Vertebrates', de Reuck A. V. S. and Knight, J. (Eds.), Churchill Ltd., London, pp. 272–287.

284. FERRIS, G. S., DAVIS, G. D., DORSEN, M. M. and HACKETT, E. R. (1967). Changes in latency and form of the photically induced averaged evoked responses in human infants. *Electroenceph. clin. Neurophysiol.*, **22**, 305–312.

285. FINKENZELLER, P. (1966). Gemittelte EEG – Potentiale bei Olfactorischer Reizung. *Pflügers Archiv.*, **292**, 76–80.

286. FIORENTINI, A. and MAFFEI, L. (1970). Electrophysiological evidence for binocular disparity detectors in the human visual system. *Science*, **169**, 208–209.

287. FLASTERHEIN, L. H. (1966). Voltage fluctuations metal-electrolyte interfaces in electrophysiology. *Med. Biol. Engn.*, **4**, 583–588.

288. FLASTERHEIN, L. H. (1966). A general analysis of voltage fluctuations of metal-electrolyte interfaces. *Med. Biol. Engn.*, **4**, 589–594.

289. FLORIS, V. and RIZZO, P. A. (1968). Studio delle riposte evocate visive nelle emianopsie. *Riv. Pat. Nerv. Ment.*, **89**, 191–206.

290. FOGARTY, T. P. and REUBEN, R. N. (1969). Light-evoked cortical and retinal responses in premature infants. *Arch. Ophthal.*, **81**, 454–459.

291. FOX, S. S. and O'BRIEN, J. H. (1965). Duplication of evoked potential waveform by curve of probability of firing of a single cell. *Science*, **147**, 838.

292. FOX, S. S. and NORMAN, R. J. (1968). Functional congruence: an index of neural homogeneity and a new measure of brain activity. *Science*, **159**, 1257–1259.

293. FOX, S. S. and RUDELL, A. P. (1969). Operant controlled neural event: formal and systematic approach to electrical coding of behaviour in brain. *Science*, **162**, 1299–1302.

293a. FOX, S. S. and RUDELL, A. P. (1970). Operant controlled neural event: functional independence in behavioural coding by early and late components of visual cortical evoked responses in cats. *J. Neurophysiol.*, **33**, 548–561.

294. FRANK, E. (1952). Electric potentials produced by two point homogeneous conducting medium. *J. Appl. Phys.*, **23**, 1225–1228.

295. FRANZÉN, O. and OFFENLOCH, K. (1969). Evoked response correlates of psychophysical magnitude. Estimates for tactile stimulation in man. *Exp. Brain. Res.*, **8**, 1–18.

296. FREEMAN, W. J. (1964). Use of digital adaptive filters for measuring prepyriform evoked potentials from cats. *Exptl. Neurol.*, **10**, 475–492.

297. FRICKER, S. J. (1962). Narrow-band filter techniques for the detection and measurement of evoked responses. *Electroenceph. clin. Neurophysiol.*, **14**, 411–413.

298. FRUHSTORFER, H., SOVERI, P. and JARVILEHTO, T. (1970). Short-term habituation of the auditory evoked response in man. *Electroenceph. clin. Neurophysiol.*, **28**, 153–161.

299. FUKADA, Y., MOTOKAWA, K., NORTON, A. C. and TASAKI, K. (1966). Functional significance of conduction velocity in the transfer of flicker information in the optic nerve of the cat. *J. Neurophysiol.*, **29**, 698–714.

300. GALAMBOS, R. and VELLUTI, R. (1968). Evoked resistance shifts in unanaesthetised cats. *Exp. Neurol.*, **22**, 243–252.

301. GARCÍA-AUSST, E. (1963). Influence of states of awareness upon sensory evoked potentials. *Electroenceph. clin. Neurophysiol., Suppl.* **24**, 76–89.

302. GARCÍA-AUSST, E., BOGACZ, J. and VANZULLI, A. (1961). Significance of the photic stimulus on the evoked response in man. In Fessard, A., Gerard, R. W. and Konorski, J. (Eds.) 'Brain mechanisms and learning', Blackwell, Oxford, pp. 603–621.

303. GARCÍA-AUSST, E., BOGACZ, J. and VANZULLI, A. (1964). Effects of attention and inattention upon visual evoked response. *Electroenceph. clin. Neurophysiol.*, **17**, 136–143.

304. GARTSIDE, I. B., LIPPOLD, O. C. J. and MELDRUM, B. S. (1966). The evoked cortical somatosensory response in normal man and its modification by oral lithium carbonate. *Electroenceph. clin. Neurophysiol.*, **20**, 382–390.

305. GASTAUT, Y. (1951). Un signe électroencéphalographique peu connu: les pointes occipitales survenant pendant l'ouverture les yeux. *Rev. Neurol.*, **84**, 640–643.

306. GASTAUT, Y. (1953). Les pointes négatives évoquées sur le vertex. Leur signification psychophysiologique et pathologique. *Rev. Neurol.*, **89**, 382–399.

307. GASTAUT, H., GASTAUT, Y., ROGER, A., CORRIOL, J. and NAQUET, R. (1951). Étude électrographique du cycle d'excitabilité cortical. *Electroenceph. clin. Neurophysiol.*, **3**, 401–428.

308. GASTAUT, H., FRANCK, G., KROLIKOWSKA, W., NAQUET, R., RÉGIS, H. and ROGER, J. (1963). Étude des potentiels évoqués visuels chez des hemianoptiques présentant des CMS'es epileptiques visuelles dans leur champ aveugle. *Rev. Neurol.*, **108**, 316–322.

309. GASTAUT, H. and RÉGIS, H. (1965). Visually-evoked potentials recorded transcranially in man. In Proctor, L. D. and Adey, W. R. (Eds.) 'The Analysis of Central Nervous System and Cardiovascular Data Using Computer Methods', Washington, NASA, pp. 7–34.

310. GASTAUT, H. and RÉGIS, H. (1967). Le potentiel évoqué visuel moyen (P.E.V.M.) chez l'homme normal dans des conditions standards. Relation avec les ondes lambda. In H. Gastaut *et al.* (Eds.) 'Les Activitiés Électriques Cérébrales Spontanées et Évoquées chez L'Homme', Gauthier-Villare, Paris, pp. 46–48.

311. GEISLER, C. D. (1960). Average responses to clicks in man recorded by scalp electrodes. Massachusetts Institute of Technology, Res. Lab. of Electronics, Tech. Rep. 380.

312. GEISLER, C. D. and GERSTEIN, G. L. (1961). The surface EEG in relation to its sources. *Electroenceph. clin. Neurophysiol.*, **13**, 927–934.

313. GERBRANDT, L. K., GOFF, W. R. and SMITH, D. B. (1970). Topography of the averaged movement potential. Presented to the American EEG Soc., Washington, D.C.

314. GESELOWITZ, D. B. (1960). Multipole representation for an equivalent cardiac generator. *Proc. IRE*, **48**, 75–79.

315. GESELOWITZ, D. B. (1965). Two theorems concerning the quadrupole applicable to electrocardiography. *IEEE Trans. Bio. Med. Engng.*, **BME-12**, 164–168.

316. GIBBS, F. A. and GIBBS, E. L. (1950). 'Atlas of Electroencephalography', Vol. 1, Addison-Wesley, Cambridge, Mass.

317. GIBLIN, D. R. (1964). Somatosensory evoked potentials in healthy subjects and in patients with lesions of the nervous system. *Ann. N.Y. Acad. Sci.*, **112**, 93–142.

318. GIBSON, J. J. (1950). 'The Perception of the Visual World', Houghton, Mifflin.

319. GILDEN, L., VAUGHAN, H. G., JR. and COSTA, L. D. (1966). Summated human electroencephalographic potentials associated with voluntary movements. *Electroenceph. clin. Neurophysiol.*, **20**, 433–438.

320. GLICKSTEIN, M. (1969). Organization of the visual pathways. *Science*, **164**, 917–926.

321. GOFF, W. R., ROSNER, B. S. and ALLISON, T. (1962). Distribution of cerebral somatosensory evoked responses in normal man. *Electroenceph. clin. Neurophysiol.*, **14**, 697–713.

322. GOFF, W. R., ALLISON, T., SHAPIRO, A. and ROSNER, B. S. (1966). Cerebral somatosensory responses evoked during sleep in man. *Electroenceph. clin. Neurophysiol.*, **21**, 1–9.

323. GOFF, W. R., ALLISON, T., MATSUMIYA, Y., STERMAN, M. B. and FAIRCHILD, M. D. (1967). Effects of 1,1-dimethylhydrazine (UDMH) on evoked cerebral neuroelectric responses. Aerospace Medical Research Labs. TR–67–67.

324. GOFF, W. R., MATSUMIYA, Y., ALLISON, T. and GOFF, G. D. (1969). Cross-modality comparisons of averaged evoked potentials. In Donchin, E. and Lindsley, D. B. (Eds.) 'Average Evoked Potentials', NASA SP–191, pp. 95–118.

325. GOFF, W. R., BOBOWICK, A. R., ALLISON, T. and LEVY, L. (1970). K-complexes evoked by somatic stimulation in patients with unilateral cerebral lesions. Presented to American EEG Soc., Sept. 1970.

326. GOFF. Personal communication.

327. GOLDSTEIN, M. H., JR. (1968). Single unit studies of cortical coding of simple acoustic stimuli. In 'Physiological and Biochemical Aspects of Nervous Integration', Carlson, F. D. (Ed.), Prentice-Hall Inc., pp. 131–151.

328. GOLDSTEIN, S. (1970). Phase coherence of the alpha rhythm during photic blocking. *Electroenceph. clin. Neurophysiol.*, **29**, 127–136.

329. GOLLA, F. L. and WINTER, A. L. (1959). Analysis of cerebral responses to flicker in patients complaining of episodic headache. *Electroenceph. clin. Neurophysiol.*, **11**, 539.

330. GON, J. J. DENIER VAN DER, STRACKEE, J. and TWEEL, L. H. VAN DER (1958). A source for modulated light. *Physics in Medicine and Biology*, **3**, 164–173.

331. GON, J. J. DENIER VAN DER and STRACKEE, J. (1966). Some aspects of EEG frequency analysis. *IEEE Trans. Bio. Med. Engng.*, **BME-13**, 120–130.

332. GOTO, A., KOSAKA, K., KUBOTA, K., NAKAMURA, R. and NARABAYASHI, H. (1968). Thalamic potentials from muscle afferents in the human. *Archiv. Neurol.*, **19**, 302–309.

333. GOURAS, P. and LINK, K. (1966). Rod and cone interaction in dark-adapted monkey ganglion cells. *J. Physiol.*, **184**, 499–510.

333a. GOURAS, P. (1970). *Invest. Opthal.*, **9**, 557–596.

334. GRAHAM, C. H. (Ed.) (1965). 'Vision and Visual Perception', Wiley, New York, pp. 637.

335. GRANIT, R. and WIRTH, A. (1953). *J. Physiol.*, **122**, 386.
GRANDA, A. M. (1961). Electrical responses of the human eye to coloured flickering light. *J. Opt. Soc. Amer.*, **51**, 648–654.

336. GRASS, A. M. and GIBBS, F. A. (1938). A Fourier transform of the electroencephalogram. *J. Neurophysiol.*, **1**, 521–526.
FISHGOLD, H., JOLIVET, G. and MATHIS, P. (1961). Analyse de frequence et integration optique en electroencephalographie. *Electroenceph. clin. Neurophysiol.*, **13**, 123–127.

WALTER, W. G., DOWEY, V. J. and SHIPTON, H. (1946). Analysis of the electric response of the human cortex to photic stimulation. *Nature* (London), **158**, 540–541.

MEISTER, M., SCHWAB, R., PETERSEN, E. and GRASS, A. (1959). Simultaneous two channel frequency analyser with non-electric (passive) filters. *Electroenceph. clin. Neurophysiol.*, **11**, 594–600.

BURCH, N. R. (1959). Automatic analysis of the encephalogram; a review and classification of systems. *Electroenceph. clin. Neurophysiol.*, **11**, 827–834.

WALTER, W. G. (1946). A new electronic analyser. *Electronic Eng.* (Nov.), 339–344.

337. GRAZIANI, L., WEITZMAN, E. D. and VELASCO, M. S. A. (1968). Neurologic maturation and auditory evoked responses in low birth weight infants. *Pediatrics*, **41**, 483–494.

338. GREEN, D. G. (1968). The contrast sensitivity of the colour mechanisms of the human eye. *J. Physiol.*, **196**, 415–429.

339. GROGINSKY, H. L., WILSON, L. R. and MIDDLETON, D. (1966). Adaptive detection of statistical signals in noise. *IEEE Trans. Info. Theory*, **IT-12**, 337–348.

340. GROSS, M. M., TOBIN, M., KISSIN, E. H. and SABOT, L. (1964). Evoked responses to clicks in delerium tremens: a preliminary report. *Ann. N.Y. Acad. Sci.*, **112**, 543–546.

341. GROSS, M. M., BEGLEITER, H., TOBIN, M. and KISSIN, B. (1965). Auditory evoked response comparison during counting clicks and reading. *Electroenceph. clin. Neurophysiol.*, **18**, 451–454.

342. GROSS, E. G., VAUGHAN, H. G. and VALENSTEIN, E. (1967). Inhibition of visual evoked responses to patterned stimuli during voluntary eye movements. *Electroenceph. clin. Neurophysiol.*, **22**, 204–209.

343. GROSSMAN, R. G., WHITESIDE, L. and HAMPTON, T. L. (1969). The time course of evoked depolarisations of cortical glial cells. *Brain Res.*, **14**, 401–415.

344. GUBISCH, R. W. (1965). Low-frequency light modulator. *J. Opt. Soc. Amer.*, **55**, 409–411.

345. HAIDER, M. (1967). Vigilance, attention, expectancy and cortical evoked potentials. *Acta Psychol.*, **27**, 246–252.

346. HAIDER, M., SPONG, P. and LINDSLEY, D. B. (1964). Attention, vigilance and cortical evoked potentials in humans. *Science*, **145**, 180–182.

347. HAIDER, M., GROLL, E. and STUDYNKA, G. (1968). Orientierungs-und Bereitschaftspotentiale bei unervarteten Reizen. *Exp. Brain Res.*, **5**, 45–54.

348. HALLIDAY, A. M. (1967). Cerebral evoked potentials in familial progressive myoclonic epilepsy. *J. Roy. Coll. Phys., London*, **1**, 123–134.

349. HALLIDAY, A. M. (1967). The electrophysiological study of myoclonus in man. *Brain*, **90**, 241–284.

350. HALLIDAY, A. M. (1967). Changes in the form of cerebral evoked responses in man associated with various lesions of the nervous system. *Electroenceph. clin. Neurophysiol., Suppl.* **25**, 178–192.

351. HALLIDAY, A. M. (1968). Computing techniques in neurological diagnosis. *Brit. med. Bull.*, **24**, 253–259.

352. HALLIDAY, A. M. and WAKEFIELD, G. S. (1963). Cerebral evoked potentials in patients with dissociated sensory loss. *J. Neurol. Neurosurg. Psychiat.*, **26**, 211–219.

353. HALLIDAY, A. M. and MASON, A. A. (1964). The effect of hypnotic anaesthesia on cortical responses. *J. Neurol. Neurosurg. Psychiat.*, **27**, 300–312.

354. HALLIDAY, A. M. and PITMAN, J. R. (1965). A digital computer averager for work on evoked responses. *J. Physiol.*, **178**, 23 P.

355. HALLIDAY, A. M. and MICHAEL, W. F. (1970). Changes in pattern-evoked responses in man associated with the vertical and horizontal meridians of the visual field. *J. Physiol.*, **208**, 499–513.

356. FIELD, J., MAGOUN, H. W. and HALL, V. E. (Eds.). (1959). 'Handbook of Physiology', Vols. 1, 2, 3, Amer. Physiological Soc., Washington, D.C.

357. HANDLER, P., VANZULLI, A., BOGACZ, J. and GARCÍA-AUSST, E. (1960). A photo-optic-electronic method for the detection and study of evoked potentials. *Acta Neurol. Latinoamer.*, **6**, 163–173.

358. HARRIS, E. K. and WOODY, C. D. (1969). Use of an adaptive filter to characterise signal-noise relationships. *Computers and Biomed. Res.*, **2**, 242–273.

359. HARTER, M. R. (1968). Effects of contour sharpness and check-size on visually evoked cortical potentials. *Vision Res.*, **8**, 701–711.

360. HARTER, M. R. (1971). Visually evoked cortical responses to on- and off-set of patterned light in humans. *Vision Res.* In press.

361. HARTER, M. R. (1971). Evoked cortical responses to checkerboard patterns: effect of check-size as a function of retinal eccentricity. *Vision Res.*, **10**, 1365–1376.

362. HARTER, M. R. and WHITE, C. T. (1967). Perceived number and evoked cortical potentials. *Science*, **156**, 406–408.

363. HARTER, M. R. and WHITE, C. T. (1969). Evoked cortical responses to checkerboard patterns: effect of check-size as a function of visual acuity. *Electroenceph. clin. Neurophysiol.*, **28**, 48–54.

364. HARTER, M. R. and SALMON, L. E. (1971). Evoked cortical responses to patterned light flashes: effects of ocular convergence and accommodation. *Electroenceph. clin. Neurophysiol.* In press.

365. HAYASH, C. (1964). 'Nonlinear Oscillations in Physical Systems', McGraw-Hill, New York.

366. HEATH, R. G. and GALBRAITH, G. C. (1966). Sensory evoked responses recorded simultaneously from human cortex and scalp. *Nature*, **212**, 1535–1537.

367. HELMHOLTZ, H. VON. (1910). 'Helmholtz's Treatise on Physiological Optics' (Ed. Southal, J. P. C.). Vol. 3, Dover, New York (1962), pp. 312–313, 388–389.
HOLTZ, E. VON. (1955). Die Beteilsgung von Konverenz und Akkommodation an der Wahrgenommenon Grozzenkonstanz. *Naturwiss.*, **42**, 444.
MCREADY, D. W. (1965). Size-distance perception and accommodation convergence micropsia – a critique. *Vision Res.*, **5**, 189–206.
RICHARDS, W. (1969). 'The Influence of Oculomotor Systems on Visual Perception', AFOSR Tech. Rep. No. 69, 1934, TR p. 121.

368. HENINGER, G. R., MCDONALD, R. K., GOFF, W. R. and SOLLBERGER, A. (1969). Diurnal variations in the cerebral evoked response and EEG. *Arch. Neurol.*, **21**, 330–337.

369. HERNÁNDEZ-PEÔN, R. (1961). Reticular mechanisms of sensory control. In Rosenblith, W. A. (Ed.) 'Sensory Communication', Wiley, New York, and M.I.T. Press, Cambridge, Mass., pp. 497–520.

370. HERNÁNDEZ-PEÔN, R. (1964). Psychiatric implications of neurophysiological research. *Bull. Menninger Clinic*, **28**, 165–185.

371. HERNÁNDEZ-PEÔN, R. (1966). Physiological mechanisms in attention. In Russell, R. W. (Ed.) 'Frontiers in Physiological Psychology', Academic Press, New York and London, pp. 121–147.

372. HERNÁNDEZ-PEÔN, R., SCHERRER, H. and JOUVET, M. (1956). Modification of electrical activity in the cochlear nucleus during attention in unanaesthetised cats. *Science*, **123**, 331–332.

373. HERNÁNDEZ-PEÔN, R., GUZMAN-FLORES, C., ALCARAZ, M. and FERNANDEZ-GUARDIOLA, A. (1957). Sensory transmission in visual pathway during 'attention' in unanaesthetised cats. *Acta Neurol. Latinoamer.*, **3**, 1–8.

374. HERNÁNDEZ-PEÔN, R. and DONOSO, M. (1959). Influence of attention and suggestion upon subcortical evoked electrical activity of the human brain. In L. van Bogaert and J. Radermecker (Eds.) 'Proceedings of the First International Congress of Neurological Sciences', Vol. III, Pergamon, London, pp. 385–396.

375. HERNÁNDEZ-PEÔN, R., CHAVEZ-IBARRA, G. and AGUILAR-FIGUEROA, E. (1963). Somatic evoked potentials in one case of hysterial anaesthesia. *Electroenceph. clin. Neurophysiol.*, **15**, 889–892.

376. HERNÁNDEZ-PEÔN, R. and STERMAN, M. B. (1966). Brain functions. *Ann. Rev. Psychol.*, **17**, 363–394.

377. HERON, T. G. (1968). Industrial deafness and the summed evoked potential. *S.A. Medical Journal*, **42**, 1176–1177.

378. HERRINGTON, R. N. and SCHNEIDAN, P. (1968). The effect of imagery of the visual evoked response. *Experientia*, **24**, 1136–1137.

379. HESS, E. H. and POLT, J. M. (1960). Pupil size as related to interest value of visual stimuli. *Science*, **132**, 349–350.

380. HILL, D. and PARR, G. (Eds.) (1963). 'Electroencephalography. A Symposium on its Various Aspects', MacDonald, London, pp. 509.

381. HILLYARD, S. Comment on Cohen's Paper. In Donchin, E. and Lindsley, D. B. (Eds.) 'Average Evoked Potentials'. NASA SP–191, Washington, D.C., pp. 188–198.

382. HIRSCH, J. F., PERTUISET, B., CALVET, J., BUISSON-FEREY, J., FISCHGOLD, H. and SCHERRER, J. (1961). Étude des résponses électrocorticales obtenues chez l'homme par des stimulations somesthésiques et visuelles. *Electroenceph. clin. Neurophysiol.*, **13**, 411–424.

383. HISHIKAWA, Y., YAMAMOTO, J., FURAYA, E., YAMADA, Y., MIYAZAKI, K. and KANEKO, Z. (1967). Photosensitive epilepsy: relationships between the visual evoked response and the epileptiform discharges induced by intermittent photic stimulation. *Electroenceph. clin. Neurophysiol.*, **23**, 320–334.

384. HODGKIN, A. L. (1964). 'The Conduction of the Nervous Impulse', Liverpool University Press, pp. 108.

385. HOF, M. W. VAN (1964). The influence of attention on the occipito-cortical responses to light flashes in man. *Docum. Ophthal.*, **18**, 238–244.

386. HOF, M. W., VAN HOF-VAN-DUIN, J., VAN MARK, F. VAN DER and RIETVELD, W. J. (1962). The effect of image formation and that of flash counting on the occipito-cortical response to light flashes. *Acta Physiol-Pharmacol. Neerl.*, **11**, 485–493.

387. HOLMES, G. (1918). Disturbances of vision by cerebral lesions. *Brit. J. Ophthal.*, **2**, 353–384.

388. HOLST, E. VON (1953). Relations between the central nervous system and the peripheral organs. *Brit. J. Animal Behaviour*, **2**, 89–94.
HOLST, E. VON and MITTELSTAEDT, H. (1950). *Naturwiss.*, **37**, 464–476.

389. HOLT, E. B. (1903). Eye movement and central anaesthesia. *Harvard Psychol. Studies*, **1**, 3–45.

391. HORN, G. (1965). Electrical activity of cerebral cortex of unanaesthetised cats during attentive behaviour. *Brain*, **83**, 57–76.

392. HORN, G. (1965). Physiological and psychological aspects of selective perception. In Lehrman and Hinde (Eds.) 'Advances in Animal Behaviour', Vol. I. Shaw Academic Press, London, pp. 155–215.

393. HORN, G. and BLUNDELL, J. (1959). Evoked potentials in the unanaesthetised cat. *Nature*, **184**, 173–174.

393a. HORVATH, R. S. (1970). Variability of cortical auditory evoked response. *J. Neurophysiol.*, **32**, 1056–1063.

394. HRBEK, A. and MARES, P. (1964). Cortical evoked responses to visual stimulation in full-term and premature newborns. *Electroenceph. clin. Neurophysiol.*, **16**, 575–581.

395. HRBEK, A., VITOVA, Z. and MARES, P. (1966). Optic evoked potentials in children, using different stimulation frequencies. *Physiol. Bohemoslov.*, **15**, 201–204.

396. HRBEK, A., VITOVA, Z. and MARES, P. (1966). The development of cortical evoked responses to visual stimulation during childhood. *Activas nervosa superior*, **8**, 39–46.

397. HRBEK, A., HRBKOVA, M. and LENARD, H. G. (1968). Somato-sensory evoked responses in newborn infants. *Electroenceph. clin. Neurophysiol.*, **25**, 443–448.

398. HRBEK, A., HRBKOVA, M. and LENARD, H. G. (1969). Somatosensory, auditory and visual evoked responses in newborn infants during sleep and wakefulness. *Electroenceph. clin. Neurophysiol.*, **26**, 597–603.

399. HUBEL, D. H. and WIESEL, T. N. (1962). Receptive fields, binocular interaction and functional architecture in the cat's visual cortex. *J. Physiol.*, **160**, 106–154.
HUBEL, D. H. and WIESEL, T. N. (1963). Receptive fields of cells in striate cortex of very young, visually inexperienced kittens. *J. Neurophysiol.*, **26**, 994–1002.
HUBEL, D. H. and WIESEL, T. N. (1965). Receptive fields and functional architecture in two non-striate visual areas (18 and 19) of the cat. *J. Neurophysiol.*, **28**, 229–289.

400. HUBEL, D. H. and WIESEL, T. N. (1967). Cortical and callosal connections concerned with the vertical meridian of visual fields in the cat. *J. Neurophysiol.*, **30**, 1561–1573.
HUBEL, D. H. and WIESEL, T. N. (1968). Receptive fields and functional architecture of monkey striate cortex. *J. Physiol.*, **195**, 215–243.

401. HUBEL, D. H. and WIESEL, T. N. (1970). Stereoscopic vision in the macaque monkey. *Nature* (London), **225**, 41–42.

402. HUMPHREY, N. K. and WEISKRANTZ, L. (1967). Vision in monkeys after removal of the striate cortex. *Nature* (London), **215**, 595–597.

403. INGLE, D. (1967/68). Two visual mechanisms underlying the behaviour of fish. SCHNEIDER, G. E. Contrasting visuomotor functions of tectum and cortex in the golden hamster. TEVARTHEN, C. B. Two mechanisms of vision in primates. HELD, R. Dissociation of visual functions by deprivation and rearrangement. Locating and Identifying: Two modes of visual processing. *Psychologische Forshung*, **31**, 1 and 4.

404. IRWIN, D. A., KNOTT, J. R., MCADAM, D. W. and REBERT, C. S. (1966). Motivational determinants of the 'contingent negative variation'. *Electroenceph. clin. Neurophysiol.*, **21**, 538–543.

405. IRWIN, D. A., REBERT, C. S., MCADAM, D. W. and KNOTT, J. R. (1966). Slow potential changes (CNV) in the human EEG as a function mof otivational variables. *Electroenceph. clin. Neurophysiol.*, **21**, 412–413.

406. IVES, H. E. (1922). Critical frequency relations in scotopic vision. *J. Opt. Soc. Amer.*, **6**, 254–268.

407. JACOBSON, J. H. and HIROSE, T. (1968). ERG and VER studies of children with poor vision. Paper presented to 73rd Ann. Session of Amer. Acad. Ophthal. and Otol., Chicago.

408. JACOBSON, J. H., HIROSE, T. and SUZUKI, T. A. (1968). Simultaneous ERG and VER in lesions of the optic pathway. *Investigative Ophthal.*, **6**, 279–292.

409. JANE, J. A., SMIRNOV, G. D. and JASPER, H. H. (1962). Effect of distraction upon simultaneous auditory and visual evoked potentials. *Electroenceph. clin. Neurophysiol.*, **14**, 344–358.

410. JASPER, H., LENDE, R. and RASMUSSEN, T. (1960). Evoked potentials from the exposed somato-sensory cortex in man. *Nerv. Ment. Dis.*, **130**, 526–537.

411. JEFFREYS, D. A. (1968). A magnetic recording method of averaging evoked biological potentials. Thesis, University of London.

412. JEFFREYS, D. A. (1969). In MacKay (Ed.) Evoked potentials as indicators of sensory information processing. *Neurosciences Res. Prog. Bull.*, **7**.

413. JEFFREYS, D. A. (1971). Cortical source locations of pattern-related VEPs (visual evoked potentials) recorded from the human scalp. *Nature*, **229**, 502–504.

414. JEFFREYS, D. A. (1971). Source locations of pattern appearance EPs. In preparation.

415. JEFFREYS, D. A. Personal communication.

416. JEFFREYS, D. A. and MACKAY, D. M. (1965). Aperiodic stimulus presentation with a closed-loop magnetic tape averaging system. *Electroenceph. clin. Neurophysiol.*, **19**, 404–406.

417. JENKINS, F. A. and WHITE, H. E. (1957). 'Fundamentals of Optics', McGraw-Hill, New York, p. 637.

418. JOHN, E. R. (1967). 'Mechanisms of Memory', Academic Press, New York, pp. 468.

419. JOHN, E. R., RUCHKIN, D. S. and VILLEGAS, J. (1963). Signal analysis of evoked potentials recorded from cats during conditioning. *Science*, **141**, 429–431.

420. JOHN, E. R., RUCHKIN, D. S. and VILLEGAS, J. (1964). Experimental background: signal analysis and behavioural correlates of evoked potential configurations in cats. *Ann. N.Y. Acad. Sci.*, **112**, 362–420.

421. JOHN, E. R., RUCHKIN, D. S., LEIMAN, A., SACHS, E. and AHN, H. (1965). Electrophysiological studies of generalisation using both peripheral and central conditioned stimuli. Proc. 23rd Int. Congr. Physiol. Sci., Tokyo; *Excepta Med. Int. Cong. Ser.*, **87**.

422. JOHN, E. R., HERRINGTON, R. N. and SUTTON, S. (1967). Effects of visual form on the evoked response. *Science*, **155**, 1439–1442.

423. JOHN, E. R. and RUCHKIN, D. S. (1967). Averaged evoked responses and learning. *Science*, **158**, 395.

424. JOHN, E. R. and MORGADES, P. P. (1969). The pattern and anatomical distribution of evoked potentials and multiple unit activity elicited by conditioned stimuli in trained cats. *Communications in Behavioural Biol.*, **A3**, 181–207.

425. JOHN, E. R. and MORGADES, P. P. (1969). Neural correlates of conditioned responses studied with multiple chronically implanted moving microelectrodes. *Exp. Neurol.*, **23**, 412–425.

426. JOHN, E. R., SHIMOKOCHI, M. and BARTLETT, F. (1969). Neural readout from memory during generalisation. *Science*, **164**, 1519–1521.

427. JONES, R. T. and CALLAWAY, E. (1969). Auditory evoked responses in schizophrenia – a reassessment. Paper presented to Society of Biological Psychiatry, Miami.

428. JONES, R. T., BLACKER, K. H. and CALLAWAY, E. (1966). Perceptual dysfunction in schizophrenia: clinical and auditory evoked response findings. *Amer. J. Psychiat.*, **123**, 639–645.

429. JONES, R. T., BLACKER, K. H., CALLAWAY, E. and LAYNE, R. S. (1969). The auditory evoked response as a diagnostic and prognostic measure in schizophrenia. *Amer. J. Psychiat.*, **122**, 33–41.

430. JONKMAN, E. J. (1967). The average cortical response to photic stimulation. Thesis, University of Amsterdam.

431. JOUVET, M. and COURJON, J. (1958). Variation of the subcortical visual response during attention in man. *Electroenceph. clin. Neurophysiol.*, **10**, 344.

432. JULESZ, B. (1960). Binocular depth perception of computer generated patterns. *Bell System Tech. J.*, **32**, 1125–1162.
JULESZ, B. (1965). Texture and visual perception. *Sci. Amer.*, **212**, 38–48.
433. JULESZ, B. Personal communication.
434. JUNG, R. (1963). Hirnpotentialwellen, Neuronentladungen und Gleichspannungs-phänomene. In Jenenser EEG-Symposium 30 Jahre Electroenzephalographie, VEB Verlag Volk und Gesundheit, Berlin, 54–81.
435. KAMP, A. (1960). Frequency analysis of the EEG. In Smyth, C. N. (Ed.) 'Medical Electronics', Iliffe, London, p. 128–131.
GOLDSTEIN, M. H. and NICOTRA, L. (1961). Spectral analyser for EEG. *Electroenceph. clin. Neurophysiol.*, **13**, 475–477.
BEKKERING, D., KAMP, A. and STORM VAN LEEUWEN, W. (1958). The EEG-spectrograph. *Electroenceph. clin. Neurophysiol.*, **10**, 555–559.
436. KAMP, A., SEM-JACOBSEN, C. W., STORM VAN LEEUWEN, W. and TWEEL, L. H. VAN DER (1960). Cortical responses to modulated light in the human subject. *Acta Physiol. Scand.*, **48**, 1–12.
437. KAMP, A., STORM VAN LEEUWEN, W. and TIELEN, A. M. (1965). A method for auto- and cross-correlation analysis of the EEG. *Electroenceph. clin. Neurophysiol.*, **19**, 91–95.
439. KAMPHUISEN, H. A. C. (1969). Average EEG response to sinusoidally modulated light in normal subjects and patients. Thesis, University of Utrecht, The Netherlands.
440. KAMPHUISEN, H. A. C. (1969). Average EEG response to sinusoidally modulated light (SML) in normal subjects and patients. EEG Conference, San Diego.
441. KANT, I. (1781). 'Critique of Pure Reason', Dent, London (1956), p. 483. Cassirer, H. W. (1954). 'Kant's First Critique', Allen & Unwin, London, p. 367. Bennet, J. (1966). 'Kant's Analytic', Cambridge University Press, p. 251.
442. KATZ, B. (1966). 'Nerve, Muscle, and Synapse', McGraw-Hill, New York.
443. KAUFMAN, L., PITBLADO, C. and MILLER, J. F., JR. (1965). Perceptual phenomena and evoked cortical potentials resulting from binocular stimulation with flickering light. Sperry Rand Research Report SRRC-RR, 65–101.
444. KAWASAKI, K., HIROSE, T., JACOBSON, J. H. and CORDELLA, M. (1970). Binocular fusion: Effect of breaking on the human visual evoked response. *Archiv. Ophthal.*, **84**, 25–28.
445. KEIDEL, W. D. (1963). Tuning between central auditory pathways and the ear. *IEEE Trans. on Military Electronics*, **MIL–7**, 131–143.
446. KEIDEL, W. D. (1965). Neuere Ergebnisse der Physiologie des Hörens. *Archiv. klin. exper. Ohren-, Nasen- und Kehlkopfheilk.*, **185**, 548–575.
447. KEIDEL, W. D. (1965). On the neurophysiological exponents of Steven's power functions electronically computed in man. 6th Int. Conf. Med. Electron. Biol. Eng., Tokyo.
448. KEIDEL, W. D. (1969). Informations physiologische Aspekte des Hörens. *Studium Generale*, **22**, 49–82.
449. KEIDEL, W. D. and SPRENG, M. (1965). Audiometric aspects and multisensory power functions of electronically averaged evoked cortical responses in man. *Acta Oto-laryng., Stockl.*, **59**, 201–208.
450. KEIDEL, W. D. and SPRENG, M. (1965). Computed audioencephalograms in man. (A technique of 'objective' audiometry.) *Internat. Audiol.*, **4**, 56–60.
451. KEIDEL, W. D. and SPRENG, M. (1965). Neurophysiological evidence for the Steven's power function in man. *J. Acoust. Soc. Amer.*, **38**, 191–195.

452. KEIDEL, W. D. and SPRENG, M. (1970). Recent status results and problems of objective audiometry in man. Parts I and II. J.F.O.R.L., XIX, No. 1.

453. KELLY, D. H. (1961). Visual signal generator. *Rev. Sci. Instr.*, **32**, 50–55.

454. KELLY, D. L., JR., GOLDRING, S. and OLEARY, J. L. (1965). Averaged evoked somatosensory responses from exposed cortex in man. *Arch. Neurol.*, **13**, 1–9.

454a. KELSEY, J. H. (1969). Electrophysiological tests of visual function. *Int. Ophthal. Clinics*, **9**(4), 883–898.

455. KENDALL, M. G. and STUART, A. (1958). 'The Advanced Theory of Statistics', Vols. I, II and III, Griffin, London.

456. KINGSLAKE, R. (Ed.) (1967). 'Applied Optics and Optical Engineering', Academic Press, New York.

457. KLIVINGTON, K. A. and GALAMBOS, R. (1967). Resistance shifts accompanying the evoked cortical response in the cat. *Science*, **157**, 211–213.

458. KLEE, M. R., OFFENLOCK, K. and TIGGES, J. (1965). Cross-correlation analysis of electroencephalic potentials and slow membrane transients. *Science*, **147**, 519.

459. KNOTT, J. R. and IRWIN, D. A. (1967). Anxiety, stress and the CNV. *Electroenceph. clin. Neurophysiol.*, **22**, 188.

460. KNOX, G. W. (1945). Investigations of flicker and fusion. IV. The effect of auditory flicker on the pronouncedness of visual flicker. *J. Gen. Psychol.*, **33**, 145–154.

SHIPLEY, T. (1964). Auditory flutter-driving of visual flicker. *Science*, **145**, 1328–1330.

461a. *Kodak Wratten Filters*, Kodak, London, p. 112.

KOELLA, W. P. and WELLS, C. H. (1963). Influence of a plasma protein fraction from schizophrenic patients upon the optic evoked response in the rabbit. *J. Neuropsychiat.*, **4**, 219–223.

461b. KÖHLER, W., HELD, R. and O'CONNEL, D. N. (1952). An investigation of cortical currents. *Proc. Amer. Phil. Soc.*, **96**, 290–330.

462. KOLMAN, I. and SHIMIZU, H. (1969). Recovery from aphasia as monitored by AER audiometry – a case report. Paper presented at 45th Annual Convention of American Speech and Hearing Assoc., Chicago.

463. KOOI, K. A. and BAGCHI, B. K. (1964). Visual evoked responses in man: normative data. *Ann. N.Y. Acad. Sci.*, **112**, 254–269.

464. KOOI, K. A., GUEVENER, A. M. and BAGCHI, B. K. (1965). Visual evoked responses in lesions of the higher optic pathways. *Neurology*, **15**, 841.

465. KOOI, K. A. and SHARBROUGH, F. W. (1966). Electrophysiological findings in cortical blindness. Report of a case. *Electroenceph. clin. Neurophysiol.*, **20**, 260–263.

466. KORN, G. A. (1966). 'Random Process Simulation and Measurements', McGraw-Hill.

466b. KORNHUBER, H. H. and DEECKE, L. (1964). Hirnpotential-änderungen beim Menschen vor und nach Willkürbewegungen, dargestellt mit Magnetband-speicherung und Rückwärtsanalyse. *Pflügers Archiv.*, **281**.

KORNHUBER, H. H. Personal communication.

468. KORNHUBER, H. H. and DEECKE, L. (1965). Hirnpotential-änderungen bei Willkürbewegungen und passivess Beuregungen des Menschen: Bereitschaftspotential und reafferente Potentiale. *Pflügers Archiv.*, **284**, 1–17.

469. KOZHEVNIKOV, V. A. (1958). Photoelectric method for the separation of weak electrical responses in the brain. *Fiziol. Z.* (*Mosk.*), **44**, 801–909.

470. KRAUSKOPF, J., GRAF, U. and GAARDER, K. (1966). Lack of inhibition during involuntary saccades. *Amer. J. Psychol.*, **79**, 73–81.

471. KREKULE, I. (1968). Zero crossing detection of the presence of evoked responses. *Electroenceph. clin. Neurophysiol.*, **25**, 175–176.

472. KUHNT, U. (1967). Visuell reaktionspotentiale an menschen und katzen in abhängigkeit von der intensität. *Pflügers Archiv.*, **298**, 82–104.

473. KURTZBURG, D. and VAUGHAN, H. G., JR. (1971). Electrocortical potentials associated with eye movement. In press.

474. LANSING, R. W. (1964). Electroencephalic correlates of binocular rivalry in man. *Science*, **146**, 1325–1327.

475. LARSON, S. J., SANCES, A. and CHRISTENSON, P. C. (1966). Evoked somatosensory potentials in man. *Arch. Neurol.*, **15**, 88–91.

476. LARSON, S. J. and SANCES, A., JR. (1968). The specific somatosensory system and dyskinesia. *Arch. Neurol.*, **18**, 543–548.

477. LASHLEY, K. S. (1942). The problem of cerebral organization in vision. *Biol. Symp.*, **7**, 301–322.

478. LATOUR, P. L. (1962). Visual threshold during eye movements. *Vision Res.*, **2**, 261–262.

479. LATOUR, P. L. (1966). Cortical control of eye movements. Institute for Perception RVO–TNO, Soesterberg, The Netherlands, pp. 93.

480. LEE, Y. W. (1950). Application of statistical methods to communication problems. Tech. Rep. 181. Res. Lab. Electron., M.I.T.

481. LEE, Y. W. (1963). 'Statistical Theory of Communication', Wiley, New York.

482. LEE, Y. W., CHEATHAM, T. P. and WIESNER, J. B. (1950). Application of correlation analysis to the detection of periodic signals in noise. *Proc. IRE*, **38**, 1165–1171.

483. LEE, Y. W. and SCHETZEN, M. (1961). Measurement of the kernels of a nonlinear system by cross correlation. *Quart. Prog. Rep. M.I.T.*, **60**, 118–130.

484. LEHMANN, D. (1971). Multichannel studies of the electrical fields of visually evoked EEG potentials in humans. Excerpta, Med. Intern. Congress Series. In press.

485. LEHMANN, D., BEELER, G. W. and FENDER, D. H. (1965). Changes in patterns of the human electroencephalogram during fluctuations of perception of stabilised retinal images. *Electroenceph. clin. Neurophysiol.*, **19**, 336–343.

486. LEHMANN, D., BEELER, G. W., JR. and FENDER, D. H. (1967). EEG responses to light flashes during the observation of stabilised and normal retinal images. *Electroenceph. clin. Neurophysiol.*, **22**, 136–142.

487. LEHMANN, D. and FENDER, D. H. (1967). Monocularly evoked electroencephalogram potentials: influence of target structure presented to the other eye. *Nature*, **215**, 204–205.

488. LEHMANN, D., KAVANAGH, R. N. and FENDER, D. H. (1969). Field studies of averaged visually evoked potentials in a patient with a split chiasm. *Electroenceph. clin. Neurophysiol.*, **26**, 193–199.

489. LETTVIN, J. Y., MATURANA, H. R., MCCULLOCH, W. S. and PITTS, W. H. (1959). What the frog's eye tells the frog's brain. *Proc. IRE*, **47**, 1940–1951.

490. LEVY, R. and BEHRMAN, J. (1970). Cortical evoked responses in hysterical hemianaesthesia. *Electroenceph. clin. Neurophysiol.*, **29**, 400–402.

491. LI, C.-L. (1963). Cortical intracellular potentials in response to thalamic stimulation. *J. Cell. Comp. Physiol.*, **61**, 165.

492. LI, C.-L., MCLENE, H. and JASPER, H. H. (1952). Brain waves and unit discharges in cerebral cortex. *Science*, **116**, 656–657.

493. LI, C.-L. and JASPER, H. (1953). Microelectrode studies of the electrical activity of the cerebral cortex in the cat. *J. Physiol.*, **121**, 117.

494. LIBERSON, W. T. (1966). Study of evoked potentials in aphasics. *Amer. J. Phys. Med.*, **45**, 135–142.

495. LIBET, B., ALBERTS, W. W., WRIGHT, E. W., JR. and FEINSTEIN, B. (1967). Responses of human somatosensory cortex to stimuli below threshold for conscious sensation. *Science*, **158**, 1597–1600.

496. LIFSHITZ, K. (1968). An analysis of information handling indicated by the AER in normal and schizophrenic subjects. Presented at the 124th Annual Meeting of the American Psychiatric Association.

497. LIFSHITZ, K. (1969). An examination of evoked potentials as indicators of information processing in normal and schizophrenic subjects. In 'Average Evoked Potentials', Methods, Results, Evaluations, Donchin, E. and Lindsley, D. B. (Eds.). NASA SP–191.

498. LIFSHITZ, K. (1969). Discussion of Callaway's paper. In 'Average Evoked Potentials', Donchin, E. and Lindsley, D. B. (Eds.). NASA SP–191, pp. 318–319.

499. LIFSHITZ, K. and KLEMM, K. (1964). Cortical evoked potentials to meaningful visual stimuli. Paper presented to American Psychiatric Assoc., Los Angeles.

500. LIPPOLD, O. C. J. (1970). Bilateral separation in alpha rhythm recording. *Nature*, **226**, 459–460.

501. LIPPOLD, O. C. J. (1970). Origin of the alpha rhythm. *Nature*, **226**, 616–618.

502. LIPPOLD, O. C. J. and NOVOTNY, G. E. K. (1968). Tremor of the extraocular muscles as the generator of alpha rhythm: cooling the orbit in man. *J. Physiol.*, **194**, 28P.

503. LODGE, A., ARMINGTON, J. C., BARNET, A. B., SHANKS, B. L. and NEWCOMB, C. N. (1969). Newborn infants' electroretinograms and evoked electroencephalographic responses to orange and white light. *Child Development*, **40**, 267–293.

504. LOMBROSO, C. T. (1969). Comment on Cohen's paper. In 'Average Evoked Potentials', Donchin, E. and Lindsley, D. B. (Eds.). NASA SP–191, pp. 171–177.

505. LOOMIS, A. L., HARVERY, N. and HOBART, G. A. (1938). Distribution of disturbance – patterns in the human electroencephalogram, with special reference to sleep. *J. Neurophysiol.*, **1**, 413–430.

506. LOPES DA SILVA, F. H. (1970). Dynamic characteristics of visual evoked potentials. Thesis, University of Utrecht.

507. LOPES DA SILVA, F. H., ROTTERDAM, A. VAN, STORM VAN LEEUWEN, W. and TIELEN, A. M. (1970). Dynamic characteristics of visual EPs in the dog. I. Cortical and subcortical potentials evoked by sine wave modulated light. *Electroenceph. clin. Neurophysiol.*, **29**, 246–259.

508. LOPES DA SILVA, F. H., ROTTERDAM, A. VAN and LANG, P. A. DE (1970). A non-linear model of cortical subharmonic responses to stimulation with sine wave modulated light. Prog. Rep. 2, Institute Med. Physics, Utrecht, The Netherlands.

509. LOW, M. D. (1969). Comment on Cohen's paper. In 'Average Evoked Potentials', Donchin, E. and Lindsley, D. B. (Eds.). NASA SP–191, pp. 163–171.

510. LOW, M. D., COATS, A. C., RETTIG, G. M. and MCSHERRY, J. W. (1967). Anxiety attentiveness – altertness: a phenomenological study of the CNV. *Neuropsychologica*, **5**, 379–384.

511. LÜCKING, C. H., CREUTZFELDT, O. D. and HEINEMANN, U. (1970). Visual evoked potentials of patients with epilepsy and of a control group. *Electroenceph. clin. Neurophysiol.* In press.

512. LUX, H. D. and KLEE, M. R. (1962). Intrazelluläre Untersuchugen über den Einfluss hemmender Potentiale in motorischen cortex. *Arch. Psychiat. Nervenkr.*, **203**, 648–666.

513. MAGNUS, O. and PONSEN, L. (1965). The influence of the phase of the alpha rhythm on the cortical evoked response to photic stimulation. *Electroenceph. clin. Neurophysiol.*, **18**, 427–428.

514. MARSHALL, W. H. and TALBOT, S. A. (1942). Recent evidence for neural mechanisms in vision leading to a general theory of sensory acuity. *Biol. Symp.*, **7**, 117–164.

515. MARTIN, J. I. (1970). Effects of binocular fusion and binocular rivalry on cortically evoked potentials. *Electroenceph. clin. Neurophysiol.*, **28**, 190–201.
516. MARTIN, L. C. (1950). 'Technical Optics', Vol. 2, Pitman, London, pp. 344.
517. MATSUMIYA, Y., GENNARELLI, T. A. and LOMBROSO, C. T. Somatosensory evoked response in the hemispherectomized man. *Electroenceph. clin. Neurophysiol.* In press.
518. MATTHEWS, B. H. C. (1931). The response of a single end organ. *J. Physiol.*, **71**, 64–110.
519. MCADAM, D., IRWIN, D. A., REBERT, C. S. and KNOTT, J. R. (1966). Conative control of the contingent negative variation. *Electroenceph. clin. Neurophysiol.*, **21**, 194–195.
520. MCADAM, D., KNOTT, J. R. and REBERT, C. S. (1969). Cortical slow potential change in man related to interstimulus interval and to pre-trial prediction of interstimulus interval. *Psychophysiology*, **5**, 349–358.
521. MCADAM, D. W. and SEALES, D. M. (1969). Bereitschaftspotential enhancement with increased levels of motivation. *Electroenceph. clin. Neurophysiol.*, **27**, 73–75.
522. MCCALLUM, W. C. and WALTER, W. G. (1968). The effects of attention and distraction on the contingent negative variation in normal and neurotic subjects. *Electroenceph. clin. Neurophysiol.*, **25**, 319–329.
523. MCCREE, K. J. (1960). Colour confusion produced by voluntary fixation. *Optica Acta*, **7**, 281–290.
RIGGS, L. A., RATLIFF, F., COMSWEET, J. C. and COMSWEET, T. N. (1953). The disappearance of steadily fixated visual test objects. *J. Opt. Soc. Amer.*, **43**, 495–501.
DITCHBURN, R. W. and GINSBORG, B. (1952). Vision with a stabilized retinal image. *Nature*, **170**, 36–37.
524. MCDONALD, H. S. (1960). Note on the use of glow modulator lamps for studies of vision. *J. Opt. Soc. Amer.*, **50**, 1138.
525. MCGEE, F. E., LEE, R. G., HARRIS, J. A., MELBY, G. and BICKFORD, R. G. (1969). Applications of interpolation and area display in EEG. *Electroenceph. clin. Neurophysiol.*, **27**, 546.
526. MACDOUGALL, W. (1904). The sensations excited by a single momentary stimulation of the eye. *Brit. J. Psychol.*, **1**, 78–113.
527. MACKAY, D. M. (1956). Towards an information-flow model of human behaviour. *Brit. J. Psychol.*, **47**, 30–43.
528. MACKAY, D. M. (1961). Interactive process in visual perception. In Rosenblith, W. A. (Ed.) 'Sensory Communication', M.I.T. Press.
529. MACKAY, D. M. (1963). Psychophysics of perceived intensity: a theoretical basis for Fechner's and Steven's Laws. *Science*, **139**, 1213–1216.
530. MACKAY, D. M. (1965). A mind's eye view of the brain. In Wiener, N. and Schadé, J. P. (Eds.) 'Progress in Brain Research', Elsevier, pp. 321–332.
531. MACKAY, D. M. (1965). Visual noise as a tool of research. *J. Gen. Psychol.*, **72**, 181–197.
532. MACKAY, D. M. (1966). Cerebral organization and the conscious control of action. In Eccles, J. C. (Ed.) 'Brain and Conscious Experience', Springer, New York, pp. 422–445.
533. MACKAY, D. M. (1967). Ways of looking at perception. In Weiant Walten-Dunn (Ed.) 'Models for the Perception of Speech and Visual Form', M.I.T. Press, Boston, pp. 25–43.
534. MACKAY, D. M. (1968). Evoked potentials reflecting interocular and monocular suppression. *Nature*, **217**, 81–83.
535. MACKAY, D. M. (1968). Neural communications: experiment and theory. *Science*, **159**, 335–353.

536. MACKAY, D. M. (Ed.) (1969). Evoked brain potentials as indicators of sensory information processing. *Neurosciences Res. Prog. Bull.*, **7**, 3.

537. MACKAY, D. M. (1970). The human touch. In 'Proc. of D.G.K. Symposium', Springer, Berlin.

538. MACKAY, D. M. (1970). Elevation of visual threshold by displacement of the retinal image. *Nature*, **225**, 90–92.

539. MACKAY, D. M. and JEFFREYS, D. A. (1960). Continuous averaging system using magnetic tape. Proc. 3rd Internat. Conf. Med. Electron.

540. MACKAY, D. M., JEFFREYS, D. A. and GLOVER, R. R. New methods of analysis of electrophysiological responses. USAF Res. Rep. AF61 (052) - 364 (1962) and AF EOAR 23–62 (1963).

541. MACKAY, D. M. and FIORENTINI, A. (1966). Evoked potentials correlated with a visual anomaly. *Nature*, **209**, 787–789.

542. MACKAY, D. M. and RIETVELD, W. J. (1968). Electroencephalogram potentials evoked by accelerated visual motion. *Nature*, **217**, 677–678.

543. MACKAY, D. M. and JEFFREYS, D. A. (1971). Visual evoked potentials and visual perception in man. In 'Central Processing of Visual Information', Handbook of Sensory Physiology, Springer Verlag.

544. MERGENHAGEN, D., CREUTZFELDT, O. D. and NEUWEILER, G. (1968). Beziehungen zwischen Aktivität corticaler neurone und EEG – wellen in motorischen cortex der Katze bei hypoglykämie. *Archiv. für Psychiatrie*, **211**, 43–62.

545. MÉZAN, I., LESÈVRE, N. and RÉMOND, A. (1968). Étude chrono-topographique de la réponse somesthésique évoquée moyen recueillie sur le scalp par stimulation électrique du nerf médian. *Rev. Neurol.*, **119**, 288–295.

546. MICHAEL, J. A. and STARK, L. (1967). Electrophysiological correlates of saccadic suppression. *Exp. Neurol.*, **17**, 233–246.

547. MILNER, B. A. (1970). The Physical Study of Bioelectric Potentials Generated in Response to Auditory Stimuli. Ph.D. Thesis, University of London.

547a. MILNER, B. A., REGAN, D. and HERON, J. R. (1971). Theoretical models of the generation of steady state evoked potentials, their relation to neuroanatomy and their relevance to certain clinical problems. 9th Internat. ISCERG Symposium, Brighton. *Vision Res.*, **11**, 1203–1204.

548. MILSUM, J. H. (1969). The role of unidirectional rate sensitivity in biological control systems stabilization. *Ann. N.Y. Acad. Sci.*, **156**, 731–739.

549. MINORSKY, N. (1962). 'Non-Linear Oscillation', D. van Nostrand Co., New York.

550. MONTAGUE, J. D. (1966). The application of electro-luminescence to photic stimulation. *Electroenceph. clin. Neurophysiol.*, **21**, 393–395.

551. MOORE, G. P., PERKEL, D. H. and SEGUNDO, J. P. (1966). Statistical analysis and functional interpretation of neuronal spike data. *Ann. Rev. Physiol.*, **28**, 493–522.

552. MOROCUTTI, C., SOMMER-SMITH, J. A. and CREUTZFELDT, O. D. (1964). Studio dei potenziali evocati visivi in soggetti mormali ed in soggetti affetti da malattie cerebrali. *Riv. Neurol.*, **34**, 57–71.

553. MOROCUTTI, C. and SOMMER-SMITH, J. A. (1966). Étude des potentiels évoqués visuels dans l'epilepsie. *Rev. Neurol. (Paris)*, **115**, 93–98.

554. MOROCUTTI, C., SOMMER-SMITH, J. A. and CREUTZFELDT, O. D. (1966). Das visuelle Reaktionspotential bei normalen Versuchspersonen und characteristische Veränderungen bei Epileptikern. *Archiv. für Psychiatrie und Zeitschrift f.g. Neurol.*, **208**, 234–254.

555. MORRELL, F. and MORRELL, L. (1965). Computer aided analyses of brain electrical activity. In Proctor, L. D. and Adey, W. R. (Eds.) 'The Analysis of Central Nervous System and Cardiovascular Data Using Computer Methods', NASA, Washington, pp. 441–478.

556. MORRELL, L. K. and MORRELL, F. (1966). Evoked potentials and reaction times: a study of intra-individual variability. *Electroenceph. clin. Neurophysiol.*, **20**, 567–575.

557. MORRISON, R. (1967). 'Grounding and Shielding Techniques in Instrumentation', Wiley, pp. 150.

558. MOUNTCASTLE, V. B. (Ed.) (1967). 'Interhemispheric Relations and Cerebral Dominance', Johns Hopkins Press, Baltimore, pp. 294.

559. MULHOLLAND, T. and EVANS, C. R. (1965). An unexpected artifact in the human electroencephalogram concerning the alpha rhythm and the orientation of the eyes. *Nature*, **207**, 36–37.

560. MULHOLLAND, T. and EVANS, C. R. (1966). Oculomotor function and the alpha activation cycle. *Nature*, **211**, 1278–1279.

561. NÄÄTÄNEN, R. (1967). Selective attention and evoked potentials. Thesis, University of Helsinki, Finland.

562. NÄÄTÄNEN, R. (1969). Anticipation of relevant stimuli and evoked potentials: a comment on Donchin's and Cohen's 'Averaged Evoked Potentials and Intramodality Selective Attention'. *Percept. Mot. Skills*, **28**, 639–646.

DONCHIN, E. and COHEN, L. (1969). Anticipation of relevant stimuli and evoked potentials: a reply to Näätänen. *Percept. Mot. Skills*, **29**, 115–117.

NÄÄTÄNEN, R. (1969). Anticipation of relevant stimuli and evoked potentials: a reply to Donchin and Cohen. *Percept. Mot. Skills*, **29**, 233–234.

DONCHIN, E. and COHEN, L. (1969). Further reply to Näätänen. *Percept. Mot. Skills*, **29**, 270.

563. NÄÄTÄNEN, R. (1970). Evoked potential, EEG, and slow potential correlates of selective attention. *Acta Psychologica*, **33**, 178–192.

564. NAGATA, M. and JACOBSON, J. H. (1966). Combined ERG and occipital response recording. *Clinical Electroretinography*, *Vision Res. Suppl.*, 249–255.

BALEN, A. T. M. VAN and HENKES, H. E. (1962). Attention and amblyopia. *Brit. J. Ophthal.*, **46**, 12–20.

565. NAMEROW, N. S. (1968). Somatosensory evoked potentials in multiple sclerosis patients with varying sensory loss. *Neurology*, **18**, 1197–1204.

566. NAMEROW, N. S. (1968). Somatosensory evoked potentials in multiple sclerosis. *Bull. Los Angeles Neurol. Soc.*, **33**, 74.

567. NAMEROW, N. S. (1969). Somatosensory evoked responses following cervical cordotomy. *Bull. Los Angeles Neurol. Soc.*, **34**, 184–188.

568. NAMEROW, N. S. (1970). Somatosensory recovery functions in multiple sclerosis patients. *Neurology* (*Minn.*), **20**, 813–817.

569. NAQUET, R., LANOIR, J., BACH-Y-RITA, G., SAIER, J. and RHODES, J. M. (1967). Induction par les mouvements oculaires de réponses évoquées dans les voies visuelles. In Ruttkay-Nedecky, I. *et al.* (Eds.) 'Mechanism of Orienting Reaction in Man', Publishing House of Slovak Academy of Sciences, Bratislava, pp. 101–113.

570. NARABAYASHI, H. Functional differentiation in and around the ventrolateral nucleus of the thalamus based on experience in human stereoencephalotomy. *John Hopkins Med. J.*, **122**, 295–300.

571. NARABAYASHI, H., NAGAOT, T., SAITO, Y., YOSHINDA, M. and NAGAHATA, M. (1963). Stereotaxic amygdalotomy for behaviour disorders. *Arch. Neurol.*, **9**, 1–16.

572. NAWRATZKI, I., AVERBACH, E. and ROWE, H. (1966). Amblyopia ex anopsia: the electrical response in retina and occipital cortex following photic stimulation of normal and amblyopic eyes. *Amer. J. Ophthal.*, **61**, 430–435.

573. NAWRATZKI, I., LANDAU, L. and AVERBACH, E. (1969). Belated visual maturation in a mentally retarded child. *J. Pediat. Ophthal.*, **6**, 39–41.

575. NICHOLSON, P. W. (1965). Specific impedance of cerebral white matter. *Exptl. Neurol.*, **13**, 386–401.

576. 'A note on the use of glow modulator lamp for studies of vision'. Memorandum, Bell Labs. (19 October 1960).

577. OESTERBERG, T. (1935). Topography of the layer of rods and cones in the human retina. *Acta Ophthal., Suppl.*, **6**, 1–102.

578. OFFENTLOCH, K. Personal communication.

579. OFFNER, F. F. (1950). The EEG as potential mapping: the value of the average monopolar reference. *Electroenceph. clin. Neurophysiol.*, **2**, 215.

580. OHBA, N. (1967). Visual evoked responses in man by localized retinal stimulation. *Jap. J. Ophthal.*, **11**, 221–226.

581. OHYE, C., KUBOTA, K., HONGO, T., NAGAO, T. and NARABAYASHI, H. (1964) Ventrolateral and subventrolateral thalamic stimulation. *Arch. Neurol.*, **11**, 427–434.

582. OOSTERHUIS, H. J. G. H., PONSEN, L., JONKMAN, E. J. and MAGNUS, O. (1969). The average visual response in patients with cerebrovascular disease. *Electroenceph. clin. Neurophysiol.*, **27**, 23–34.

583. ORKAND, R. K., NICHOLLS, J. G. and KUFFLER, S. W. (1966). Effect of nerve impulses on the membrane potential of glial cells in the central nervous system of amphibia. *J. Neurophysiol.*, **29**, 788.

584. ORNITZ, E. M. (1969). A note on the AEP of autistic children recorded during sleep. In Donchin, E. and Lindsley, D. B. (Eds.) 'Average Evoked Potentials', NASA SP–191, pp. 355–356.

585. ORNITZ, E. M., RITVO, E. R., EVERETT, M. C., LA FRANCHI, S. and WALTER, R. D. (1967). The effect of sleep onset on the auditory averaged evoked response. *Electroenceph. clin. Neurophysiol.*, **23**, 335–341.

586. ORNITZ, E. M. and RITVO, E. R. (1968). Perceptual inconstancy in early infantile autism. The syndrome of early infantile autism and its variants including certain cases of childhood schizophrenia. *Arch. Gen. Psychiat.*, **18**, 76–98.

587. ORNITZ, E. M., RITVO, E. R., LEE, Y. H., PANMAN, L. M., WALTER, R. D. and MASON, A. (1969). The auditory evoked response in babies during REM sleep. *Electroenceph. clin. Neurophysiol.*, **27**, 195–198.

588. ORNITZ, E. M., RITVO, E. R., TANGUAY, P. E. and WALTER, R. D. (1969). EEG spikes and the averaged evoked response to clicks and flashes. *Electroenceph. clin. Neurophysiol.*, **27**, 387–391.

589. OSGOOD, C. E. (1953). 'Method and Theory in Experimental Psychology', Oxford University Press, New York, pp. 43–59.
STEVENS, S. S. (Ed.) (1951). 'Handbook of Experimental Psychology', Wiley, New York, pp. 1–50.

590. PAGNI, C. A. (1967). Somatosensory evoked potentials in thalamus and cortex of man. *Electroenceph. clin. Neurophysiol., Suppl.*, **26**, 147–155.

591. PAGNI, C. A., ETTORRE, G., MAROSSERO, F., INFUSO, L. and CASSINARI, V. (1964). Primary visual potentials in man during repetitive photic stimulation. *Experientia (Basel)*, **20**, 641–643.

592. PAICER, P. L., SANCES, A. and LARSON, S. J. (1967). Theoretical evaluation of cerebral evoked potentials. Proc. 20th ACEMB (Boston, Mass.) paper 14.1.

593. PALESTININ, M., DAVIDOVITCH, A. and HERNÁNDEZ-PEÓN, R. (1959). Functional significance of centrifugal influences upon the retina. *Acta Neurol. Latinoamer.*, **5**, 113–131.

594. PALMER, D. A. (1966). A system of mesopic photometry. *Nature*, **209**, 276–281.

595. PALMER, D. A. (1967). The definition of a standard observer for mesopic photometry. *Vision Res.*, **7**, 619–628.

596. PALMER, D. A. (1968). Standard observer for large-field photometry at any level. *J. Opt. Soc. Amer.*, **58**, 1296–1299.

597. PANOFSKY, W. K. H. and PHILLIPS, M. (1955). 'Classical Electricity and Magnetism', Addison-Wesley, Reading, Mass.

598. PASIK, P. and PASIK, T. (1968). Further studies on extrageniculostriate vision in the monkey. *Trans. Am. Neurol. Assoc.*, **93**, 262–264.

599. PATTON, H. D. (1961). Spinal reflexes and synaptic transmission. In Ruch, T. C., Patton, H. D., Woodbury, J. W. and Towe, A. L. 'Neurophysiology', W. B. Saunders, Philadelphia and London, pp. 521.

600. PEACOCK, S. M. (1970). Averaged 'after activity' and the alpha regeneration cycle. *Electroenceph. clin. Neurophysiol.*, **28**, 287–295.

601. PEREZ-BORJA, C., CHATRIAN, C. E., TICE, F. A. and RIVERS, N. H. (1962). Electrographic patterns of the occipital lobe in man. A topographic study based on the use of implanted electrodes. *Electroenceph. clin. Neurophysiol*, **14**, 171–182.

602. PENFIELD, W. and BOLDREY, E. (1937). Somatic motor and sensory representation in the cerebral cortex of man as studied by electrical stimulation. *Brain*, **60**, 389–443.

603. PERKEL, D. H. and BULLOCK, T. H. (Eds.) (1968). Neurel coding. *Neurosciences Res. Prog. Bull.*, **6** (3).

604. PERRY, N. W., JR. and CHILDERS, D. G. (1968). Cortical potentials in normal and amblyopic binocular vision. In 'Advances in electrophysiology and pathology of the visual system', Georg Thieme, Leipzig.

605. PERRY, N. W. and CHILDERS, D. G. (1969). 'The Human Visual Evoked Response', Thomas, Springfield, Illinois, p. 187.

606. PETERS, J. F., KNOTT, J. R., MILLER, L. H., VAN VEEN, W. J. and COHEN, S. I. (1970). Response variables and magnitude of the contingent negative variation. *Electroenceph. clin. Neurophysiol.*, **29**, 608–611.

607. PETTIGREW, J. D., NIKARA, T. and BISHOP, P. O. (1968). Binocular interaction on single units in cat striate cortex: simultaneous stimulation by single moving slit with receptive fields in correspondence. *Exp. Brain. Res.*, **6**, 391–410.

BARLOW, H. B., BLAKEMORE, C. and PETTIGREW, J. D. (1967). The neural mechanism of binocular depth perception. *J. Physiol.*, **193**, 327–342.

NIKARA, T., BISHOP, P. O. and PETTIGREW, J. D. (1968). Analysis of retinal correspondence by studying receptive fields of binocular single units in cat striate cortex. *Exp. Brain Res.*, **6**, 353–372.

PETTIGREW, J. D., NIKARA, T. and BISHOP, P. O. (1968). Responses to moving slits by single units in cat striate cortex. *Exp. Brain Res.*, **6**, 373–390.

608. PIÉRON, H. (1952). 'The Sensations', Mueller, London.

609. PLANE, C. (1969). Potentiels évoqués visuels chez le sujet normal et dans les atteintes du nerf optique. Thesis, University of Clermont.

610. PLATTIG, K.-H. (1968). Über den electrischen Geschmack. *Zeitschrift für Biologie*, **116**, 162–211.

611. POLYAK, S. (1957). 'The Vertebrate Visual System', University of Chicago Press, p. 1390.

612. POLYANSKII, V. B. Connection between spike discharges and evoked potentials in rabbit visual cortex.

613. POTTS, A. M. and NAGAYA, T. (1965). Studies on the visual evoked response. I. The use of a 0·06 degree red target for evaluation of foveal function. *Invest. Ophthal.*, **4**, 303–309.

614. POTTS, A. M. and NAGAYA, T. (1967). Studies on the visual evoked response. II. The effect of special cortical activity. *Invest. Ophthal.*, **6**, 657–665.

615. POTTS, A. M. and NAGAYA, T. (1969). Studies on the visual evoked response. III. Strabismus amblyopia and hysterical amblyopia. *Docum. Ophthal.*, **26**, 394–402.

616. PRITCHARD, J. W., CHIMIENTI, J. and GALAMBOS, R. (1965). Evoked responses from extracranial sites in the cat. *Electroenceph. clin. Neurophysiol.*, **18**, 493–499.
617. PURPURA, D. P. (1959). Nature of electrocortical potentials and synaptic organizations in cerebral and cerebellar cortex. In Pfeiffer, C. C. and Smythies, J. R. (Eds.), *Int. Rev. Neurobiol.*, Academic Press, New York, pp. 47–163.
618. PURPURA, D. P. and GRUNDFEST, H. (1956). *J. Neurophysiol.*, **19**, 573.
619. PURPURA, D. P. and COHEN, B. (1962). Intracellular recording from thalamic neurons during recruiting responses. *J. Neurophysiol.*, **25**, 621.
620. RALL, W. (1960). Membrane potential transients and membrane time constant of motoneurons. *Exptl. Neurol.*, **2**, 503–532.
621. RALL, W. (1967). Distinguishing theoretical synaptic potentials computed for different soma-dendritic distributions of synaptic input. *J. Neurophysiol.*, **30**, 1138–1168.
622. RALL, W. (1968). Synaptic activity at dendritic locations: theory and experiment. In Caianiello, E. R. (Ed.) 'Neural Networks', Springer Verlag, Berlin, pp. 1–5.
623. RALL, W. (1969). Distributions of potential in cylindrical coordinates and time constants for a membrane cylinder. *Biophys. J.*, **9**, 1509–1541.
624. RALL, W., Electrophysiology of a dendritic neuron model. In 'Mathematical Models of Biophysical Mechanisms'.
625. RALL, W., SHEPHERD, G. M., REESE, T. S. and BRIGHTMAN, M. W. (1966). Dendrodendritic synaptic pathway for inhibition in the olefactory bulb. *Exptl. Neurol.*, **14**, 44–56.
626. RAPIN, I., SCHIMMEL, H., TOURK, L. M., KRASNEGOR, N. A. and POLLAK, C. (1966). Evoked responses to clicks and tones of varying intensity in waking adults. *Electroenceph. clin. Neurophysiol.*, **21**, 335–344.
627. RAPIN, I. and GRAZIANI, L. J. (1967). Auditory evoked responses in normal, brain damaged and deaf infants. *Neurology* (*Minn.*), **17**, 881–894.
628. RAPIN, I., RUBEN, R. J. and LYTTLE, M. (1970). Diagnosis of hearing loss in infants using auditory evoked responses. Paper presented to Amer. Laryng. Rhin. and Otol. Soc. (Eastern), Boston.
629. RATCLIFFE, F. and RIGGS, L. A. (1950). Involuntary motions of the eye during monocular fixation. *J. Exptl. Psychol.*, **40**, 687–701.
630. RAU, R.-M. (1968). Über die Abhängigkeit der objectiv ermittelten Intensitätsfunktion des meschlichen Gehörs von der Tonfolgefrequenz. *Archiv. klin. exper. Ohren-, Nasen- und Kehlkopfheilk*, **190**, 133–145.
631. REBERT, C. S. and KNOTT, J. R. (1970). The vertex non-specific evoked potential and latency of the contingent negative variation. *Electroenceph. clin. Neurophysiol.*, **28**, 561–565.
632. REESE, T. S. (1966). Further studies on dendrodendritic synapses in the olefactory bulb. *Anat. Rec.*, **154**, 408.
633. 'A Reference Zero for the Calibration of Pure-Tone Audiometers', BS 2497 Part I; 'An Artificial Ear', BS 2042; 'Pure Tone Audiometers', BS 2980; 'Performance of Loudspeakers', BS 2498. British Standards Institution, 2 Park St., London W.1.
634. REGAN, D. (1966). Some characteristics of average steady-state and transient responses evoked by modulated light. *Electroenceph. clin. Neurophysiol.*, **20**, 238–248.
635. REGAN, D. (1966). An effect of stimulus colour on average steady-state potentials evoked in man. *Nature*, **210**, 1056–1057.
636. REGAN, D. (1968). A high frequency system which underlies visual evoked potentials. *Electroenceph. clin. Neurophysiol.*, **25**, 231–237.

637. REGAN, D. (1968). Evoked potentials and sensation. *Percept. Psychophys.*, **4**, 347–350.
638. REGAN, D. (1968). Chromatic adaptation and steady-state evoked potentials. *Vision Res.*, **8**, 149–158.
639. REGAN, D. (1970). An objective method of measuring the relative spectral luminosity curve in man. *J. Opt. Soc. Amer.*, **60**, 856–859.
640. REGAN, D. (1970). Evoked potential and psychophysical correlates of changes in stimulus colour and intensity. *Vision Res.*, **10**, 163–178.
641. REGAN, D. Evoked potentials specific to spatial patterns of luminance and colour. In preparation.
642. REGAN, D. Unpublished observations.
643. REGAN, D. and HERON, J. R. (1969). Clinical investigation of lesions of the visual pathway: a new objective technique. *J. Neurol. Neurosurg. Psychiat.*, **32**, 479–483.
644. REGAN, D. and CARTWRIGHT, R. F. (1970). A method of measuring the potentials evoked by simultaneous stimulation of different retinal regions. *Electroenceph. clin. Neurophysiol.*, **28**, 314–319.
645. REGAN, D. and HERON, J. R. (1970). Simultaneous recording of visual evoked potentials from the left and right hemispheres in migraine. In 'Background to Migraine', Heinemann, London, pp. 66–77.
646. REGAN, D. and SPEKREIJSE, H. (1970). Electrophysiological correlate of binocular depth perception in man. *Nature*, **225**, 92–94.
647. REGAN, D. and SPERLING, H. G. (1971). A method of evoking contour-specific scalp potentials by chromatic checkerboard patterns. *Vision Res.*, **11**, 173–176.
648. REGAN, D. and BEVERLEY, K. (1971). Evoked potentials and flicker perception at and above subjective threshold. In press.
649. REGAN, D. and RICHARDS, W. A. (1971). Independence of evoked potentials and apparent size. *Vision Res.* **11**, 679–684.
650. REGAN, D. and TYLER, C. W. (1971). Wavelength-modulated light generator. *Vision Res.*, **11**, 43–56.
651. RÉMOND, A. (1960). Le Phasotron pour l'analyse la sélection et l'integration des phases en EEG. In Smyth, C. N. 'Medical Electronics', Thomas, Springfield, pp. 108–112.
652. RÉMOND, A. (1964). Level of organization of evoked responses in man. *Ann. N.Y. Acad. Sci.*, **112**, 143–159.
653. RÉMOND, A. (1964). Surface electrical fields as displayed by digital computer. In 'Electrophysiology of the Heart', Pergamon Press, London.
654. RÉMOND, A. (1965). A method of electrode placement with a view to topographical research. *Electroenceph. clin. Neurophysiol.*, **19**, 187–189 and **17**, 577–578.
655. RÉMOND, A. (1965). Topological aspects of the organization processing and presentation of data. In Proctor, L. D. and Adey, W. R. (Eds.) 'The Analysis of Central Nervous System and Cardiovascular Data Using Computer Methods', NASA, Washington, pp. 73–93.
656. RÉMOND, A. (1968). The importance of topographic data in EEG phenomena, and an electrical model to reproduce them. *Electroenceph. clin. Neurophysiol.*, *Suppl.*, **27**, 27–49.
657. RÉMOND, A., LÈSEVRE, N. and TORRES, F. (1965). Étude chronotopographiques de l'activité occipitale moyenne recueillie sur le scalp chez l'homme en relation avec les déplacements de regard (complex lambda). *Rev. Neurol. (Paris)*, **113**, 195–226.
658. RENSHAW, B., FORBES, A. and MORISON, B. R. (1940). *J. Neurophysiol.*, **3**, 74.
659. RHODES, J. M., LANOIR, J., SAIER, J. and NAQUET, R. (1962). Étude des

responses évoqués par les mouvements des yeux le long de la voie visuelle. *Rev. Neurol.*, **107**, 177–187.

661. RICE, S. O. (1948). *Bell System Tech. J.*, **27**, 109–157.

662. RICHARDS, W. (1969). Saccadic suppression. *J. Opt. Soc. Amer.*, **59**, 617–623.

663. RICHARDS, W. (1970). Streopsis and stereoblindness. *Exp. Brain Res.*, **10**, 380–388.

664. RICHARDS, W. Personal communication.

665. RICHEY, E. T., KOOI, K. A. and WAGGONER, R. W. (1966). Visually evoked response in migraine. *Electroenceph. clin. Neurophysiol.*, **21**, 23–27.

666. RIETVELD, W. J. (1963). The occipitocortical response to light flashes in man. *Acta Physiol. Pharmacol. Neerl.*, **12**, 373–407.

667. RIETVELD, W. J. (1966). Contributions of various retinal areas to the visual evoked potential in the human cortex. *Acta Physiol. Pharmacol. Neerl.*, **14**, 1.

668. RIETVELD, W. J. and TORDOIR, W. E. M. (1965). The influence of flash intensity upon the visual evoked response in the human cortex. *Acta Physiol. Pharmacol. Neerl.*, **13**, 160–170.

669. RIETVELD, W. J., TORDOIR, W. E. M. and DUYFF, J. W. (1965). Contribution of fovea and parafovea to the visual evoked response. *Acta Physiol. Pharmacol. Neerl.*, **13**, 330–339.

670. RIETVELD, W. J., TORDOIR, W. E. M., HAGENOUW, J. R. B. and VAN DONGEN, K. J. (1965). Contribution of fovea-parafoveal quadrants to the visual evoked response. *Acta Physiol. Pharmacol. Neerl.*, **13**, 340–347.

671. RIETVELD, W. J., TORDOIR, W. E. M., HAGENOUW, J. R. B., LUBBERS, J. A. and SPOOR, TH. A. C. (1967). Visual evoked responses to blank and to checkerboard patterned flashes. *Acta Physiol. Pharmacol. Neerl.*, **14**, 259–285.

672. RIGAL, D. (1970). Potentiels évoqués visuels chez l'enfant normal et dans les troubles de la fonction visuelle. Thesis, University of Clermont.

673. RIGGS, L. A. Personal communication.

674. RIGGS, L. A., JOHNSON, E. P. and SCHICK, A. M. L. (1966). Electrical responses of the human eye to changes in wavelength of the stimulating light. *J. Opt. Soc. Amer.*, **56**, 1621–1627.

675. RIGGS, L. A. and WHITTLE, P. (1967). Human occipital and retinal potentials evoked by subjectively faded visual stimuli. *Vision Res.*, **7**, 441–451.

676. RIGGS, L. A. and STERNHEIM, C. E. (1969). Human retinal and occipital potentials evoked by changes of the wavelength of the stimulating light. *J. Opt. Soc. Amer.*, **59**, 635–640.

677. RITTER, W. and VAUGHAN, H. G., JR. (1969). Averaged evoked potentials in vigilance and discrimination: a reassessment. *Science*, **164**, 326–328.

678. RITTER, W., VAUGHAN, H. G., JR. and COSTA, L. D. (1968). Orienting and habituation to auditory stimuli: a study of short-term changes in average evoked potentials. *Electroenceph. clin. Neurophysiol.*, **25**, 550–556.

679. RITVO, E. R., ORNITZ, E. M. and WALTER, R. D. (1967). Clinical application of the auditory averaged evoked response at sleep onset in the diagnosis of deafness. *Pediatrics*, **40**, 1003–1008.

680. RODIN, E. (1969). Comment on Callaway's paper. In Donchin, E. and Lindsley, D. B. (Eds.) 'Average Evoked Potentials', NASA SP–191, Washington, D.C., p. 324.

681. RODIN, E., GRISELL, J. and GOTTLIER, J. (1968). Some electrographic differences between chronic schizophrenic patients and normal subjects. In Wortis, J. (Ed.) 'Recent Advances in Biological Psychiatry', Vol. X, Plenum Press, New York, p. 194.

682. ROSE, D. E. and RITTMANIC, P. A. (1968). Evoked response tests with mentally retarded. *Arch. Otolaryng.*, **88**, 495–498.

683. ROSE, J. E. and MOUNTCASTLE, V. B. (1959). Touch and kinesthesis. In Field, J., Magoun, H. W. and Hall, V. E. (Eds.) 'Handbook of Physiology', Sect. 1, Amer. Physiol. Soc., Washington.

684. ROSE, G. H. and LINDSLEY, D. B. (1965). Visually evoked electrocortical responses in kittens: development of specific and nonspecific systems. *Science*, **148**, 1244–1246.

ROSE, G. H. and LINDSLEY, D. B. (1968). Development of visually evoked potentials in kittens: specific and nonspecific responses. *J. Neurophysiol.*, **31**, 607–623.

684a. ROSENFELD, J. P., RUDELL, A. P. and FOX, S. S. (1969). Operant control of neural events in humans. *Science*, **165**, 821–823.

685. ROSNER, B. S. and GOFF, W. R. (1967). In 'Contributions to Sensory Physiology', Vol. 2, Academic Press, New York, pp. 169–221.

686. ROTHMAN, H. H. and DAVIS, H. (1969). The amplitude of the slow evoked cortical responses in relation to temporal features of stimulation. Paper presented to EEG Conference, San Diego.

687. ROTTERDAM, A. VAN (1970). Limitations and difficulties in signal processing by means of principal-component analysis. *IEEE Trans. Bio. Med. Eng.*

688. ROUHER, F., PLANE, C. and SOLÉ, P. (1969). Intéret des potentials évoqués visuels dans les affections du nerf optique. *Arch. Opht.* (*Paris*), **29**, 555–564.

689. RUCH, T. C., PATTON, H. D., WOODBURY, J. W. and TOWE, A. L. (Eds.) (1962). 'Neurophysiology', Saunders, Philadelphia.

690. RUCHKIN, D. S. (1965). An analysis of average response computations based upon aperiodic stimuli. *IEEE Trans. Bio. Med. Engng.*, **BME–12**, 87–94.

691. RUCHKIN, D. S. (1968). Analysis of nonhomogeneous sequences of evoked potentials. *Exp. Neurol.*, **20**, 275–284.

692. RUCHKIN, D. S. (1969). Discussion of Donchin's paper. In Donchin, E. and Lindsley, D. B. (Eds.) 'Average Evoked Potentials', NASA SP–191, Washington, D.C., 229–230.

693. RUCHKIN, D. S. and JOHN, E. R. (1966). Evoked potential correlates of generalisation. *Science*, **153**, 209–211.

694. RUCHKIN, D. S., VILLEGAS, J. and JOHN, E. R. (1964). An analysis of averaged evoked potentials making use of least mean squares techniques. *Ann. N.Y. Acad. Sci.*, **115**, 799–826.

695. RUSH, S. and DRISCOLL, D. A. (1968). Current distribution in the brain from surface electrodes. *Anesthesia and Anelgesia*, **47**, 717–723.

696. RUSH, S. and DRISCOLL, D. A. (1969). EEG electrode sensitivity – an application of reciprocity. *IEEE Trans. Bio. Med. Engng.*, **BME–16**, 15–22.

697. RUSHTON, W. A. H. (1961). Peripheral coding in the nervous system. In Rosenblith, W. A. (Ed.) 'Sensory Communication', M.I.T. press, pp. 169–181.

698. SANCES, A., JR. and LARSON, S. J. (1967). Evoked potential recording: an adjunct to human stereotactic surgery. *IEEE Trans. Bio. Med. Engng.*, **BME–14**, 162–166.

699. SANDT, W. VAN DER (1969). Clinical applications of evoked-response audiometry. *S.A. Medical Journal*, **43**, 33–35.

700. SATTERFIELD, J. H. (1965). Evoked cortical response enhancement and attention in man. A study of responses to auditory and shock stimuli. *Electroenceph. clin. Neurophysiol.*, **19**, 470–475.

701. SATTERFIELD, J. H. and CHEATUM, D. (1964). Evoked cortical potential correlates of attention in human subjects. *Electroenceph. clin. Neurophysiol.*, **17**, 456.

702. SCHADÉ, J. P. and FORD, D. H. (1965). 'Basic Neurology', Elsevier, Amsterdam, London, New York, pp. 371.

703. SCHADÉ, O. H., SR. (1956). Optical and photoelectric analogy of the eye. *J. Opt. Soc. Amer.*, **46**, 721–739.

704. SCHILLER, P. H. and CORDOVER, S. L. (1966). Metacontrast: Its relation to evoked potentials. *Science*, **153**, 1398–1400.

705. SCHIMMEL, H. (1967). The (±) reference: accuracy of estimated mean components in average response studies. *Science*, **157**, 92–94.

706. MARK, F. VAN DER. In Schipperheyn, J. J. (1965). Contrast detection in the frog's retina. *Acta Physiol. Pharmacol. Neerl.*, **13**, 231–277.

707. SCHNEIDER, G. E. (1969). Two visual systems. *Science*, **163**, 895–902.

708. SCHREINEMACHERS, H. P. and HENKES, H. E. (1968). Relation between localised retinal stimuli and the visual evoked response in man. *Ophthalmologica*, **155**, 17–27.

709. SCHWARTZ, M. (1959). 'Information Transmission, Modulation and Noise', McGraw-Hill.

710. SCOTT, D. F. and BICKFORD, R. G. (1967). Electrophysiologic studies during scanning and passive eye movements in humans. *Science*, **155**, 101–102.

711. SCOTT, D. F., GROETHYSEN, U. C. and BICKFORD, R. G. (1967). Lambda responses in the human electroencephalogram. *Neurology*, **17**, 770–778.

712. SEAL, H. L. (1964). 'Multivariate Statistical Analysis for Biologists', London, Methuen, pp. 207.

713. SHAGASS, C. (1962). In Roessler, R. and Greenfield, N. S. (Eds.) 'Physiological Correlates of Psychological Disorder', University of Wisconsin Press, Madison.

714. SHAGASS, C. (1968). Cerebral evoked responses in schizophrenia. *Condit. Reflex*, **3**, 205–216.

715. SHAGASS, C. (1968). Averaged somatosensory evoked responses in various psychiatric disorders. In Wortis, J. (Ed.) 'Recent Advances in Biological Psychiatry', **10**, 205–219. Plenum Press, New York.

716. SHAGASS, C. and OVERTON, D. A. (1968). An evoked potential approach to measurement of central inhibitory and excitatory reactivity in man. *Excerpta Medica Internat. Congr. Series*, **180**, 401–403.

717. SHAGASS, C. and SCHWARTZ, M. (1961). Reactivity cycle of somatosensory cortex in humans with and without psychiatric disorder. *Science*, **134**, 1757–1759.

718. SHAGASS, C. and SCHWARTZ, M. (1963). Psychiatric correlates of evoked cerebral cortical potentials. *Amer. J. Psychiat.*, **119**, 1055–1061.

719. SHAGASS, C. and SCHWARTZ, M. (1963). Psychiatric disorder and deviant cerebral responsiveness to sensory stimulation. In Wortis, J. (Ed.) 'Recent Advances in Biological Psychiatry', **5**, 321, Plenum Press, New York.

720. SHAGASS, C. and SCHWARTZ, M. (1965). Age, personality and somatosensory cerebral evoked responses. *Science*, **148**, 1359–1361.

721. SHAGASS, C. and STRAUMANIS, J. J. (1969). Evoked potentials and psychopathology. In 'Neurobiological Aspects of Psychopathology', Grune and Stratton Inc.

722. SHAGASS, C., OVERTON, D. A. and BARTOLUCCI, G. (1968). Evoked responses in schizophrenia. In Siva Sankar, D. V. (Ed.) 'Schizophrenia – Current Concepts and Research', PJD Publications, Hicksville, New York, pp. 220–235.

723. SHAKOW, D. (1963). Psychological deficit in schizophrenia. *Behav. Sci.*, **8**, 275–305.

724. SHAW, J. C. and ROTH, M. (1955). Potential distribution analysis. I. A new technique for the analysis of electrophysiological phenomena. *Electroenceph. clin. Neurophysiol.*, **7**, 273–284.

725. SHAW, J. C. and ROTH, M. (1955). Potential distribution analysis. II. A theoretical consideration of its significance in terms of electrical field theory. *Electroenceph. clin. Neurophysiol.*, **7**, 285–292.

726. SHEATZ, G. C. and CHAPMAN, R. M. (1969). Task relevance and auditory evoked responses. *Electroenceph. clin. Neurophysiol.*, **26**, 468–475.
727. SHIMIZU, H. (1968). Evoked response in VIIIth nerve lesions. *Laryngoscope*, **78**, 2140–2152.
728. SHIMIZU, H. (1969). AER in the severely retarded. Paper presented at 9th Internat. Congress of Otorhinolaryngology, Mexico City.
729. SHIMIZU, H. Some methodological considerations in EEG audiometry.
730. SHIMIZU, H. and GLACKIN, R. (1967). Comparison of graphic and computer averaging methods of EEG. *J. Speech Hearing Res.*, **10**, 373–376.
731. SHIPLEY, T. (1969). The visually evoked occipitogram in strabismic amblyopia under direct-view ophthalmoscopy. *J. Pediat. Ophthal.*, **6**, 97–112.
732. SHIPLEY, T. (1970). Evoked brain potentials and sensory interaction in the retarded child. *Am. J. Ment. Defic.*, **74**, 517–523.
733. SHIPLEY, T. Personal communication.
734. SHIPLEY, T., JONES, R., WAYNE and FRY, A. (1965). Evoked visual potentials. and human colour vision. *Science*, **150**, 1162–1164.
735. SHIPLEY, T., JONES, R., WAYNE and FRY, A. (1966). Intensity and the evoked occipitogram in man. *Vision Res.*, **6**, 657–667.
736. SHIPLEY, T., JONES, R., WAYNE and FRY, A. (1968). Spectral analysis of the visually evoked occipitogram in man. *Vision Res.*, **8**, 409–431.
737. SHIPTON, H. W. (1960). Photographic averaging technique for the study of evoked cortical potentials in man. In Smythe, C. N. (Ed.) 'Medical Electronics', Iliffe, London, pp. 186–187.
738. SIEGFRIED, J. B. (1970). The relationship between stimulus wavelength and the wavelength of averaged visual evoked cortical potentials. *Amer. J. Optometry and Archiv. of Am. Acad. Optom.*, **47**, 282–287.
739. SIEGFRIED, J. B., TEPAS, D. I., SPERLING, H. G. and HISS, R. H. (1965). Evoked brain potential correlates of psychophysical responses: heterochromatic flicker photometry. *Science*, **149**, 321–323.
740. SLATTER, K. A. (1968). Some clinical and EEG findings in patients with migraine. *Brain*, **91**, 85–98.
741. SMITH, D. B. D., DONCHIN, E., COHEN, L. and STARR, A. Auditory averaged evoked potentials in man during selective binaural listening. *Electroenceph. clin. Neurophysiol.*, **28**, 146–152.
742. SMITH, D. B., ALLISON, T. and GOFF, W. R. (1970). Effects of destruction of the trigeminal or olefactory nerve on the human cerebral evoked response to odorous stimuli. U.S. Eastern EEG Soc., Ste. Marguerite, Canada.
SMITH, D. B., ALLISON, T., GOFF, W. R. and PRINCIPATO, J. J. (1971). Human odorant evoked responses: effects of trigeminal or olefactory deficit. *Electroenceph. clin. Neurophysiol.* In press.
743. SMITH, R. A. (1970). Adaptation of visual contrast sensitivity to specific temporal frequencies. *Vision Res.*, 275–279.
744. SMYTH, V. O. G. and WINTER, A. L. (1964). The EEG in migraine. *Electro enceph. clin. Neurophysiol.*, **16**, 194.
745. SMYTHE, W. R. (1950). 'Static and Dynamic Electricity', McGraw-Hill, New York.
746. SPECK, L. B., DIM, B. and MERCER, M. (1966). Visual evoked responses of psychiatric patients. *Arch. gen. Psychiat.*, **15**, 59–63.
747. SPEHLMANN, R. (1965). The averaged electrical response to diffuse and to patterned light in the human. *Electroenceph. clin. Neurophysiol.*, **19**, 560–569.
748. SPEKREIJSE, H. (1966). 'Analysis of EEG Responses in Man', Junk Publishers, The Hague, The Netherlands.
749. SPEKREIJSE, H. (1969). Rectification in the goldfish retina: analysis by sinusoidal and auxilliary stimulation. *Vision Res.*, **9**, 1461–1472.

SPEKREIJSE, H. and NORTON, A. L. (1970). The dynamic characteristics of colour coded S potentials. *J. Gen. Physiol.*, **56**, 1–15.

750. SPEKREIJSE, H. Personal communication.

751. SPEKREIJSE, H. and OOSTING, H. (1970). Linearizing, a method for analysing and synthesizing nonlinear systems. In press.

752. SPEKREIJSE, H. and TWEEL, L. H. VAN DER (1965). Linearization of evoked responses to sinusoidally modulated light by noise. *Nature*, **205**, 913.

753. SPEKREIJSE, H. and TWEEL, L. H. VAN DER (1966). Flicker and noise. In Burian, H. M. and Jacobson, J. H. (Eds.) 'Clinical Electroretinography', Oxford, Pergamon, pp. 275–280.

754. SPEKREIJSE, H., TWEEL, L. H. VAN DER and REGAN, D. (1971). Interocular sustained suppression: correlation with evoked potential amplitude and distribution. In press.

755. SPERRY, R. W. (1950). Neural basis of the spontaneous optokinetic response produced by visual inversion. *J. Comp. Physiol. Psychol.*, **43**, 482–489.

756. SPONG, P., HAIDER, M. and LINDSLEY, D. B. (1965). Selective attentiveness and cortical evoked responses to visual and auditory stimuli. *Science*, **148**, 395–397.

757. SPRAGUE, J. M. (1966). Interaction of cortex and superior colliculus in mediation of visually guided behaviour in the cat. *Science*, **153**, 1544–1547.

758. SPRENG, M. (1966). Neurophysiological evidence for the critical bandwidth in audition. Bionics Symposium, Dayton, Ohio.

759. SPRENG, M. (1969). Problems in objective cerebral audiometry using short sound stimulation. *Internat. Audiol.*, **8**, 424–429.

760. SPRENG, M. (1970). Detection of influence of latency variability upon the averaged evoked responses. *Internat. Audiol.* In press.

761. SPRENG, M. and ICHIOKA, M. (1964). Langsame Rindenpotentiale bei Schmertzreizung am Menschen. *Pflüger's Arch. Ges. Physiol.*, **279**, 121–132.

762. SPRENG, M. and KEIDEL, W. D. (1967). Separierung von Cerebroaudiograium (CAG), Neuroaudiogramm (NAG) and Otoaudiogramm (OAG) in der objectiven Audiometrie. *Archiv. klin. exper. Ohren-, Nasen- und Kehlkopfheilk.*, **189**, 225–246.

763. SPRENG, M. and KEIDEL, W. D. (1969). New aspects of evoked potential research concerning objective audiometry. Scand. Symp. on ER audiometry, Copenhagen.

764. SPRENG, M. and KEIDEL, W. D. (1970). Recent status results and problems of objective audiology in man. Parts I and II. *J.F.O.R.L.*, **19**, 45–60.

765. 'Standard Reference Zero for the Calibration of Pure-Tone Audiometers', R 389; 'Expression of the power and intensity levels of sound or noise', R 357; 'Expression of the physical and subjective magnitudes of sound or noise', R 131. International Organisation for Standardisation; Physikalisch-Technische Bundesanstalt, Braunschweig, Germany; National Physical Laboratory, Teddington, England; National Bureau of Standards, Washington, U.S.A.; UNIIM Laboratory, Leningrad, U.S.S.R.; Centre National d'Etudes des Telecommunications, Paliseau, France.

766. STEVENS, S. S. (1961). The psychophysics of sensory function. In Rosenblith, W. A. (Ed.) 'Sensory Communication', John Wiley & Sons, pp. 1–33.

767. STEVENS, S. S. (1970). Neural events and the psychophysical law. *Science*, **170**, 1043–1050.

768. STILES, W. S. and CRAWFORD, B. H. (1933). The luminous efficiency of rays entering the eye pupil at different points. *Proc. Roy. Soc.* (Lond.), **B112**, 428–450.

769. STOHR, P. E. and GOLDRING, S. (1969). Origin of somatosensory evoked scalp responses in man. *J. Neurosurg.*, **31**, 117–127.

770. STONE, G. C. (1968). Temporal properties in cognitive processing of the child. Paper presented to American Psychological Assoc., San Francisco.

771. STRAUMANIS, J. J., SHAGASS, C. and SCHWARTZ, M. (1965). Visually evoked cerebral response changes associated with chronic brain syndromes and ageing. *J. Gerontol.*, **20**, 498–506.

772. STRAUMANIS, J. J., SHAGASS, C. and OVERTON, D. A. (1969). Problems associated with application of the contingent negative variation to psychiatric research. *N. Nerv. Ment. Dis.*, **148**, 170–179.

773. STREETER, D. N. and RAVIV, J. Research on advanced computer methods for biological data processing. Defence Documentation Centre, Clearinghouse for Federal Scientific and Technical Information, Springfield, Va., Rept. ASTIA, Doc. AD 637–452.

774. STRELETS, V. B. (1968). Investigations of brain bioelectrical activity in schizophrenic patients by evoked potentials. *Zh Nevropat Psikhiat Korsakov*, **68**, 82–89 (Russian, English summary).

775. SUTTON, S. (1969). The specification of psychological variables in an average evoked potential experiment. In Donchin, E. and Lindsley, D. B. (Eds.) 'Average Evoked Potentials', NASA SP–191, Washington, D.C.

776. SUTTON, S. (1970). The sensitivity of the evoked potential to psychological variables. Presented at meeting of EEG Soc., Washington, D.C.

777. SUTTON, S. (1970). Correspondence between psychological and physiological thresholds. Presented to American Psychological Assoc., Miami.

778. SUTTON, S., BRAREN, M. and ZUBIN, J. (1965). Evoked potential correlates of stimulus uncertainty. *Science*, **150**, 1187–1188.

779. SUTTON, S., TUETING, P., ZUBIN, J. and JOHN, E. R. (1967). Information delivery and the sensory evoked potential. *Science*, **155**, 1436–1439.

780. SUZUKI, T. and TAGUCHI, K. (1965). Cerebral evoked responses to auditory stimuli in waking man. *Ann. Otol.* (*St. Louis*), **74**, 128–139.

781. SWETS, J. A., TANNER, W. P., JR. and BIRDSALL, T. G. (1964). Decision processes in perception. In Swets, J. A. (Ed.) 'Signal Detection and Recognition by Human Observers', Wiley, pp. 3–57.

782. SCHWARTZ, S. and SHAGASS, C. (1961). *J. Neuropsychiat.*, **2**, 262.

783. TASAKI, I., POLLEY, E. H. and ORREGO, F. (1954). *J. Neurophysiol.*, **17**, 454.

784. The ten-twenty electrode system of the international federation (1958). *Electroenceph. Clin. Neurophysiol.*, **10**, 371–375.

785. TEPAS, D. I. and ARMINGTON, J. C. (1962). Evoked potentials in the human visual system. In 'Biological Prototypes and Synthetic Systems', Vol. 1, Plenum Press, New York, 13–21.

786. TEUBER, H.-L. (1960). Perception. In Field, T., Magoun, H. W. and Hall, V. E. (Eds.) 'Handbook of Physiology', Section I. American Physiological Society, Washington, D.C., pp. 1595–1669.

787. TEUBER, H.-L. (1964). Alterations of perception after brain injury. In Eccles, J. C. (Ed.) 'Brain and Conscious Experience', Springer-Verlag, New York.

788. TEUBER, H.-L., BATTERSBY, W. S. and BENDER, M. B. (1960). 'Visual Field Defects after Penetrating Missile Wounds of the Brain', Harvard Univ. Press, Cambridge, Mass.

789. THOMPSON, R. F. and SPENCER, W. A. (1966). Habituation: a model phenomenon for the study of neuronal substrates of behaviour. *Psychol. Rev.*, **73**, 16–43.

790. TOWNSEND, N. R. A. (1967). The EEG in migraine. In 'Background to Migraine', Heinemann, London.

791. TREVARTHEN, C. B. (1968). Two mechanisms of vision in primates. *Psychologische Forschung*, **31**, 299–337.

792. TSUTSUI, J. (1968). The electroencephalic response evoked by binocular vision. *Acta Soc. Ophthal. Jap.*, **71**, 785–790.

793. TUETING, P., SUTTON, S. and ZUBIN, J. Qualitative evoked potential correlates of the probability of events. *Psychophysiology*. In press.
794. TWEEL, L. H. VAN DER (1961). Some problems in vision regarded with respect to linearity and frequency response. *Ann. N.Y. Acad. Sci.*, **89**, 829–856.
795. TWEEL, L. H. VAN DER (1964). Relation between psychophysics and electrophysiology of flicker. In Henkes, H. E. and Tweel, L. H. van der (Eds.), *Flicker, Docum. Ophthal.* (Den Haag), **18**, 287–304.
796. TWEEL, L. H. VAN DER. Personal communication.
797. TWEEL, L. H. VAN DER and VERDUYN LUNEL, H. F. E. (1965). Human visual responses to sinusoidally, modulated light. *Electroenceph. clin. Neurophysiol.* **18**, 587–598.
798. TWEEL, L. H. VAN DER and SPEKREIJSE, H. (1966). Visual evoked responses. ISCERG Symp. Ghent, pp. 83–94 (Karger, Basel/New York).
799. TWEEL, L. H. VAN DER and SPEKREIJSE, H. (1969). Signal transport and rectification in the human evoked-response system. *Ann. N.Y. Acad. Sci.*, **156**, 678–695.
800. TWEEL, L. H. VAN DER, SPEKREIJSE, H. and REGAN, D. (1970). A correlation between evoked potentials and point-to-point interocular suppression. *Electroenceph. clin. Neurophysiol.*, **28**, 209–212.
801. TWEEL, L. H. VAN DER, REGAN, D. and SPREKREIJSE, H. (1970). Some aspects of potentials evoked by changes in spatial brightness contrast. ISCERG Symposium, Istanbul.
802. TWEEL, L. H. VAN DER, SPEKREIJSE, H. and ZUIDEMA (1970). The eye as a differential amplifier. ISCERG Symposium, Istanbul.
803. TWEEL, L. H. VAN DER and SPEKREIJSE, H. Personal communication.
804. TYBERGHEIN, J. and FORREZ, G. (1969). Cortical audiometry in normal hearing subjects. *Acta Otolaryngologica*, **67**, 24–32.
805. UMEZAKI, H. and MORRELL, F. (1970). Developmental study of photic evoked responses in premature infants. *Electroenceph. clin. Neurophysiol.*, **28**, 55–63.
806. Units and Standards of Measurement. II. Light. Her Majesty's Stationery Office.
807. UNO, M., KUBOTA, K., OHYE, C., TOMONORI, N. and NARABAYASHI, H. (1967). Topographical arrangement between thalamic ventro-lateral nucleus and precentral motor cortex in man. *Electroenceph. clin. Neurophysiol.*, **22**, 437–443.
808. UTTAL, W. R. (1960). The IBM biophysical research system. IBM Research Report RC–195.
809. UTTAL, W. R. (1965). Do compound evoked potentials reflect psychological codes? *Psychol. Bull.*, **64**, 377–392.
810. UTTAL, W. R. (1967). Evoked brain potentials: signs or codes? *Perspect. Biol. Med.*, **10**, 627–639.
811. UTTAL, W. R. and COOK, L. (1964). Systematics of the evoked somatosensory cortical potential: A psychophysical–electrophysiological comparison. *Ann. N.Y. Acad. Sci.*, **112**, 60–80.
812. VAN HEEL, A. C. S. (1946). Correcting the spherical and chromatic aberration of the eye. *J. Opt. Soc. Amer.*, **36**, 237–239.
813. VAN HOF, M. W. (1960). The relation between the cortical responses to flash and flicker in man. *Acta Physiol. Pharmacol. Neerl.*, **9**, 210–224.
814. VASTOLA, E. F. (1968). Localisation of visual functions in the mammalian brain: A review. *Brain Behav. Evol.*, **1**, 420–471.
815. VAUGHAN, H. G., JR. (1966). The perceptual and physiologic significance of visual evoked responses recorded from the scalp in man. In 'Clinical Electroretinography', Supp. Vision Res., 203–223.

816. VAUGHAN, H. G. (1969). The relationship of brain activity to scalp recording of event-related potentials. In Donchin, E. and Lindsley, D. B. (Eds.) 'Average Evoked Potentials', NASA SP–191, Washington, D.C.

817. VAUGHAN, H. G., JR. New physiological approaches to psychopathology. In Kietzman, M. L., Sutton, S. and Zubin, J. (Eds.) 'Experimental Approaches to Psychopathology', Academic Press, New York, in press.

818. VAUGHAN, H. G., JR. (1971). The motor potentials. In 'EEG Journal Handbook on CNS Evoked Potentials'. In press.

819. VAUGHAN, H. G., JR. (1971). Psychological correlates of association cortex potentials. In 'EEG Journal Handbook on CNS Evoked Potentials'. In press.

819a. VAUGHAN, H. G., JR. (1971). The role of stimulus pattern in suppression of vision during eye movements. In press.

820. VAUGHAN, H. G., JR., COSTA, D. and RITTER, W. (1968). Topography of the human motor potential. *Electroenceph. clin. Neurophysiol.*, **25**, 1–10.

821. VAUGHAN, H. G., JR. and GROSS, C. G. (1969). Cortical responses to light in unanaesthetized monkeys and their alteration by visual system lesions. *Exp. Brain Res.*, **8**, 19–36.

822. VAUGHAN, H. G., JR. and HULL, R. C. (1965). Functional relation between stimulus intensity and photically evoked cerebral responses in man. *Nature*, **206**, 720–722.

823. VAUGHAN, H. G., JR., KATZMAN, R. and TAYLOR, J. (1963). Alterations of visual evoked responses in the presence of homonymous field defects. *Electroenceph. clin. Neurophysiol.*, **15**, 737–746.

824. VAUGHAN, H. G., JR. and KATZMAN, R. (1964). Evoked responses in visual disorders. *Ann. N.Y. Acad. Sci.*, **112**, 305–319.

825. VAUGHAN, H. G., JR. and KATZMAN, R. Detection of visual defects in man with average responses from retina and visual cortex.

826. VAUGHAN, H. G., JR. and RITTER, W. (1969). The sources of auditory-evoked responses recorded from the human scalp. *Electroenceph. clin. Neurophysiol.*, **28**, 360–367.

827. VAUGHAN, H. G., JR. and SILVERSTEIN, L. (1968). Metacontrast and evoked potentials: A reappraisal. *Science*, **160**, 207–208.

828. VERZEANO, M. (1961). Neuronal interaction and synchronization of the EEG. Excerpta Medica, Int. Cong. 37, paper 43.

829. VERZEANO, M. (1963). Las functiones del sistema nervioso; correlaciones entre estructura bioquimica y electrofisiologica. *Acta. Neurol. Latinoamer.*, **9**, 297–307.

830. VERZEANO, M. (1967). The nature of brainwaves. 20th Ann. Conf. Eng. Med. Biol., Boston.

831. VERZEANO, M. (1970). Evoked responses and network dynamics. In 'The Neural Control of Behaviour', Academic Press, New York.

832. VERZEANO, M. and CALMA, I. (1954). Unit activity in spindle bursts. *J. Neurophysiol.*, **17**, 417–428.

833. VERZEANO, M. and NEGISHI, K. (1960). Neuronal activity in cortical and thalamic networks. *J. Gen. Physiol.*, **43**, Suppl. 6, 177–195.

834. VERZEANO, M., LAUFER, J., SPEAR, P. and MCDONALD, S. (1965). The activity of neuronal networks in the thalamus of the monkey. *Actualites Neurophysiol.*, **6**, 223.

835. VOITINSKY, E. YA. and ERMOLAEVA, R. YA. (1968). An analysis of evoked potentials in patients with atrophia of the visual nerves with the help of computers. *Zh Nervropat Psikhiat Korsakov*, **68**, 1716–1719 (Russian, English summary).

836. VOLKMAN, F. C. (1962). Vision during voluntary saccadic eye movements. *J. Opt. Soc. Amer.*, **52**, 571–578.

837. WALKER, A. E. and MARSHALL, C. (1964). The contribution of depth recording to clinical medicine. *Electroenceph. clin. Neurophysiol.*, **16**, 88–99.

838. WALRAVEN, P. L. and LEEBECK, H. J. (1964). Phase shift of sinusoidally alternating coloured stimuli. *J. Opt. Soc. Amer.*, **54**, 78–82.

839. WALSH, J. W. T. (1953). 'Photometry', Constable, London.

840. WALTER, D. O. (1963). Spectral analysis for electroencephalograms: mathematical determination of neurophysiological relationships from records of limited duration. *Exp. Neurol.*, **8**, 155.

841. WALTER, D. O. (1968). *A Posteriori* 'Wiener filtering' of averaged evoked responses. *Electroenceph. clin. Neurophysiol., Suppl.*, **27**, 61–70.

842. WALTER, D. O. and ADEY, W. R. (1965). Analysis of brain-wave generators as multiple statistical timeseries. *IEEE Trans. Bio. Med. Engng.*, **BME–12**, 8–13.

843. WALTER, D. O., RHODES, J. M., BROWN, D. and ADEY, W. R. (1966). Comprehensive spectral analysis of human EEG generators in posterior cerebral regions. *Electroenceph. clin. Neurophysiol.*, **20**, 224–237.

844. WALTER, D. O. and BRAZIER, M. A. B. (Eds.) (1969). Advances in EEG Analysis. *Electroenceph. clin. Neurophysiol.*, Suppl. 27.

845. WALTER, W. G. (1953). Toposcopy. *Electroenceph. clin. Neurophysiol., Suppl.*, **4**, 7–16.

WALTER, W. G. (1953). 'The Living Brain', W. W. Norton Co.

846. WALTER, W. GREY. (1963). Specific and non-specific responses and autonomic mechanisms in human subjects during conditioning. *Prog. in Brain Res.*, **1**, 395–401.

847. WALTER, W. GREY. (1964). The convergence and interaction of visual, auditory and tactile responses in human nonspecific cortex. *Ann. N.Y. Acad. Sci.*, **112**, 320–361.

848. WALTER, W. GREY. (1964). Slow potential waves in the human brain associated with expectancy, attention and decision. *Arch. Psychiat. Nervenkr.*, **206**, 309–322.

849. WALTER, W. GREY. (1965). Brain responses to semantic stimuli. *J. Psychosom. Res.*, **9**, 51–61.

850. WALTER, W. GREY. (1967). Slow potential changes in the human brain associated with expectancy, decision and intention. *Electroenceph. clin. Neurophysiol., Suppl.*, **26**, 123–130.

851. WALTER, W. GREY., COOPER, R., ALDRIDGE, V. J., MCCALLUM, W. C. and WINTER, A. L. (1964). Contingent negative variation: an electric sign of sensorimotor association and expectancy in the human brain. *Nature*, **203**, 380–384.

852. WARREN, R. M. (1958). A basis for judgements of sensory intensity. *Am. J. Psychol.*, **71**, 675–687.

WARREN, R. M. and WARREN, R. P. (1963). A critique of S. S. Steven's 'New Psychophysics'. *Percept. Mot. Skills*, **16**, 797–810.

853. WATANABE, S., KONISHI, M. and CREUTZFELDT, O. D. (1966). Postsynaptic potentials in the cat's visual cortex following electrical stimulation of afferent pathways. *Exp. Brain Res.*, **1**, 272–283.

854. WATSON-WATT, R. (1946). The evolution of radiolocation. *J. Inst. Elect. Eng.* **93**, part IIIA, 11–19.

855. WEBER, D. S. and BUCHWALD, J. S. (1965). A technique for recording and integrating multiple unit activity simultaneously with the EEG in chronic animals. *Electroenceph. clin. Neurophysiol.*, **19**, 190–192.

856. WEINMAN, J. and MAHLER, J. (1964). An analysis of electrical properties of metal electrodes. *Med. Electron Biol. Eng.*, **2**, 299.

857. WEINMANN, H., CREUTZFELDT, O. D. and HEYDE, G. (1965). Die entwicklung der visuellen reizantwort bei kindern. *Archiv. für Psychiatrie u. Zeitschift. f. ges. Neurol.*, **207**, 323–341.

858. WEINSTEIN, S. (1967). Differences in effects of brain wounds implicating right and left hemispheres. In Mountcastle, V. B. (Ed.) 'Interhemispheric Relations and Cerebral Dominance', Johns Hopkins Press, Baltimore, pp. 159–176.

859. WEISKRANTZ, L. (1963). Contour discrimination in a young monkey with striate cortex ablation. *Neuropsychologica*, **1**, 145–164.

860. WEITZMAN, E. D., FISHBEIN, W. and GRAZIANI, L. J. (1965). Auditory evoked responses obtained from the scalp electroencephalograms of the full-term human neonate during sleep. *Pediatrics*, **35**, 458–462.

861. WEITZMAN, E. D. and KREMEN, H. (1965). Auditory evoked responses during different stages of sleep in man. *Electroenceph. clin. Neurophysiol.*, **18**, 65–70.

862. WEITZMAN, E. D., RÉMOND, A. and LESÈVRE (1965). Étude chrono-topographique des potentiels évoqués auditifs recueillis sur le scalp chez l'homme normal au cours du sommeil et de l'état de veille. *Rev. Neurol.*, **113**, 253–261.

863. WEITZMAN, E. D. and GRAZIANI, L. J. (1968). Maturation and topography of the auditory-evoked response of the prematurely born infant. *Developmental Psychobiology*, **1**, 79–89.

864. WERNER, G. and MOUNTCASTLE, V. B. (1965). Neural activity in mechano-receptive cutaneous afferents: stimulus-response relations, Weber functions and information transmission. *J. Neurophysiol.*, **28**, 359–397.

865. WERRE, P. F. and SMITH, C. J. (1964). Variability of responses evoked by flashes in man. *Electroenceph. clin. Neurophysiol.*, **17**, 644–652.

866. WESTHEIMER, G. (1966). The Maxwellian View. *Vision Res.*, **6**, 669–682.

867. WEYER, E. M. and FEDER, W. (Eds.) (1968). Bioelectronics. *Ann. N.Y. Acad. Sci.*, **148**.

868. WHITE, C. T. and EASON, R. G. (1966). Evoked cortical potentials in relation to certain aspects of visual perception. *Psycholog. Monogr.*, **80**, No. 24.

869. WHITE, C. T. (1969). Evoked cortical responses and patterned stimuli. *Am. Psychol.*, **24**, 212–214.

870. WICKE, J. D., DONCHIN, E. and LINDSLEY, D. B. (1964). Visual evoked potentials as a function of flash luminance and duration. *Science*, **146**, 83–85.

871. WILCOCK, A. H. and KIRSNER, R. L. G. (1969). A digital filter for biological data. *Med. and Biol. Engng.*, **7**, 653–660.

872. WILKINSON, R. T. (1967). Evoked response and reaction time. *Acta Psychol.*, **27**, 235–245.

873. WILKINSON, R. T. and MORLOCK, H. C. (1967). Auditory evoked response and reaction time. *Electroenceph. clin. Neurophysiol.*, **23**, 50–56.

874. WILLIAMSON, P. D., GOFF, W. R. and ALLISON, R. (1970). Somatosensory evoked responses in patients with unilateral cerebral lesions. *Electroenceph. clin. Neurophysiol.*, **28**, 566–575.

875. WILSON, F. N. and BAYLEY, R. H. (1950). The electric field of an eccentric dipole in a homogeneous spherical conducting medium. *Circulation*, **1**, 84–92.

876. WINANS, S. S. (1967). Visual form discrimination after removal of visual cortex in cats. *Science*, **158**, 944–946.

877. WOHLBARSHT, M. L. and SPEKREIJSE, H. (1968). Interference and noise in biological instrumentation. In Levine, S. N. (Ed.) 'Advances in Biomedical Engineering and Medical Physics', Interscience, New York, pp. 205–242.

878. WOODBURY, J. W. (1961). The cell membrane: Ionic and potential gradients and active transport. In Ruch, T. C., Patton, H. D., Woodbury, J. W. and Towe, A. D. 'Neurophysiology', W. B. Saunders, Philadelphia and London, pp. 521.

879. WOODWORTH, R. S. (1906). Vision and localisation during eye movements. *Psychol. Bull.*, **3**, 68–70.

880. WOODY, C. D. (1967). Characterization of an adaptive filter for the analysis of variable latency neuroelectric signals. *Med. and Biol. Engng.*, **5**, 539–553.

881. WOOTEN, B. R. (1968). Photopic and scotopic contributions to the human visual evoked cortical response. Unpublished. M.Sc. Thesis, Brown University.

882. WRIGHT, W. D. (1946). Researches on Normal and Defective Colour Vision. Kimpton, London.

883. YOSHIDA, M., YANAGISAWA, N., SHIMAZU, H., GIVRE, A. and NARABAYASHI, H. (1964). Physiological identification of the thalamic nucleus. *Arch. Neurol.*, **11**, 435–443.

884. ZANGWILL, O. L. (1960). 'Cerebral Dominance and its Relation to Psychological Function', Oliver and Boyd, Edinburgh.

884a. ZERLIN, S. and DAVIS, H. (1967). The variability of single evoked vertex potentials in man. *Electroenceph. clin. Neurophysiol.*, **23**, 468–472.

885. ZUBER, B. L., STARK, L. and LORBER, M. (1966). Saccadic suppression of the pupillary light reflex. *Exp. Neurol.*, **14**, 351–370.

SUPPLEMENTARY REFERENCES

886. BERLYNE, D. E. (1969). The development of the concept of attention in psychology. In Evans, C. R. and Mulholland, T. B. (Eds.) 'Attention in Neurophysiology', Butterworths, London, pp. 1–26.

887. BIZZI, E. (1966). Discharge patterns of single geniculate neurons during the rapid eye movements of sleep. *J. Neurophysiol.*, **29**, 1087–1095.

888. BIZZI, E. (1967). Discharge of frontal eye field neurons during eye movements in unanaesthetized monkeys. *Science*, **157**, 1588–1590.

889. BIZZI, E. (1968). Discharge of frontal eye field neurons during saccadic and following eye-movements in unanaesthetized monkeys. *Exp. Brain Res.*, **6**, 69–80.

890. BLACKWELL, H. R. (1946). Contrast thresholds of the human eye. *J. opt. Soc. Amer.*, **36**, 624–643.

891. BOSTOCK, H. and JARVIS, M. J. (1970). Changes in the form of the cerebral evoked response related to the speed of simple reaction time. *Electroenceph. clin. Neurophysiol.*, **29**, 137–145.

892. BOURNE, J. R., CHILDERS, D. G. and PERRY, N. W., Jr. (1971). Topological characteristics of the visual evoked response in man. *Electroenceph. clin. Neurophysiol.*, **30**, 423–436.

893. BRACEWELL, R. N. (1965). The Fourier Transform and Its Applications. McGraw-Hill, New York.

894. BUCHSBAUM, M. and SILVERMAN, J. (1968). Stimulus intensity control and the cortical response. *Psychosomat. Medicine*, **30**, 12–22.

895. BUTLER, R. A., SPRENG, M. and KEIDEL, W. D. (1969). Stimulus repetition rate factors which influence the auditory evoked potential in man. *Psychophysiol.*, **5**, 665–672.

896. CAMPBELL, F. W. (1968). The human eye as an optical filter. *Proc. IEEE*, **56**, 1009–1014.

897. CAVONIUS, C. R. and STERNHEIM, C. E. The temporal modulation transfer function of the human ERG and VECR. IUPS–ISCERG Symposium, Brighton 1971. *Vision Res.*, **11**, 1201.

898. COHN, R. (1971). Differential cerebral processing of noise and verbal stimuli. *Science*, **172**, 599–601.

899. CORNSWEET, T. N. (1962). The staircase-method in psychophysics. *Am. J. Psychol.*, **75**, 485–491.

900. CREUTZFELDT, O. D. and KUHNT, U. (1971). Electrophysiology and topographical distribution of visual evoked potentials in animals. Handbook of Sensory Physiology. Springer.

901. DONALD, M. W., Jr. and GOFF, W. R. (1971). *Science*, 1163.

902. DONCHIN, E. and LINDSLEY, D. B. (1965). Visually evoked response correlate of perceptual masking and enhancement. *Electroenceph. clin. Neurophysiol.*, **19**, 325–335.

903. DOTY, R. W., KIMURA, D. S. and MORGENSON, J. (1964). Photically and electrically elicited responses in the central visual system of the squirrel monkey.

904. EVANS, C. R. and MULHOLLAND, T. B. (1969). Attention in Neurophysiology. Butterworths, London, pp. 190–191.

905. FEHMI, L. G., ADKINS, J. W. and LINDSLEY, D. B. (1969). Electrophysiological correlates of visual perceptual masking in monkeys. *Exp. Brain Res.*, **7**, 299–316.

906. GABOR, D., KOCK, W. E. and STROKE, G. W. (1971). Holography. *Science*, **173**, 11–23.

907. GARCIA AUSTT, E. (1969). Relationship between visual evoked response and some psychological processes. In Evans, C. R. and Mulholland, T. B. (Eds.) 'Attention in Neurophysiology'. Butterworths, London, pp. 258–280.

908. GOFF, W. R. (1969). Evoked potential correlates of perceptual organisation in man. In Evans, C. R. and Mulholland, T. B. (Eds.) 'Attention in Neurophysiology'. Butterworths, London, pp. 169–193.

909. GROVES, P. M. and THOMPSON, R. F. (1971). Habituation: a dual-process theory. *Psychol. Rev.*, **77**, 419–450.

910. HARTER, M. R. and SUITT, C. D. Visually evoked cortical response and pattern vision in the infant: a longitudinal study. In press *Psychonom. Sci.*

911. HAYASHI, Y., SUMITOMO, I. and IWAMA, K. (1967). Activation of lateral geniculate neurons by electrical stimulation of superior colliculus in cats. *Jap. J. Physiol.*, **17**, 638–651.

912. HEINEMANN, E. G. (1961). The relation of apparent brightness to the threshold for differences in luminance. *J. exp. Psychol.*, **61**, 389–399.

912a. HESS, E. H. (1965). Attitude and pupil size. *Scientific American*, **212**, 46–54.

913. HILLYARD, S. A., SQUIRES, K. C., BAUER, J. W. and LINDSAY, P. H. (1971). Evoked potential correlates of auditory signal detection. *Science*, **172**, 1357–1360.

914. HOFFMAN, K. P. and STRASCHILL, M. (1970). Eye movements and single unit responses in the superior colliculus of the cat. *Proc. Aust. Physiol. Pharmacol. Soc.*, **1**, 65.

915. HOPKINS, H. H. (1953). On the diffraction theory of optical images. *Proc. Roy. Soc.*, **217A**, 408–432.

916. HOPKINS, H. H. (1955). The frequency response of a defocused optical system. *Proc. Roy. Soc.*, **231A**, 91–103.

917. HOPKINS, H. H. (1957). *Proc. Phys. Soc.* BLXX, 1002.

918. HORN, G. (1969). Novelty, attention and habituation. In Evans, C. R. and Mulholland, T. B. (Eds.) 'Attention in Neurophysiology'. Butterworths, London, pp. 230–246.

919. HUBEL, D. H. and WIESEL, T. N. (1965). Binocular interaction in striate cortex of kittens reared with artificial squint. *J. Neurophysiol.*, **28**, 1041–1059.

WIESEL, T. N. and HUBEL, D. H. (1965). Comparison of effects of unilateral and bilateral eye closure on cortical unit responses in kittens. *J. Neurophysiol.*, **28**, 1029–1040.

WIESEL, T. N. and HUBEL, D. H. (1965). Extent of recovery from the effects of visual deprivation in kittens. *J. Neurophysiol.*, **28**, 1060–1072.

HUBEL, D. H. and WIESEL, T. N. (1971). The period of susceptibility to the physiological effects of unilateral eye closure in kittens. *J. Physiol.*, **206**, 419–436.

DEWS, P. B. and WIESEL, T. N. (1971). Consequences of monocular deprivation on visual behaviour in kittens. *J. Physiol.*, **206**, 437–455.

920. JAMI, L., FOURMENT, A., CALVET, J. and THIEFFRY, M. (1968). Étude sur modèle des méthodes de détection EEG. *Electroenceph. clin. Neurophysiol.*, **24**, 130–145.

921. JASPER, H. H. (1969). In Evans, C. R. and Mulholland, T. B. (Eds.) 'Attention in Neurophysiology'. Butterworths, London, p. 189.

921a. JEWETT, D. L., ROMANO, M. N. and WILLISTON, J. S. (1970). Human auditory evoked potentials; possible brain stem components detected on the scalp. *Science*, **167**, 1517–1518.

922. JEFFREYS, D. A. and AXFORD, J. G. Source locations of pattern-specific components of human visual evoked potentials: I. Component of striate cortical origin. II. Component of extrastriate cortical origin. Submitted to *Exp. Brain Res.*

923. JOHNSTONE, J. R. and MARK, R. F. (1971). The efference copy neurons. *J. Exp. Biol.*, **54**, 403–414.

924. KARLIN, L., MARTY, M. J. and MORDKOFF, A. M. (1970). Motor performance and sensory evoked potentials. *Electroenceph. clin. Neurophysiol.*, **28**, 307–313.

925. KOOI, K. A., SHAFII, M. and RICHEY, E. T. (1968). Differentiation between visually evoked F and V potentials. *Electroenceph. clin. Neurophysiol.*, **24**, 482–485.

926. KORNHUBER, H. H. (1971). Motor functions of cerebellum and basal ganglia: the cerebellocortical saccadic (ballistic) clock, the cerebellonuclear hold regulator, and the basal ganglia ramp (voluntary speed smooth movement) generator. *Kybernetik*, **8**, 157–162.

927. LEISSNER, P., LINDHOLM, L.-E. and PETERSÉN, I. (1970). Alpha amplitude dependence on skull thickness as measured by ultrasonic technique. *Electroenceph. clin. Neurophysiol.*, **29**, 392–399.

928. MACKAY, D. M. (1971). Visual stability during voluntary eye movements. In 'Central Processing of Visual Information', Handbook of Sensory Physiology, Springer Verlag.

929. MAY, J. G., FORBES, W. B. and PIANTANIDA, T. P. (1971). The visual evoked response obtained from an alternating barred pattern: rate, spatial frequency and wavelength. *Electroenceph. clin. Neurophysiol.*, **30**, 222–228.

930. MCADAM, D. W. and WHITTAKER, H. A. (1971). Language production: electroencephalic localisation in normal human brain. *Science*, **172**, 499–502.

931. MICHAEL, W. F. and HALLIDAY, A. M. (1971). Differences between the occipital distribution of upper and lower field pattern-evoked responses in man. *Brain Res.*, **32**, 311–324.

932. MILNER, B. A., REGAN, D., HERON, J. R., WEINER, M. and CARTWRIGHT, R. F. An attempt to develop the use of steady-state evoked potential techniques as a method of detecting brain lesions. *Presented to Autumn 1971 meeting of British EEG Society*. In press *Electroenceph. clin. Neurophysiol.*

933. POLLEN, D. A., LEE, J. R. and TAYLOR, J. H. (1971). How does the striate cortex begin the reconstruction of the visual world? *Science*, **173**, 74–77.

934. REGAN, D. (1964). A study of the visual system by the correlation of light stimuli and evoked electrical responses. Ph.D. Thesis, Imperial College, University of London.

935. REGAN, D. (1970). Colour vision and evoked potentials. ISCERG Symposium, Istanbul. Published by Medical Faculty, University of Istanbul.

936. REGAN, D. (1971). Evoked potentials to changes in the chromatic contrast and to changes in the luminance contrast of checkerboard stimulus patterns. *Vision Res.*, **11**, 1203.

937. RICHARDS, W. Personal communication.

937a. ROTH, W. T., KOPELL, B. S. and BERTOZZI, P. E. (1970). The effect of attention on the averaged evoked response to speech sounds. *Electroenceph. clin. Neurophysiol.*, **29**, 38–46.
938. SCOTT, D. F., HOFFMANN, H. J. and BICKFORD, R. G. (1969). Evoked potential (lambda waves) relating to the nonadditive properties of visual sensory inflow. *Perceptual and Motor Skills*, **29**, 307–314.
939. SCOTT, D. F., LIGHTERHELD, F. R. and BICKFORD, R. G. (1968). Lambda wave studies on the EEG of animals. *Archiv. Neurol.*, **18**, 574–582.
940. SIMONS, L. A., DUNLOP, C. W., WEBSTER, W. R. and AITKIN, L. M. (1966). Acoustic habituation in cats as a function of stimulus rate and the role of temporal conditioning of the middle ear muscles. *Electroenceph. clin. Neurophysiol.*, **20**, 485–493.
941. SKINNER, J. E. and LINDSLEY, D. B. (1971). Enhancement of visual and auditory evoked potentials during blockade of the non-specific thalamocortical system. *Electroenceph. clin. Neurophysiol.*, **31**, 1–6.
942. SOKOLOFF, Y. N. (1963). Perception and the Conditioned Reflex. Pergamon, New York.
942a. SPEKREIJSE, H., TWEEL, L. H. VAN DER and KHOE, L. (1971). Electrophysiology and psychophysics in a case of amblyopia. IUPS–ISCERG, Symposium, Brighton 1971. *Vision Res.*, **11**, 1201.
943. SPILKER, B. and CALLAWAY, E. (1969). 'Augmenting' and 'reducing' in averaged visual evoked responses to sine wave light. *Psychophysiol.*, **6**, 49–57.
944. SPILKER, B. and CALLAWAY, E. (1969). Effects of drugs on 'augmenting' 'reducing' in averaged visual evoked responses in man. *Psychopharmacologia* (*Berl.*), **15**, 116–124.
945. SPILKER, B., KAMIYA, J., CALLAWAY, E. and YEAGER, C. (1969). Visual evoked responses in subjects trained to control alpha rhythm. *Psychophysiol.*, **5**, 683–695.
946. STARK, L., VOSSIUS, G. and YOUNG, L. R. (1962). *Trans. Inst. Radio Engrs.* HFE-3, 52–57.
946a. SWETS, J. A. (1961). Is there a sensory threshold? *Science*, **134**, 168–177.
947. TAYLOR, M. M. (1971). On the efficiency of psychophysical measurement. *J. Acoust. Soc. Amer.*, **49**, 505–508.
948. TAYLOR, M. M. and CREELMAN, C. D. (1967). PEST: Efficient estimates on probability functions. *J. Acoust. Soc. Amer.*, **41**, 782–787.
949. WEBSTER, W. R. (1971). The effects of repetitive stimulation on auditory evoked potentials. *Electroenceph. clin. Neurophysiol.*, **30**, 318–330.
949a. WOOD, C. C., GOFF, W. B. and DAY, R. S. (1971). Auditory evoked potentials during speech perception. *Science*, **173**, 1248–1251.
950. WOODWORTH, R. S. and SCHLOSBERG, H. (1954). Experimental Psychology. Holt and Reinhard, New York.
951. WURTZ, R. H. (1968). Visual cortex neurons. Responses to stimuli during rapid eye movements. *Science*, **162**, 1148–1150.
952. WURTZ, R. H. (1969). Response of striate cortex neurons to stimuli during rapid eye movements in the monkey. *J. Neurophysiol.*, **32**, 975–986.
953. WURTZ, R. H. (1969). Comparison of effects of eye movements and stimulus movements on striate cortex neurons in the monkey. *J. Neurophysiol.*, **32**, 987–994.

Supplementary footnotes

S1. (p. 15). Note additional references [922, 931] see supplementary footnote No. 47.

S2. (p. 16). The currents generated by the sources of EPs flow through the resistive tissues of the head and result in IR potential differences on the scalp. It is these potential differences which are recorded as EPs. The electric field within the head can be described by equipotentials. There is some analogy between these equipotentials and rays of light. A simple example is their 'refraction' at the series of surfaces where conductivity changes abruptly between the cortex, cerebrospinal fluid, dura, skull and scalp.[312, 592, 695, 696, 816] Perhaps a further analogy might be the focusing effects of concave and convex mirrors (see for example[920]). By drawing the equipotentials and adding the contributions of, say, ten dipoles arranged along a curved surface it is easy to show that by arranging dipoles along a concave surface the equipotentials are 'focused' in such a way as to produce a greater electric field strength at some specific distance than would be produced by similar dipoles arranged along a flat sheet. Conversely, a convex array causes the equipotentials to diverge; at all distances the electric field is weaker than that due to similar dipoles arranged on a flat sheet.

The convexity of the upper half of the occipital lobe[931] would consistently tend to reduce the resultant electric field strength at the scalp produced by EP generators in that part of the cortex (on the assumption that the generators could be regarded as being equivalent to a surface distribution of dipoles arranged at right angles to the cortex). On the other hand, the shape of the corresponding part of the lower lobe is quite different and more complex than the shape of the upper part. The 'focusing' effects due to the different bendings of the upper and lower parts of the lobe would presumably be quite different, and the difference might be subject to marked intersubject variations. Such 'focusing' effects might contribute to Halliday and Michael's[355] anomaly that the scalp responses due to the more distant (lower lobe) generators were no smaller than the scalp responses due to the nearer (upper lobe) generators. If 'focusing' effect did contribute to this anomaly, it would be confounded with other suggested effects of (*a*) non-indifference of the reference electrode[931] and (*b*) different orientations of equivalent dipoles.[413] However, the question whether 'focusing' effects could (at least partially) explain a particular subject's characteristic anomaly might be open to experimental test by investigating the equipotentials not only along the two-dimensional surface of the scalp, but also in three dimensions. Following a suggestion by Manfred Clynes,[248] the extracellular currents which lead to EP recordings would flow through the scalp and onwards into the space beyond if the scalp were surrounded by a medium whose conductivity were equal to that of the scalp. For example, a box held on to the back of the head could be filled with a jelly of suitable conductivity. It might then be possible to detect and quantify such a 'focusing' effect by comparing records made from electrodes placed on the scalp, and from electrodes located above them in the conducting jelly.

S3. (p. 18). There is some evidence that brain stem activity can be recorded from scalp electrodes and can contribute to the auditory EP.[921a]

S4. (p. 23). Creutzfeldt and Kuhnt[900] have recently discussed the model illustrated in Fig. 1.9 in a review of evoked potential recording in animals. Again, though, the discussion is almost entirely restricted to EPs elicited by flashed, spatially-unstructured stimuli.

S5. (p. 24). Evoked potentials elicited by stimulation of the visual pathway are more sensitive to barbiturate anaesthesia in primate (squirrel monkey) than in cat.[900] In squirrel monkey, barbiturate anaesthesia has been reported to reduce the number of primary positive deflections and to suppress the negative potential.

S6. (p. 34). Inhibition of visual units by voluntary movement has been found in the lateral geniculate body of sleeping cat[887] (but not of alert monkey),[888] and in the visual cortex of monkey.[951] Bizzi,[889] recording from the frontal eye fields of monkeys found units which fired only during an eye saccade in a particular direction, and during the fast phase of nystagmus which was in that direction. Recording from the tectal commisure of carp, Johnstone and Mark[923] found units which fired simultaneously with saccades, but only for saccades in a particular direction. The activities of these units were not directly related to sensory input. On two occasions a unit of this type was recorded simultaneously with a tonically-firing, 'presumably visual'[923] unit whose activity was suppressed during each burst of firing by the non-visual unit. Johnstone and Mark suggested that their non-visual units were 'efference copy neurons' responsible for the maintenance of perceptual stability during eye movements. Wurtz, however, has found single units which are suppressed by movement of a spatially-structured retinal image both when the movement is due to eye movement and when it is due to moving the image across a stationary retina. Wurtz considered that this would not be expected if suppression were due to a corollary discharge from the oculomotor system.

S7. (p. 34). In a recent review of the problem of visual stability[928] Mackay points out that the notion of *subtraction* of a neural 'efference copy' from the sensory inflow is effective in accounting for the maintenance of sensorimotor coordination, although he argues against its relevance to the problem of perceptual stability.

S8. (pp. 37, 55, 62, 64, 114, 146, 167, 175). This discussion is restricted to contrast (contour) specific EP components elicited by stimulation of a normally-sighted subject with checkerboard patterns whose individual checks subtend less than some 15′. The EPs elicited by stimulation with such small checks are predominantly due to foveal stimulation. This has been reported for both steady-state EPs to pattern reversal[748] (Fig. 2.9*B*) and for transient EPs[671] to 'the pattern-specific components of the EPs to flash-presented patterns' (Fig. 2.9*A* – but see pages 52, 51[750] for criticisms of the 'subtraction' method). For foveal stimulation by flashed pattern[359, 671] or pattern-appearance[415] a check size of 10′ to 20′ gives contrast (contour) specific EP components of greatest amplitudes, although a 100 msec component has been reported to be insensitive to check size.[359] Contrast (contour) specific components of steady-state EPs to pattern-reversal of check patterns give EPs of maximal amplitude for 11′ to 18′ checks[748, 649] (Fig. 2.8) especially when the stimulus field size does not greatly exceed foveal dimensions. In contrast, extra-foveal stimuli give EPs of greatest amplitudes when check sizes are considerably larger than 15′[361] (page 62; note that flashed patterns were used).

This suggests that the contrast (contour) specific EP components elicited by patterns of checks considerably larger than 15′ and which stimulate appreciably more than the central 3° might well include important contributions due to extra-foveal stimulation. In fact Michael and Halliday[931] recently reported that (for lower field responses) pattern-reversal EPs elicited by a stimulus falling on to the central 4° (diameter) were of roughly similar amplitudes to those elicited by 50′ checks falling within an annular region whose internal diameter was 4° and external diameter 16°. [Michael and Halliday stimulated one quadrant only of the visual field and measured the peak to peak amplitude between a 75–85 msec wave and the following wave of opposite polarity (90–110 msec to peak).] For upper-field stimulation the EP measure described above showed even less proportional contribution due to central stimulation than the lower-field responses.

This précis does grossly simplify Michael and Halliday's account. The balance between responses to central and peripheral stimulation depended both on recording site *and on the site of the reference electrode*, moreover these factors did not have the same importance for upper- and lower-field responses. (Michael and Halliday's paper provides a clear illustration and explanation of the importance of allowing for non-indifference of the 'reference' electrode.) Such complications were incorporated into Michael and Halliday's suggested model.

One purpose of my present remarks is to point out that check size may also be an important parameter when responses to stimulation of different retinal regions are being compared – even though some effects of check size may predominantly reflect retinal function. In any case the fact that the subjective (psychophysical) acuity of daylight vision is greatest in the fovea and declines rapidly as stimulus eccentricity is increased suggests that the EPs to patterns made up of checks which are appreciably larger than 15′ (e.g. 50′) would be less affected by defocusing the reginal image than patterns made up of checks smaller than 15′ or so (and it is worth noting that such an effect of check size could reflect little more than the characteristics of *retinal* organisations). It is quite possible that similar arguments would apply to Spekreijse's test for contrast (contour) specificity of placing a fine opaque grid over the borders within a checkerboard pattern (page 55). A further argument that large fields of large checks would be expected to include a relatively smaller contribution due to foveal stimulation than large fields made up of small checks is that very few checks fall on a central 2° to 3° region when the check size is large (e.g. approaching 1°).

For bar or grating patterns the situation is, in many respects, quite different from the situation for check patterns. Campbell and Maffei's finding that the amplitudes of pattern-reversal EPs for a grating pattern declined monotonically (and steeply) as the spatial frequency of the grating pattern was increased above roughly 2 cycles/degree (i.e. each light or dark part of a grating subtended 15′) implies that defocusing a bar pattern which initially had sharp edges would have less effect on EP amplitude than comparable defocusing of a checkerboard pattern [assuming that the check size was such as to ensure that the EPs were predominantly of the contrast (contour) specific type, see page 54]. The argument runs along the following lines: defocusing is equivalent to attenuating the higher spatial frequencies. A bar pattern can be described by a fundamental spatial frequency plus contributions due to multiples of this spatial frequency (harmonics). Since the plot of EP amplitude *versus* spatial frequency falls off steeply and monotonically, only the fundamental spatial frequency is important so that the attenuation of higher spatial frequencies has little effect. Now a sharp-edged checkerboard pattern is described, in spatial frequency terms, in such a way that higher harmonics are relatively more important than for a bar pattern. Therefore, when the higher spatial frequencies of a checkerboard pattern are attenuated by defocusing, the resulting attenuation of the EP is greater than when a bar pattern is defocused. [See supplementary footnote No. 30 for the fundamental notions which underlie the use of spatial frequency analysis to investigate the performance of an optical system.]

To give an example, this argument would apply to the results of defocusing bar and check patterns which had been chosen so as to give optimal responses to foveal stimulation.

It is worth pointing out that for a 2° stimulus, the amplitudes of pattern-reversal EPs can be *increased* by moderate defocusing. This occurs for check sizes exceeding 22′ or so. The expected attenuation due to defocusing occurs only for checks smaller than 15′ or so (Fig. 2.8). Analogous effects seem to occur for transient pattern EPs (page 57).

A final point is that the results and interpretation of different studies where pattern stimulation has been used are difficult to compare, contrast and generalise from. One reason for this is the use of different electrode placements, bipolar *versus* referential recording, the different locations of reference electrodes, and different methods of measuring EP amplitudes. Quite distinct, and equally implacable problems arise from the use of different stimuli. Some workers have used small checks, some large checks and others bar or grating patterns. A few suggestions as to what common ground might underlie the results of these different investigations is discussed above and in Section 2.4. There is real difficulty, however, in comparing the results of studies in which pattern reversal, pattern appearance and disappearance, and flashed patterns have been used as stimuli. A pattern reversal can be regarded physically as a pattern disappearance followed instantaneously by a pattern appearance. Unfortunately the visual system behaves nonlinearly. The little evidence that is available suggests that pattern-reversal EPs are more akin to pattern-disappearance than to pattern-appearance EPs. But what is the effect of the transition time in pattern reversal? Little is known except that the rate of change of spatial contrast exerts a strong effect on pattern-appearance and pattern-disappearance EPs, and that the effect is stronger for pattern-disappearance EPs (Fig. 2.6). When the patterned-mirror stimulator is used, pattern reversal may be instantaneous. In contrast, when pattern reversal is achieved by using vibrators or pen motors to displace the patterned stimulus through one square's width, the transition time may be 3 msec to 8 msec. Whether this transition time is an influential factor is not known. However if pattern-reversal EPs are regarded as the limiting case of motion EPs for infinitely rapid motion then the evidence for a relationship between the acceleration of the retinal image and EP amplitude would suggest that transition time might be important in pattern reversal. On the other hand if pattern-reversal and motion EPs proved to be inherently different, a too-long transition time might be expected to introduce motion-EP components and result in contamination of the pattern-reversal EP.

S9. (p. 41). This view implies the improbability that a short-latency 'timing' neural signal (whose latency was comparatively unaffected by stimulus intensity) might precede the later neural signal which gives rise to the EP.

S10. (p. 42). Donchin and Lindsley[902] recorded the EPs to double flash stimuli where the initial brief test flash (TF) was closely followed by a second brief, but brighter flash (BF). It is well known that for sufficiently brief interflash intervals the first flash (TF) cannot be perceived; it is masked by the second flash (BF). For long interflash intervals there is no interaction between the neural signals elicited by the flashes. For intermediate interflash intervals, the apparent brightness of the first flash (TF) is enhanced. Donchin and Lindsley reported EP correlates of these well-known psychophysical observations. For long interflash intervals the EPs to the TF and to the BF were quite separate and resembled the EPs recorded when TF or BF respectively was presented by itself. In the 'brightness enhancement' range of interflash intervals the EP pattern resembled neither the EP to the TF alone nor the EP to the BF alone; nevertheless when the EP to the BF (recorded alone) was subtracted from this combined EP, the residual resembled the EP to the TF alone. Finally, when perceptual masking of the TF occurred, the form of the EP elicited by the pair of flashes resembled the EP characteristic of the BF alone.

Donchin and Lindsley drew interesting conclusions from their psychophysiological-EP correlation on the assumption that the correlation directly reflected physiological activities common to their subjective and EP observations. One query which might be raised concerns the possible effect of EP saturation. Saturation (i.e. a levelling off of response amplitude as stimulus 'strength' is increased – stimulus 'strength' being for example either absolute or percentage intensity change) occurs both for transient and for steady-state EPs (Section 2.33 and [152, 648]). In other words the relation between, for example, the absolute energy change of a stimulus and EP amplitude is grossly nonlinear in many cases, so that the addition of extra intensity to a flash changes the EP very little when the total flash intensity is sufficiently high. In some cases the saturation of EPs clearly does not correlate with perception since EP amplitude levels off (or even falls) with increasing stimulus 'strength', although the magnitude of the resulting sensation continues to grow.[637, 640, 648, 749] In such cases it seems that there is no direct relation between EP amplitude and the neural activities which underlie sensation. In the retroactive masking paradigm used by Donchin and Lindsley it could be argued that for short interflash intervals the EP would to some extent reflect the time-integrated intensity of the flash pair (as it must do completely for a zero interflash interval). Since the second flash is bright the first flash will, due to saturation contribute little to the EP and the attenuation of the EP due to the first flash will decrease as interflash interval is decreased. This, it could be argued, would be expected as a result of EP saturation so that some correlation between EP and subjective measures would be expected without postulating any direct common physiological basis. It is difficult to estimate how large an effect, if any saturation might have had in Donchin and Lindsley's experiment. However, recordings from wires implanted in optic nerve, tract, lateral geniculate body and visual cortex of monkey suggest that any effect of saturation was sufficiently small that it did not influence their interpretation. Fehmi *et al.*[905] found in agreement with Donchin and Lindsley that when the 'perception' of TF was (behaviourally) masked by BF, then only the EP characteristic of BF could be recorded. Significantly, however, a behavioural response to the TF was possible when the interflash interval was such that only the initial segment of the EP to TF could be recorded.

S11. (p. 42). In 1966 Spekreijse reported that the amplitudes of pattern-reversal EPs to checks depended little on mean luminance within the photopic range.[748] In contrast, the phase and 'apparent latency' (page 76) of the response were strongly influenced by mean luminance. The percentage change in stimulus contrast (modulation depth) exerted a strong influence on EP amplitude, but had little effect on response phase. Spekreijse's findings are in accord with our own subsequent results. May *et al.*[929] reported similar phenomena when they used bar rather than check patterns.

S12. (p. 42). Milner[547] has recorded the averaged auditory vertex response from two subjects to pure tone pulses with the following parameters; 1 KHz modulated frequency, a pulse duration of 350 mS to ensure no interaction of ON and OFF responses and a pulse rise time of 10 mS. Twenty stimuli each of different intensity ranging from 5 dB to 105 dB (B.S. Zero) in 5 dB steps, were presented randomly at seven-second intervals to the subject in one experimental run. This was repeated thirty times each run having a different random arrangement of intensities. The ongoing EEG was recorded and analysed off-line, so that all the responses to one intensity were averaged together.

The resulting intensity function [amplitude (μV) *v.* intensity (dB)] was not monotonic. It consisted of three parts; a sensitive portion (approx. linear) between 5 dB and 50 dB, a flat portion between 50–70 dB with little sensitivity to intensity changes and a second sensitive portion (a further linear increase) between 70–105 dB.

S13. (p. 38). There is certainly no sharply-defined sensory threshold in the same sense as the all-or-nothing firing threshold of a single neuron. The very existence of a sensory threshold has been questioned. In a brief and lucid discussion of the question Swets concluded that the existence of a sensory threshold has neither been demonstrated nor disproved. What is certain, though, is that it is easy to confound the effects of a subject's sensitivity and his response criterion, and that the response criterion may vary considerably for any individual subject when the experimental design is altered. As a result, the measured threshold will depend on the subjects' instructions. Response criteria also vary widely between individuals. Methods of conducting psychophysical experiments and of presenting data so as to distinguish between the effects of sensitivity and response criterion have been developed.[946a] Forced-choice methods have some advantageous features.[890, 946a, 950] The staircase ('up and down') and double staircase methods have the feature of high efficiency[899] in converging upon a specified probability for the accuracy of the final measure.[947] Taylor and Creelman[948] have attempted to quantify an experimenter's practical requirement in their definition of the 'sweat factor' – a combined measure of effort and precision. They have described a psychophysical method which has a particularly low sweat factor (PEST).[948]

S14. (p. 47). A further point is that unstructured-field stimuli whose repetition frequencies are high are likely to elicit EPs that include less contributions from retinal rods than EPs to stimuli of lower frequencies [it is difficult to be quantitative, since the necessary EP data are not available, but a (questionable) analogy with ERG findings points to a lower limit of roughly 20 Hz]. The combination of fairly high stimulus repetition frequency and a steady adapting background of greater than 5000 trolands retinal illumination would seem likely to minimise complications due to the different ratios of cones to rods in the fovea and parafovea.

S15. (pp. 52, 148, 172). It has been claimed that certain EP features correlate with a behavioural measure ('augmenting' *v.* 'reducing') which can distinguish between different subjects.[894, 943] 'Augmenters' were reported to show little or no saturation of EP amplitude to sinusoidally modulated light (Section 2.3.3). In contrast, 'reducers' showed saturation or even oversaturation (paradoxical diminution). These EP findings paralleled the 'augmenters' tendency to overestimate the size of an object to a greater extent than a 'reducer' in a specific experimental situation which inclined a subject to overestimate.[943] The effect of depressant drugs was both to increase the tendency of the EP to saturate and also to move a subject's behavioural results towards the 'reducing' end of the 'augmenting' – 'reducing' continuum.[944] Unexpectedly, drug stimulants did not produce the opposite effect on the EP.

At first sight it is not straightforward to relate the above EP findings to the effects on EP saturation of (*a*) stimulus colour, (*b*) the frequency of the EP component recorded or (*c*) electrode site. A single subject can show, in the same experimental session saturation (or oversaturation) when yellow light is modulated, but no saturation when red light is modulated. This behaviour occurs for 'medium-frequency' EP components.[640] At the same time, and from the same electrode, second harmonic 'high-frequency' EP components can be recorded which show similar saturation behaviour for red and yellow modulations.[935, 640, 639] In these studies the stimulus light was a yellow patch superposed on a red patch; subjects found great difficulty in discriminating between modulations of the yellow and the red components.

The shape of the saturation characteristic to stimulation with sinusoidally modulated white light depends on the position of the active electrode in referential recordings.[648] For 'high-frequency' components the saturation curve recorded from some (but not all) electrode sites showed an initial rapid rise, then a fall at medium modulation depths and finally a rise as the modulation depth reached 80–100%. 'Medium-frequency' components recorded simultaneously from the same electrodes did not saturate.[648]

S16. (pp. 53, 61, 62, 113, 114, 168, 175). The first component (latency to peak roughly 80 msec) of the EP to pattern appearance can be larger in amplitude than the second component (latency to peak roughly 120 msec). This depends both on the particular subject and on the retinal location of the stimulus (Jeffreys and Axford, personal communication). The second component seems to be mainly due to stimulation of the fovea; for upper-field stimulation mainly the central 1° while for lower field stimulation mainly the central 3°. The first component seems to be mainly due to extrafoveal stimulation, between 2° and the extreme limit of the stimulus used (6°).[922] These remarks apply with varying force to different subjects.[922]

It is difficult to compare Jeffreys and Axford's results with Eason *et al.*'s[259] report that different check sizes were optimal for stimulation of upper and lower half-fields, since Eason *et al.* did not compare foveal and parafoveal responses, while Jeffreys and Axford reported mainly on the responses to one size of pattern element.

S17. (pp. 63, 111, 113, 167, 175, 227). The reservation should be made that the activity of the 'indifferent' reference electrode is likely to be different for the EPs to pattern stimulation of the upper and the lower retinal half-fields since the active cortical areas are differently located and orientated relative to the reference electrode[931] (see footnote No. 8).

S18. (pp. 63, 65). A good estimate of psychophysical threshold is obtained also for EPs to: (*a*) luminance contrast reversal of monochromatic (red or green) 2° check patterns (12′ checks); (*b*) chromatic contrast reversal of constant-luminance, red-green patterns of checks (2° subtence, 12′ checks); (*c*) luminance contrast reversal of a monochromatic (red or green) bar patterns (2° subtence, bars 11′ wide); (*d*) chromatic contrast reversal of constant-luminance red-green bar patterns (2° subtence, bars 11′ wide). In these experiments the plot of EP amplitude *versus* contrast was no longer a straight line for contrasts in excess of 30% to 40%. The curves tended to 'level-out' to an extent which (for luminance contrast reversal of monochromatic patterns) was different for red and green. Similar results were found for bars and checks. The stimulus frequency was six reversals per second and the amplitude of the 6 Hz Fourier component was recorded between electrodes located 1 cm and 9 cm from the inion along the midline.[936]

S20. (pp. 73, 129). It has been suggested that lambda waves (Section 2.6.3) might reflect the operation of a neuronal 'shutter' mechanism that prevents blurring of the visual image when the direction of gaze is voluntarily shifted. Lambda waves can be recorded in monkey, cat and dog (though not in rat, guinea-pig and rabbit). The latency of these responses, Scott *et al.*[939] suggested, was sufficiently long to render the neuronal 'shutter' hypothesis less attractive, since the main movement component would be completed before the peak lambda wave response was reached.

S21. (pp. 78, 221). Spilker *et al.* have recorded visual EPs in subjects trained to control their alpha rhythms.[945] They found that steady-state EPs to light sinusoidally modulated at 10 Hz were of greater amplitudes when there was high or abundant alpha in the EEG than when alpha was low. They reported similar findings for 7 Hz and 13 Hz stimulation and cited this as evidence against 'driving' (see pages 77, 237, 250). Two early waves of the flash EP showed similar effects. In contrast, two peaks of the auditory EP showed no such effects.

Spilker *et al.*'s report is in accord with van der Tweel and Spekreijse's earlier findings that near the alpha frequency the shape of the amplitude *versus* frequency curve for EPs to sinusoidally modulated light is similar to the amplitude spectrum of the spontaneous EEG (Section 2.8.2 and Figs. 2.13, 5.12*F*). The close relationship between high amplitude of 'low-frequency' EP components and alpha amplitude (interpreted in terms of changes in the Q factor of the 10 Hz filter in Fig. 2.13 upper) was exploited by the Amsterdam group in their use of diffuse-field stimulus when studying 'low-frequency' EPs. Similarly, a change in the Q factor of the 10 Hz filter is assumed to be the reason for the flattening of the 10 Hz 'low-frequency' peak when yellow light is used.[635, 748] The effects reported by Spilker *et al.* of alpha on visually evoked transient EPs might be due to manifestations of changes in filter Q factor in the time domain rather than the frequency domain.

It is worth noting that a close relation between the amplitude *versus* stimulus frequency curve for steady-state EPs and the amplitude distribution of the EEG is far from being a universal rule. It holds for 'low-frequency' and 'high-frequency' components of unstructured-field EPs, but not for 'medium-frequency' components of unstructured-field EPs nor for EPs to pattern-reversal (Sections 2.8.2, 2.8.3, 2.8.4 and 2.8.5). The reasons for these differences are not clear. One oddity might be worth investigating. This is that van der Tweel and Spekreijse (in the Netherlands) and Regan (in England) find that, although there is considerable inter-individual variability in the centre frequencies of the 'high-frequency' peak, this peak is often not more than 8 Hz or so removed from 50 Hz. Now 50 Hz is the frequency of the a.c. supply both in the Netherlands and in England. With a Fourier Analyser it is a simple matter to demonstrate that mains interference could not possibly account for 'high-frequency' EPs. Nevertheless it would be interesting to know whether the median frequency of the 'high-frequency' peak is higher in the U.S.A. than in Europe.

S22. (p. 85). The situation would seem to be more complicated. Cavonius and Sternheim used a different kind of stimulus (broad bars, pattern reversal – see Section 2.9.5). They extrapolated plots of EP amplitude *versus* log modulation depth to obtain the modulation depths for zero EP amplitude as a function of stimulus repetition frequency. They found the shapes of these 'extrapolated threshold' *versus* frequency curves to be similar to the shapes of the De Lange curves.[897]

S23. (pp. 107, 121, 167). This last remark should be qualified by pointing out that EPs to bars or gratings are rather less sensitive to ocular accommodation than are the EPs to checks smaller than 15′ or so[748] (see also supplementary footnote No. 8).

S24. (pp. 111, 117). Kooi, Tipton and Marshall[925] were unable to confirm the generality of Vaughan's report of a zero equipotential along the line of the Sylvian fissure (Fig. 2.33). They claimed that the location of a zero equipotential along the line of the Sylvian fissure was an artifact due to non-indifference of the nasal reference electrode (see Section 5.4.7).

S25. (pp. 123, 192). The correlation between the amplitudes of steady-state pattern-reversal EPs and a stable, non-adapting subjective suppression of pattern vision reported by van der Tweel, Spekreijse and Regan[800] holds also for transient EPs to pattern appearance (van der Tweel, Spekreijse and Regan, *Vision Res.* – in press). This interocular suppression effect of pattern vision may have some analogy with the suppression of pattern vision in amblyopia. Hubel, Wiesel and Dews[912] have studied the single-cell basis for losses of pattern perception produced both by artificially-induced squint and by eye closure, and have reported neurophysiological evidence for enhanced susceptibility to losses of pattern vision between certain ages (in cat). They also investigated single-cell correlates of recovery from such impairments of visual function. Van der Tweel, Spekreijse and Regan's report suggests that pattern EPs might in this instance provide a bridge between single-unit studies of the effects of squint in animals and the subjective losses of visual function produced by squint in children; there is some evidence that amblyopia is accompanied by abnormalities in the interocular EP suppression effect.[942a]

S26. (pp. 131, 172). Wood, Goff and Day[949a] claimed that EPs elicited by similar speech signals were of different amplitudes in tasks which required discrimination of linguistic *versus* non-linguistic stimulus parameters. Furthermore, these differences occurred at electrode locations over the left hemisphere but not over the right hemisphere (for right-handed subjects). Wood *et al.* interpreted this finding as a reflection of different neural events (in the left hemisphere) during the analysis of linguistic *versus* non-linguistic parameters in similar auditory signals [EPs were recorded from locations T3 and C3 (left) and T4 and C4 (right) relative to a linked-ear reference (10–20 system)].

On the other hand, Roth, Kopell and Bertozzi[937a] reported no significant differences in vertex EPs elicited by 'sense' and 'non-sense' monosyllables; the use of different electrode placements render comparison of the two reports difficult.

S27. (p. 78). The optic radiations (in cat) include cortico-geniculate fibres which originate in area 18.[900] Whether such connections exist in man is an interesting question.

S28. (pp. 39, 126). Quite apart from the question of movement-related potentials (Section 3.4), the EPs to sensory stimuli have been reported to be affected both by the occurrence of a motor response[924] and by the speed of the response.[891]

S29. (p. 99). Provided that the EP component remained in the 'medium-frequency' region, the fundamental components of the EPs to modulation of the red or the yellow components of a red-plus-yellow stimulus light had a phase difference which did not vary with stimulus repetition frequency over a range of frequencies whose end points lay some 28 Hz apart. The absolute phase of both fundamental EP components changed by roughly 900° while the *difference* in the phases of the 'red' and 'yellow' responses remained constant to within $\pm 10°$. This surprising finding does not seem easy to model. The phase difference between the 'red' and 'yellow' EP components cannot be due to a latency difference (although, as would be expected, when the luminances of the yellow and red components were made unequal, some additional phase shifts appeared; these additional phase shifts were proportional to frequency and were therefore most probably due to latency differences). The difference in response phase between EP components to different colours (of equal luminances) depends strongly on stimulus colour.

This finding of an EP feature which depends strongly and stably on colour suggests that phase might reflect the neural activities which underlie our discrimination of different hues. Since it seems difficult to model a frequency-invariant phase shift in any way which is physiologically plausible, the question has rested at this point for some three years (Regan, unpublished observations).

It has been reported that the latencies of EPs to equiluminant stimuli of different colours correlate with the shape of the relative spectral luminosity curve. Regan reported that the 'apparent latency' (page 77) of the 'medium-frequency' EPs to stimuli of different wavelengths had a deep minimum in the yellow.[934] This suggested that apparent latency was not a correlate of hue (since red and blue responses had similar latencies); Regan speculated that 'apparent latency' might correlate with the saturation of a colour, since saturation is least in the yellow.

S30. (p. 63). Until recently the classical way of investigating the performance of an optical system was by either computing or measuring the various kinds of aberrations in the imaging of a point source of light. The criterion for a good optical system was its capacity to image a point source as a point image. It became clear that this criterion was not always satisfactory when it was required to design a lens to image real scenes, particularly scenes such as railway marshalling yards which contained many straight lines and parallel lines. Fourier analysis, translated from the temporal to the spatial domain, was found to provide a more appropriate criterion of optical performance. The performance could be investigated by using as a target, not a point source of light, but a grating pattern whose luminance was modulated sinusoidally.[915, 916, 917]

This approach has since been extensively used in assessing the optical performance of the human visual system by psychophysical[119, 896] and by EP means.[120]

S31. (pp. 131, 149). Slow potentials have been reported to occur before speech production. Interestingly, their amplitudes were larger at electrodes located over the left than at electrodes located over the right hemisphere for polysyllabic words, whereas symmetrically-distributed potentials were found before the production of control non-speech sounds.

S32. (p. 149). Slow potentials have been reported to occur before voluntary eye movements (see last paragraph, Section 2.6.3).

S33. (pp. 33, 144, 151). A neural 'model' hypothesis has been suggested by Sokoloff[942] in order to account for habituation of the orienting reaction (see supplementary footnote S. 39 and Section 3.4). He suggested that a neuronal 'model' of a stimulus is built up during its repeated presentations. When complete, the model is equivalent to a full description of the stimulus. If a match occurs between the incoming sensory signals and the neural 'model', then inhibitory impulses pass to other regions in the CNS and cut off the neural signals reaching them from sensory receptors. Any mismatch between 'model' and sensory inflow causes cells in these 'other regions' to fire, and to fire more strongly the greater the mismatch.

On this view, the 'response' to the omission of a stimulus from a long train of auditory stimuli (Fig. 3.1) might be regarded as a 'mismatch' response. For visual stimuli also Garcia Ausst reported that the *absence* of a stimulus can result in a vertex response (the latency of the visual response was some 350 msec whereas the latency of the click response was 260 msec – the difference was attributed to a shorter auditory transmission time).[907]

S34. (p. 134). Jonkman[430 p. 145] stated that when he ensured that his subjects remained fully alert there was *no habituation* to flash stimuli even for large numbers of flashes.

S35. (pp. 39, 140, 144, 160, 192). The task of Hillyard *et al.*'s subjects[913] was to decide on each trial whether or not an acoustic signal had been added to a continuous background noise. The EPs were averaged separately for: (*a*) detected signals (hits), (*b*) failures to detect signals (misses), (*c*) incorrect reports of signal presence (false alarms) and (*d*) correct reports of signal absences (correct rejections). Recordings were made from vertex referred to right mastoid, dc to 200 Hz; eye movements were monitored.

The CNV was consistently larger *before correct detection* of near-threshold signals than for other responses (*b*, *c*, *d* above).

In the period following the signal, a large P300 component was recorded *only* for hits. An important finding was that psychophysical detection threshold (chance performance) correlated well with EP 'extrapolation threshold' (footnote on p. 163) – see Hillyard *et al.*'s Fig. 2.

When the experiment was repeated with the subject sitting passively there was no evidence of P300 enhancement – Hillyard *et al.* pointed out that when their 'detection' paradigm was used, P300 waves were visible in the AEP at intensity levels some 6 to 8 db less than the levels where any component of the vertex AEP was detectable when he conventtional *passive* AEP audiometry method was used.

Hillyard *et al.* interpreted their finding as an indication that the P300 wave was enhanced 'only when stimulus information was being actively processed, and was uniquely associated with the occurrence of a signal and its correct detection'. If they are correct in this interpretation, they have added weight to the hypothesis that the vertex P300 wave (*recorded when the subject is actively making psychophysical discriminations*) can be used as an objective index of the subject's detection of a sensory signal. This contrasts with other scalp-recorded potentials (e.g. Sections 2.3.4, 2.8.6, 2.9.3) which are quite dissociated from perception. Hillyard *et al.*, pointed out that their finding that P300 amplitude depended on the specific stimulus-response outcome and that it declined when performance neared chance levels was at variance with Ritter and Vaughan's[677] interpretation of the P300 component as reflecting 'cognitive evaluation of stimulus significance' since this would predict a P300 whenever a difficult decision was made. Hillyard *et al.* suggested that their P300 wave 'indexes the observer's degree of confidence or certainty that a signal has occurred'.

In order to account for a decline in P300 amplitude on hit trials for detection beyond 90% correct they invoked an influence of the '*a priori* improbability of an event'. It might, however, be possible to account for this small anomaly in terms of lower-level rather than entirely in terms of 'higher central' activities. For example, a high hit rate might possibly be regarded as a strong stimulus for the P300. A fall-off in response amplitude at high stimulus levels is well known in studies where higher neural functioning is never invoked in interpretations since EP effects can be attributed to comparatively low-level neural processing.

S36. (p. 150). Kornhuber has suggested that: cerebellar cortex generates short bursts of impulses which initiate rapid pre-programmed movements; the function of cerebellar nuclei is to hold the positions reached by rapid movements; the basal ganglia (strio-nigro-pallidum) generate slow smooth movements of voluntary speed (i.e. function as ramp generators). Kornhuber speculated that the function of motor cortex was to 'make appropriate use of the movement and posture patterns generated by the cerebellum and basal ganglia with respect to the mechanical properties of the things which are analysed by the somatosensory system'.[926] Movement-related potentials reflect these various sub-activities.

S37. (p. 141). See Reference [912a].

S38. (p. 162). Kooi *et al.*[925] reported the occurrence of a wave (F wave) which followed closely upon the vertex potential, but could be distinguished from it on grounds of topographical distribution and on latency to peak (150–200 msec and 110–160 msec respectively).

S39. (p. 151). In some circumstances a subject (or animal) decides whether or not he (or it) will respond to a stimulus. In other circumstances, or when certain stimuli are used, the stimulus forces a response. The orienting reaction is a behavioural response to such response-determining stimuli.[942] The gradual waning of the orienting reaction to a repeated stimulus is known as habituation. It has been defined operationally in terms of nine characteristics.[789] Habituation is generally specific to a particular stimulus. A demonstration of dishabituation is an important indicator that a decline in response amplitude is really due to habituation (dishabituation is the renewal of stimulus effectiveness. This can sometimes be produced by interpolating different stimuli between the stimuli to which the subject has become habituated.) Habituation of the responses of individual neurons to repeated stimulation is well known.[918]

Simons *et al.*[940] suggested that long-lasting neural inhibitory mechanisms could account for a large part of the response decrements observed in the auditory pathway (of cat) during repetitive stimulation. If this process were cumulative, then the amount of EP depression would increase as stimulus frequency was increased – as they found to be the case. Their results were confirmed by Webster.[949]

S40. (p. 43). Jasper has observed that EPs cortically-recorded in man during surgery, can be much larger to a mild 'physiological' touch stimulus than to strong 'unphysiological' electrical stimulation of the nerve.[921]

S41. (pp. 148, 151, 153, 184). McCallum observed CNVs with interstimulus intervals of 0·5 to 13 secs. while Grey Walter had seen CNVs with interstimulus intervals as long as 30 secs.

On the possible relation between CNV and EP Grey Walter pointed out that: (*a*) competition between stimuli attenuates all EP components, but spares the CNV; (*b*) conversely 'the CNV can be attenuated by equivocation and the evoked response remains'.

Grey Walter reported that recordings from electrodes implanted subdurally in human frontal cortex showed that CNV depolarisation occurs in patches over the cortex.

Jung pointed out that d.c. changes in scalp potential are critically dependent on CO_2 level; a reduction of CO_2 concentration in the blood increased surface negativity, and more CO_2 resulted in surface positivity. He suggested that some contribution to CNV recorded from schizophrenic subjects might be due to the effect of overbreathing.

Grey Walter reported that children who were autistic but suffered from no other disorder had no CNV. Respiration was monitored routinely[pp. 58–60, 190–191] The youngest age at which a recognisable CNV has been recorded is six years. The CNV is fully developed by twenty years.

S42. (p. 220). An eyeblink artifact may be much larger (e.g. 100 times larger) than an EP so that a single eyeblink artifact could seriously contaminate a summated EP, even though 100 responses were summated. Suggested solutions include: (*a*) run the recording equipment near saturation (Offner); (*b*) record the EEG and compare summations of, say, each of the groups of twenty-five responses comprising the 100 total (Goff); (*c*) directly record eyeblinks by a photoelectric method (Stark).[946]

S43. (p. 12). Fenwick stated that vibration of the eye did not alter the alpha frequency. Grey Walter described a patient with 'jelly nystagmus' who could cause his eye to wobble at about 16 Hz. There was no component at this frequency recordable from the back of the head, although eye-movement potentials were clear.[904 p. 346]

S44. (p. 138). See Reference.[886]

S45. (p. 154). McCallum has observed that while conditioning eye-blink in human subjects, CNV appeared during the acquisition phase but tended to disappear when the response was well established.[904 p. 59]

S46. (p. 221). See Reference [904] for fuller discussions.

S47. (pp. 72, 169, 171, 175). In our own clinical work we have so far found that a 1.5:1 criterion for 'abnormal' asymmetry is satisfactory both for unstructured-field flicker stimuli and for pattern reversal (although we have not yet examined such a large population as Cohn).

Cooper *et al.*[175] found experimentally that in man the attenuation of slow waves between cortical and scalp electrodes could vary between 2:1 and 5000:1 depending on whether the cortical activity was widespread and coherent or local (see Section 1.2.1). The evidence is that the skull is not the major contributor to this attenuation (Section 1.2.1). Nevertheless, asymmetries in skull thickness might add to the neurally-determined asymmetries of scalp EPs. Leissner *et al.* found that nine of their twenty-seven subjects had asymmetries of skull bone thickness exceeding 33%.[927] In these subjects, alpha amplitudes were 20–70% smaller on the side with the thicker bone. Interestingly, skull thickness was more often greater on the left than on the right side (52 to 28) Leissner *et al.* suggested that this might account for reports that alpha amplitude is greater on the right.

What all this might mean in terms of EPs is difficult to say, since such an effect would depend on the coherence and geometry of the neural sources. It is clear, though, that skull thickness measurements might set tighter limits on 'abnormal' asymmetry criteria, and also might be useful as a control measurement in patients.

S48. (pp. 171, 175, 193). Cortical lesions in different locations have different effects on 'low-frequency' and 'medium-frequency' EPs. Pattern-reversal stimulation can detect a lesion which produces a quadrantic field defect extending to no more than 2° from the central fovea.[547a]

S49. (pp. 167, 190). Harter and Suitt investigated the maturation of EPs to checkboard-patterned light flashes in one subject (Harter junior) between post-natal ages of 21 to 156 days. The latencies of the major positive and negative components decreased from 160 msec (21–30 days) to 90 msec (137–150 days), and from 250 to 130 msec respectively. Perhaps their most interesting finding was that as the subject grew older, progressively smaller check sizes evoked the largest responses. By roughly 70 days the relationship between check size and P2 amplitude resembled the normal adult U-shaped function (N2 amplitude was more variable). Harter and Suitt interpreted their interesting findings in terms of a progressive improvement of visual acuity with increasing age. They were able to implicate retinal development, since the low EP acuity at one and three months could only partially be explained by refractive errors.

S50. (p. 168). There is electrophysiological evidence that some optic tract fibres bifurcate, giving one branch to the lateral geniculate body and the other branch to the superior colliculus (in cat); there is further evidence for connections which run *from* colliculus to geniculate.[911]

S51. (p. 194). Skinner and Lindsley[941] have reported that (reversible) cryogenic blocking of the non-specific thalamo-cortical system in cats produces *enhancement* of EPs. Their EPs were elicited by electrical stimulation within the auditory and visual pathways. Skinner and Lindsley[941] pointed out that their EP changes correlated with behavioural deficits in response inhibition and directed attention.

S52. (pp. 167, 239). A commercial device is currently being developed for use in both clinical and fundamental work which, although envisaged to be markedly cheaper (channel for channel) than commercial summation devices will have the following advantages: (*a*) steady-state EPs will be Fourier analysed. A digital readout will give phase and amplitude measures of required harmonic components and in addition a numerical indication of the statistical reliability of the measurements; (*b*) the device will be capable of measuring much smaller EP components than are presently within the scope of conventionally-used summation devices; (*c*) the device will be much less affected by alpha and other noise than summation computers as normally used; (*d*) it will be possible to use the simultaneous stimulation/recording method on-line for two, three or four simultaneous stimuli. This technique drastically reduces the effect of variability when comparing EPs elicited by stimulating different sites, and therefore much reduces the time required to carry out an EP investigation (page 173 and supplementary footnote No. 48); (*e*) the device is designed so that it can be operated by other than research personnel; (*f*) it will be cheap and straightforward to add extra channels and to couple the device to a wide range of stimulators.

S53. (p. 213). A continuous variation of retinal disparity (and hence of perceived depth) can be produced by viewing with one eye an unvarying reference pattern (e.g. two vertical bars, one on each side of a central fixation point) and a similar pattern with the right eye. The left and right images are fused, and (in this example) the right-hand bar of one pair is moved sideways by means of a vibrator. The bar then appears to move continuously in depth relative to the fixation mark.[937]

A method of generating apparent depth using two CROs was described by Florentini and Maffei.[286]

S54. (p. 224). Bourne *et al.*[892] have described a computer method of displaying both topographical distribution and amplitude on a single sheet of paper.

S55. (p. 166). One reason for these differences between the responses to small spots of light and the EPs to large, spatially-unstructured, stimulus fields might be that the *edges* of the small light spot contributes relatively more to the EP than do the edges of the large light patch. Two factors which would suggest this are: (*a*) the edge of the small spot falls on the macula which has high acuity and is particularly important in the eliciting of contour (contrast) specific EP components (Sections 2.4.1, 2.4.4 and footnotes 8, 16); (*b*) the ratio of circumference to area for a small spot is larger than for a large spot. For example, in Copenhauer, Perry and Childers' experiments the ratio of circumference to area would be eight times greater for the 2·5° spot than for the 20° spot, and furthermore, the edge of the 20° spot would fall on a retinal region of comparatively poor acuity. This question of contour (contrast) specific EP components *versus* areal (luminance change) EP components is of particular importance in studies of amblyopia where the visual defect seems to be predominantly of pattern vision, but is also of importance in basic research (see Section 2.3.1) especially in view of possible nonlinear interactions between the two types of EP component (Section 2.3.1).

S56. (pp. 36, 63, 192). For many years there has been a great deal of informal discussion as to the relations between the spatial frequency description of the psychophysics of human pattern vision (developed by Campbell, Kulikowsky, Robson and Cooper[119] – see supplementary footnotes 8 and 30) and the properties of those single cortical neurons which are most effectively stimulated by bars of particular orientations.[399, 400] Pollen, Lee and Taylor[933] have given a succinct account of a number of current issues. They explicitly bring out one basic point that since a Fourier transform expresses the relation between any temporal waveform (or spatial amplitude distribution) and its frequency spectrum (temporal or spatial respectively);[893, 915–917] the Fourier transform re-expresses the information represented by a spatial pattern in terms of the spatial frequency domain. A fundamental property of the spatial frequency description of visual images is that the Fourier transform is (except for a phase term) *translationally invariant*; this would carry clear advantages in pattern-recognition. Pollen, Lee and Taylor explicitly argued that 'the striate cortex transforms the topographical representation of visual space in the lateral geniculate body into a Fourier transform or spatial frequency representation at the complex cell level via the intermediary simple cell stage of strip integration'. They presented neurophysiological data to support the notion that the necessary phase information might be coded in terms of the latencies of complex cell responses. However in partial support of their argument they cited the 'alpha gating' hypothesis; this is the subject of controversy (Section 1.2).

Pollen, Lee and Taylor cited their evidence for Fourier transform processes within the visual pathway in support of the notion that information may be stored holographically.[906] Whether or not it proves to be the case that the brain utilises the peculiar advantages of the Fourier transform it seems, to this author, both astonishing and comical how the most ingenious developments in physics and mathematical physics are so often closely followed by suggestions or demonstrations that these principles and techniques are basic to the functioning of the brain – and, no doubt, have been so for several million years. Unless, as seems hardly likely, this common sequence of events reflects no more than the influence of scientific fashion, it would seem that a fruitful occupation for control systems engineers and mathematical physicists might well be research on the brain, where solutions to many of their present and future problems are waiting to be recognised.

Index

Page numbers in bold refer to diagrams in the text